Physical Education, Exercise Science and Sports

Physical Education, Exercise Science and Sports

Editor: Patrick Clinton

Callisto Reference
www.callistoreference.com

Callisto Reference,
118-35 Queens Blvd., Suite 400,
Forest Hills, NY 11375, USA

Visit us on the World Wide Web at:
www.callistoreference.com

ISBN: 978-1-63239-960-1(Hardback)

The publisher's policy is to use permanent paper from mills that operate a sustainable forestry policy. Furthermore, the publisher ensures that the text paper and cover boards used have met acceptable environmental accreditation standards.

Printed in China.

Cataloging-in-Publication Data

Physical education, exercise science and sports / edited by Patrick Clinton.
p. cm.
Includes bibliographical references and index.
ISBN 978-1-63239-960-1
1. Physical education and training. 2. Exercise. 3. Sports. 4. Medicine, Physical.
5. Sports medicine. I. Clinton, Patrick.
RM700 .P49 2018
613.7--dc23

Table of Contents

Preface VII

Chapter 1 **Disciplinary integration of digital games for science learning** 1
Douglas B Clark, Pratim Sengupta, Corey E Brady, Mario M Martinez-Garza and Stephen S Killingsworth

Chapter 2 **Exploring variation in measurement as a foundation for statistical thinking in the elementary school** 22
Lyn D English and Jane M Watson

Chapter 3 **An exploratory study of informed engineering design behaviors associated with scientific explanations** 42
Şenay Purzer, Molly Hathaway Goldstein, Robin S Adams, Charles Xie and Saeid Nourian

Chapter 4 **The landscape of PreK-12 engineering online resources for teachers: global trends** 54
Aikaterini Bagiati, So Yoon Yoon, Demetra Evangelou, Alejandra Magana, Garene Kaloustian and Jiabin Zhu

Chapter 5 **STEM education K-12: perspectives on integration** 69
Lyn D English

Chapter 6 **Incorporating effective e-learning principles to improve student engagement in middle-school mathematics** 77
Kevin Mulqueeny, Victor Kostyuk, Ryan S. Baker and Jaclyn Ocumpaugh

Chapter 7 **The effects of using exploratory computerized environments in grades 1 to 8 mathematics** 91
Andrzej Sokolowski, Yeping Li and Victor Willson

Chapter 8 **Teachers' perceptions of students' mathematical work while making conjectures: an examination of teacher discussions of an animated geometry classroom scenario** 108
Wendy R Aaron and Patricio G Herbst

Chapter 9 **On understanding and improving the teaching of university mathematics** 121
Alan H. Schoenfeld, Mike Thomas and Bill Barton

Chapter 10 ***Standards*-based mathematics curricula and the promotion of quantitative literacy in elementary school** 138
Jesse L. M. Wilkins

Chapter 11 **Mathematical practices and mathematical modes of enquiry: same or different?** 151
Hamsa Venkat

Chapter 12 **Developing preservice elementary teachers' specialized content knowledge: the case of associative property** **163**
Meixia Ding

Chapter 13 **Get a room: the role of classroom space in sustained implementation of studio style instruction** **182**
Alexis V. Knaub, Kathleen T. Foote, Charles Henderson, Melissa Dancy and Robert J. Beichner

Permissions

List of Contributors

Index

Preface

Exercise and sports are important aspects of human life. Exercise science studies the impact of exercise and diet on the physical fitness of an individual and helps in developing a better understanding of human health. Physical education and exercise play a significant role in sports. They help in enhancing athletic performance. Some of the areas which overlap with the subject of physical education, sports and exercise science are physiology, anatomy and biokinetics. Different approaches, evaluations, methodologies and advanced studies on physical education, exercise science and sports, have been included in this book. It will prove to be immensely beneficial to students and researchers in this field.

Various studies have approached the subject by analyzing it with a single perspective, but the present book provides diverse methodologies and techniques to address this field. This book contains theories and applications needed for understanding the subject from different perspectives. The aim is to keep the readers informed about the progresses in the field; therefore, the contributions were carefully examined to compile novel researches by specialists from across the globe.

Indeed, the job of the editor is the most crucial and challenging in compiling all chapters into a single book. In the end, I would extend my sincere thanks to the chapter authors for their profound work. I am also thankful for the support provided by my family and colleagues during the compilation of this book.

Editor

1

Disciplinary integration of digital games for science learning

Douglas B Clark[1*], Pratim Sengupta[1], Corey E Brady[2], Mario M Martinez-Garza[1] and Stephen S Killingsworth[1]

Abstract

Background: In this paper, we investigate the relationship between theory and design in the context of creating digital games to support children's development of scientific expertise.

Synthesis: Theoretically, we consider two frameworks: Knowledge in Pieces (or KiP) and Science as Practice (or SaP). While KiP is a theory about the structure of human knowledge, SaP is a theoretical perspective about the development of scientific expertise that emphasizes the deeply intertwined nature of conceptual development and the development of epistemic and representational practices. We then synthesize research on modeling and games from our research group and others to create a composite argument and theoretical framing for the importance of *disciplinary integration* in the design of digital games for science learning.

Conclusions: We show how shifting from KiP to SaP as the underlying theoretical anchor in our designs results in shifting from focusing on *conceptual integration* to focusing on *disciplinary integration*. We first present our initial framing and design around conceptual integration. We then trace the evolution and rationale for disciplinary integration across our development and research on four game platforms. Finally, we discuss the implications and generalizability of disciplinary integration across the design of digital games for science learning.

Keywords: Digital games; Learning; Science education; Learning technologies

Background

Digital games provide a promising medium for science education (Clark et al. 2009; Honey and Hilton 2010; National Research Council 2009). The potential of digital games as a genre of educational technologies for fostering scientific expertise has been noted not only by educators but also by scientists (Federation of American Scientists 2006; Hines et al. 2009). There is now a growing body of research that shows that digital games can indeed be productively used to support science learning in K-12 classrooms (Clark et al. 2014a; Martinez-Garza et al. 2013; Wouters et al. 2013).

In this paper, we focus on theorizing the design of digital games to support the learning of core scientific concepts and representational practices. Theoretically, we consider two frameworks: Knowledge in Pieces (or KiP) (diSessa 1993; Hammer 1996; Sherin 2001; Clark et al. 2009) and Science as Practice (or SaP) (Pickering 1995; Lehrer and Schauble 2006a; Duschl et al. 2007). While KiP is a theory about the structure of human knowledge, SaP is a theoretical perspective about the development of scientific expertise. Grounded in the history of science, SaP argues that the development of scientific concepts is deeply intertwined with the development of epistemic and representational practices (e.g., modeling). We report how these theoretical frameworks have shaped the design of our digital games for learning Newtonian dynamics across an extended design experiment. We show how shifting from KiP to SaP as the underlying theoretical anchor has enabled a shift from designing games that focus on *conceptual integration* (Clark and Martinez-Garza 2012) to games that focus on *disciplinary integration*. Whereas conceptually integrated games integrate the targeted conceptual relationships directly into the mechanics of the core game environment, disciplinary integration extends conceptual integration by incorporating disciplinary practices as well as conceptual relationships into the mechanics of interacting with, manipulating, or navigating the core game environment.

* Correspondence: doug.clark@vanderbilt.edu
[1]College of Education, Vanderbilt University, Box 230, 230 Appleton Place, Nashville, Tennessee 37203-5721, USA
Full list of author information is available at the end of the article

Knowledge in pieces as the theoretical anchor for conceptual integration

The Knowledge-in-Pieces perspective frames conceptual change as a gradual process that relies on bootstrapping ideas that students bring to the instructional setting (diSessa 1988, 1993; Hammer 1996; Smith et al. 1993; Amin 2009; Jeppsson et al. 2013). In this perspective, human knowledge consists of many, loosely organized, fragmented pieces of knowledge (Clark 2006; diSessa 1993; Hammer et al. 2005). In framing this perspective, diSessa (1993) postulated that the building blocks of understanding are phenomenological primitives (p-prims). P-prims are small knowledge elements whose origins stem from repeated abstractions of familiar events. Cued upon recognition of contextual features, p-prims are used to construct intuitive understandings of the physical world. According to this perspective, naïve understanding is highly sensitive to context, with predictions and explanations depending in subtle ways on the particular knowledge elements that are triggered in particular reasoning situations.

According to the Knowledge-in-Pieces perspective, conceptual change involves a gradual development of coherence that typically involves altering *structured priorities* (diSessa 1993) of relevant knowledge elements. Conceptual change, in this perspective, involves altering the structured priorities of knowledge elements - i.e., altering the likelihood that particular pieces of knowledge will be activated upon recognition of specific contextual cues. In this view, misconceptions cannot easily be 'removed and replaced' because they are productive pieces of knowledge that are valid in certain contexts. In order to develop coherent understanding from pieces of knowledge, these naïve conceptions must be reorganized and refined into more stable, expert-like knowledge structures (Clark 2006; diSessa 1993; diSessa et al. 2004). As diSessa (1983) pointed out, physics learners tend to make errors because they overgeneralize - i.e., they use certain p-prims to make sense of situations in a manner that leads to erroneous explanations of the underlying physical mechanisms. Through instruction and experience, the student learns to activate different, more productive p-prims when presented with the same situation. Over time, similar contexts cue the more productive p-prims, thus modifying the structured priority of p-prim activation and building a more expert-like knowledge structure (diSessa et al. 2004).

From a KiP perspective, digital games can provide a context to support students in refining their structured priorities around targeted disciplinary relationships. An example of a disciplinary relationship that a digital game could target would be the shift from an emphasis on the *Force as Mover* p-prim to the *Force as Deflector* p-prim (diSessa 1988, 1993; White 1984). The *Force as Mover* p-prim assumes that a force causes motion in the direction of the force, ignoring the effect of previous motion (diSessa 1988; 1993). diSessa (1983) explains that 'the most commonplace situation involving forces, pushing on objects from rest, becomes abstracted as the highest priority p-prim that one will use to predict motion in general circumstances' (diSessa 1983, p 30). diSessa also pointed out that even experts likely use this p-prim to explain situations such as this one. However, the difference between novice and expert use of this p-prim is that the expert priority system 'knows' much better when and when not to use that intuition (diSessa 1993, p 130). diSessa argued that development of a more expert understanding involves raising the priority of a competing p-prim, *Force as Deflector*. Similar restructuring of priorities is critical to understanding other Newtonian relationships between force, mass, and acceleration as well as the interaction of multiple objects (diSessa 1993; diSessa et al. 2004). Designing games around conceptual integration focuses on supporting students in restructuring these cueing priorities through experiences in the games. Such designs can be informed by microgenetic analyses of student thinking and learning from a KiP perspective (and can leverage a long history of developing simulations and microworlds toward these goals).

The science as practice perspective: games as model-based learning

The Science as Practice (or SaP) perspective (Pickering 1995; Lehrer and Schauble 2006a; Duschl et al. 2007) argues that the development of scientific concepts is deeply intertwined with the development of epistemic and representational practices (e.g., modeling). Modeling is generally recognized as *a*, if not *the*, core disciplinary practice in the development of scientific expertise (Giere 1988; Nersessian 2002; Lehrer and Schauble 2006b; Duschl et al. 2007). Modeling involves the iterative generation and refinement of inscriptions (Latour 1990; Lehrer et al. 2000). As Latour (1990) originally explained, inscriptions refer to marks on a medium, such as paper or an electronic screen, and scientists *design* inscriptions in order to represent salient aspect(s) of the phenomenon under inquiry. Philosophers of science have pointed out that the central activity of science is the generation and testing of these models (Giere 1988; Hesse, 1974).

Models in science are explanatory in nature - i.e., they provide mechanistic explanations of natural phenomena (Giere 1988; Nersessian 2008; Lehrer and Schauble 2002). We can define models as fictive representations of real things (e.g., planes, cars, or buildings) or of systems (e.g., atomic structure, weather patterns, traffic flow, ecosystems, or social systems) that are simpler than the real objects and systems they represent but preferentially highlight certain properties of the referent (Rapp and Sengupta 2012). Giere argues that scientific explanations are constructed with models that have been developed in the sciences: 'Little can be learned ... about science that could not be learned more directly by examining the nature of scientific models and how they are developed' (Giere 1988; p. 105).

Specifically in the domain of kinematics, which is the focal domain of our own research, Hestenes (1993) argued that 'modeling is the name of the game' (p. 1) and that 'modeling is the main activity of scientists' (p. 6). Furthermore, Hestenes (1992) explains that modeling in kinematics involves three practices: development of a model; exploring the ramifications of the model in order to investigate the complex interactions in the phenomena; and deployment of the model in order to iteratively match it to empirical phenomena and data. According to Hestenes, the games of scientific explanation and prediction are key facets of model deployment. 'A physical phenomenon can be explained by a theory only to the extent that it can be modeled within the theory. Thus, the model is the explanation! [...] In a prediction game, the model is usually more explicit, because it is needed to generate some trend in simulated data' (Hestenes 1992, p 736–737).

Science and math education researchers have shown that engaging in modeling and progressively refining one's representation of some aspect of the world (e.g., a model or an inscription) can contribute to a deeper understanding of mathematical and scientific knowledge and practices (Gravemeijer et al. 2000; Hall and Stevens 1995; Lehrer and Pritchard 2002; Lehrer and Schauble, 2002). Enyedy (2005) refers to this process as 'progressive symbolization'. Lehrer (2009) makes clear that, while students need to see and handle models of abstract concepts in order for meaningful conceptual change to happen, the nature of the model is key. Not only do representations capture essential dynamic features of the relationships they describe but they also edit those relationships, foregrounding some elements and obscuring or omitting others (Lehrer and Schauble 2002; Lynch 1990). This 'editing' can potentially result in desirable as well as undesirable consequences for learners in terms of the structures and relationships recognized and interpreted by the learners as salient.

Can digital games as a medium support productive modeling and progressive symbolization? Gee (2008) discusses two characteristics supporting an affirmative answer: (1) games can enable the player to take on an *empathetic* perspective and (2) games can engage students using models and modeling as supports toward mastering relevant content knowledge. These two characteristics represent important meeting points between games and science education. The first characteristic, empathetic perspective, refers to a point of view a person can take in which they 'think like' the objects that they are investigating. Gee (2008) pointed out that taking the perspective of objects being investigated often plays a crucial role in the development of scientific understanding. A well-known example of this perspective in action can be found in Fox-Keller's biography of Barbara McClintock, in which the Nobel-prize winner describes how she achieved a major breakthrough in her research by learning to think like the DNA molecules that she was investigating (Fox-Keller 1983). Wilensky and Reisman (2006) and Dickes and Sengupta (2013) demonstrated that the ability to take on the perspective of thinking *like* the individual elements in a complex system can enable novice science learners to develop a deep understanding of the system. Gee argues that well-designed games accomplish exactly that

> Video games, under the right circumstances, may well be able to encourage (and actually help players to enact) an 'attitude' or 'stance' similar to the one taken by scientists studying complex systems. This stance involves a sort of 'embodied empathy for a complex system' wherein a person seeks to enter imaginatively into a system, all the while seeing and thinking of it as a system, rather than as a group of local or random events. (Gee 2008, p 32).

Gee's second point pertains to the use of models and modeling as key interactive elements in games. Gee points out that 'models and modeling allow specific aspects of experience to be interrogated and used for problem solving in ways that lead from concreteness to abstraction' (Gee 2008, pp 30). However, as Gee (2008) points out, the fact that a game deploys models does not automatically imply that the game play will necessitate modeling or the use of models. In some cases, for example, models within games are used primarily to drive and manage the context within which players themselves act (e.g., *World of Warcraft*). Focusing on disciplinary integration is intended to move students beyond acting within models to instead engage students in modeling as a means of predicting, controlling, and reflecting on actions and events in the game environment.

Early focus on conceptual integration

We began our own work on digital games and science learning with the goal of helping students integrate intuitive and formal understandings of Newtonian dynamics. We initially conceptualized the design as integrating (1) disciplinary representations and formal relationships of Newtonian dynamics with (2) popular recreational game mechanics from games such as *Mario Galaxy* and *Switchball* that include marble motion. The first game we developed and studied, *SURGE Classic,* takes places in an outer-space environment (Figure 1). Students use the arrow keys to navigate a rocket-powered spaceship (piloted by the 'Surge' avatar) around barriers and through corridors in search of non-player characters in need of rescue. Overlaid on the screen are different read-outs of information for players, including their ship's current speed, velocity vectors, the number of impulses used, the number of collisions with the walls, and elapsed time on a given game level. Players must minimize collisions, level completion time, and number of impulses used in order to earn a high score. Some levels also include a motion map region, where students must maintain a constant velocity, increase their speed, or decrease their speed in order to continue onward.

SURGE Classic (and subsequent *SURGE* designs) are 'conceptually integrated games' for learning (Clark and Martinez-Garza 2012), as opposed to merely 'conceptually embedded games'. This means that the science to be learned is integrated directly into the mechanics as the central focus of navigating or manipulating the game world, rather than being embedded as an activity to be visited at some location in the game environment (i.e., isolated from the process of navigating or manipulating the overall game word and confined to challenges experienced at particular moments in time and/or special locations in the game world). The latter structure is typical of many virtual worlds designed for science learning. Note that both conceptually integrated and conceptually embedded games can represent intrinsic, as opposed to extrinsic, game design (c.f., Habgood and Ainsworth 2011). As an example, the intrinsic version of Habgood and Ainsworth's *Zombie Division* game is conceptually embedded rather than conceptually integrated

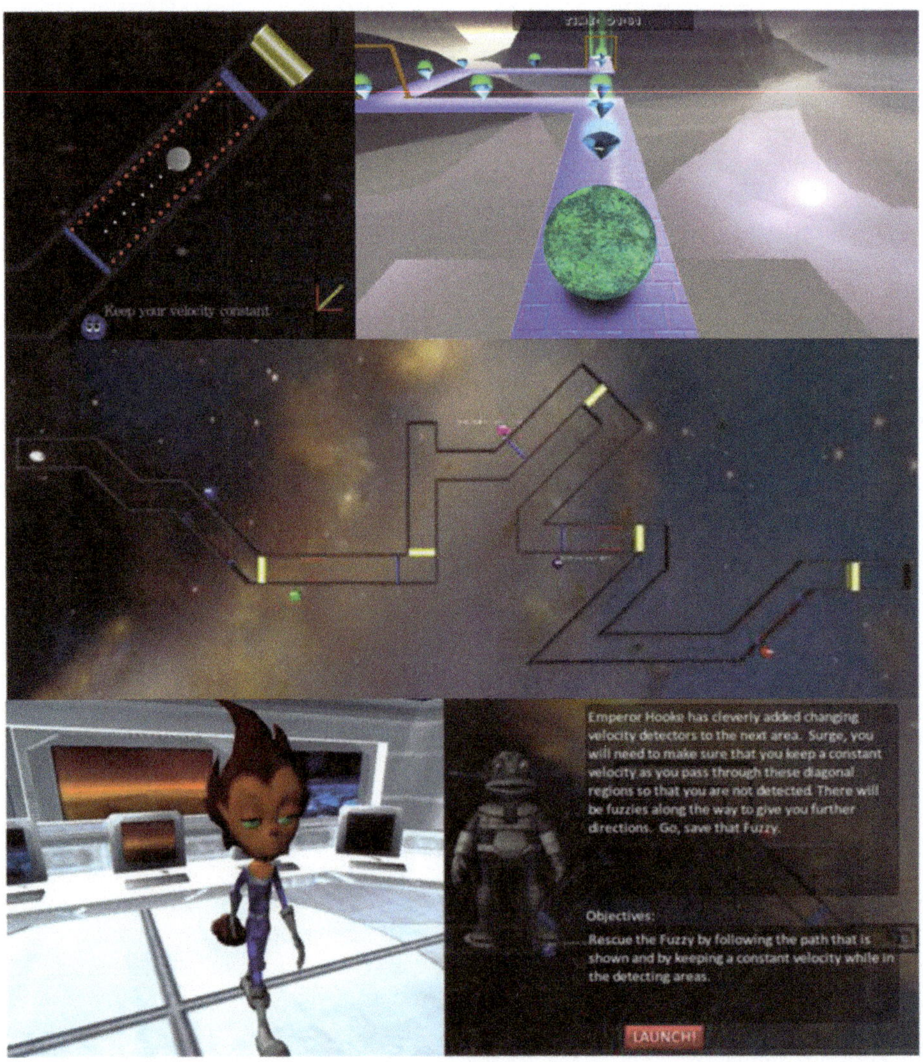
Keep your velocity constant
Emperor Hooke has cleverly added changing velocity detectors to the next area. Surge, you will need to make sure that you keep a constant velocity as you pass through these diagonal regions so that you are not detected. There will be fuzzies along the way to give you further directions. Go, save that Fuzzy.
Objectives:
Rescue the Fuzzy by following the path that is shown and by keeping a constant velocity while in the detecting areas.
LAUNCH!

Figure 1 Screenshots from an impulse level in SURGE. Students must guide Surge in her spherical spaceship through maze-like prisons to rescue Fuzzies.

in the sense that, while the math solution activity is intrinsic in the game, it is embedded rather than integrated into the fabric of navigating the world.

Conceptual integration required a two-pronged design approach: (1) designing levels around popular game-play mechanics from appropriate game genres, while also (2) designing challenges that directly explore, rather than merely contain, targeted physics relationships. Along the first dimension, *SURGE Classic* adopted core ideas from recreational game design conventions including (a) supporting engagement and approachable entry (Koster 2004; Squire 2011), (b) situating the player with a principled stance and perspective (McGonigal 2011), (c) providing context and identification for the player with a role and narrative (Gee 2007a; Pelletier 2008), (d) monitoring and providing actionable feedback for the player (Annetta et al. 2009; Garris et al. 2002; Munz et al. 2007), and (e) using pacing and gatekeeping to guide the player through cycles of performance (Squire 2006).

Along the second dimension, *SURGE Classic* game levels were designed to require students to apply and coordinate many principles related to Newtonian dynamics to complete levels (e.g., impulse, inertia, vector addition, elasticity of collisions, gravity, velocity, acceleration, free-fall, mass, force, and projectile motion). Physics ideas and terminology were built into pre-level and post-level story and feedback screens and within the levels of the game itself. The levels were designed so that physics concepts built upon one another and gradually introduced the student to new ideas and ways of interacting with the game world. For example, a student would first navigate through an orthogonal maze (which students could solve by using impulses to bring Surge to a stop in one direction before initiating movement in the perpendicular direction) before having to pass through mazes with diagonal corridors (requiring students to achieve states of motion that have non-zero velocities in both coordinate dimensions at once). Each level highlighted one or two topics, and levels allowed students to connect the concepts together and to see the relationships among the topics.

Throughout the levels, we attempted to minimize frustration for novice players. We learned, however, that protecting students from failure must not outweigh requiring mastery for progress. Clark et al. (2011) elaborate on these *SURGE Classic* design approaches in greater detail, but the descriptions here are sufficient to ground our discussion of the implications of lessons learned from *SURGE Classic* for subsequent phases of our game design, as well as for games for science learning more generally.

Students playing versions of *SURGE Classic* demonstrated high engagement and modest but statistically significant learning gains on items based on the Force Concept Inventory (FCI), which is a widely known benchmark assessment for conceptual understanding of Newtonian dynamics at the undergraduate level (Hestenes and Halloun 1995; Hestenes et al. 1992). A study with seventh and eighth grade students in Taiwan and the United States (Clark et al. 2011) showed significant pre-post gains with modest effect sizes. Furthermore, students of both genders in both counties liked playing the game. Similar findings were obtained in four further studies conducted with US undergraduate physics students (D'Angelo et al. 2010), US Title I sixth grade students, and US undergraduate educational psychology students (Slack et al. 2010, 2011). Students' gains and increased mastery, however, focused on intuitive understanding (which is what the FCI largely measures) rather than competence with formal terminology or notations. Essentially, players could more accurately predict the results of various actions, impulses, and interactions (which improves performance in the game and on FCI questions), but players were not being supported in explicitly articulating the intuitive relationships in terms of formal disciplinary representations and concepts.

Toward modeling and science as practice: prediction, reflection, and articulation

Building on the findings from *SURGE Classic*, we began to explore ways to incentivize prediction and explanation to enhance conceptual integration in our next two game platforms, *SURGE Next* and *Fuzzy Chronicles*. A growing body of research and scholarship on games and cognition emphasizes informal cycles of prediction, explanation, and refinement at the core of game-play processes (Games-to-Teach Team 2003; Salen and Zimmerman 2004, Wright 2006). Research in science education has demonstrated that prediction and explanation can scaffold students in reflecting more consciously and deliberately about the underlying physics models (e.g., Scott et al. 1992). Prediction and explanation can also promote metacognition, learning, and reflection (e.g., Champagne et al. 1982) as well as conceptual change (Tao and Gunstone, 1999; Kearney 2004). We have found, however, that design principles from research on learning often require adaptation for the digital game medium in a manner that is synergistic with, rather than disruptive to, the conventions and affordances of the medium.

Integrating prediction into game play

As in *SURGE Classic*, players in *SURGE Next* and *Fuzzy Chronicles* navigate their avatar through the play area to rescue game characters and deliver them to safe locations while avoiding obstacles and enemies. We changed the mechanisms of navigation, however, to emphasize prediction/anticipation rather than reaction. *SURGE Classic* employed a real-time reactive navigation structure where

(a) pressing an 'arrow key' resulted in immediate application of an impulse or constant thrust in the direction of the arrow key and (b) motion in a desired direction often required continual split-second adjustments. In contrast, *SURGE Next* and *Fuzzy Chronicles* explored approaches to incentivize prediction by (a) creating challenges that required players to make fewer but higher impact decisions and (b) requiring players to spatially place all of these commands in advance. First, we reduced the total number of commands players initiate in a given level (thereby increasing the salience and impact of each individual command) to encourage players to think more carefully about the outcomes and implications of each action. Additionally, we required players to pre-place their solution rather than enact it in real time. Thus, in order to move along a particular path, the learner creates a predictive model of the trajectory by placing impulses along the target path (Figure 2). The learner then deploys his or her model by 'launching' the level to 'run' the plan. Players watch their plans unfold and then revise them accordingly.

Microgenetic outcomes and implications

In order to investigate the students' sense-of-mechanism (diSessa 1993) of the underlying physics, we conducted a microgenetic study in a ninth grade classroom in a Mid-Southern US public school with an early version of *SURGE Next* (Krinks et al. 2013; Sengupta, Krinks, and Clark: Conceptual Change in Physics through Use of Digital Games, revised and resubmitted). The data took the form of semi-structured clinical interviews that were conducted with each student upon successful completion of each level. We observed one particular conceptual

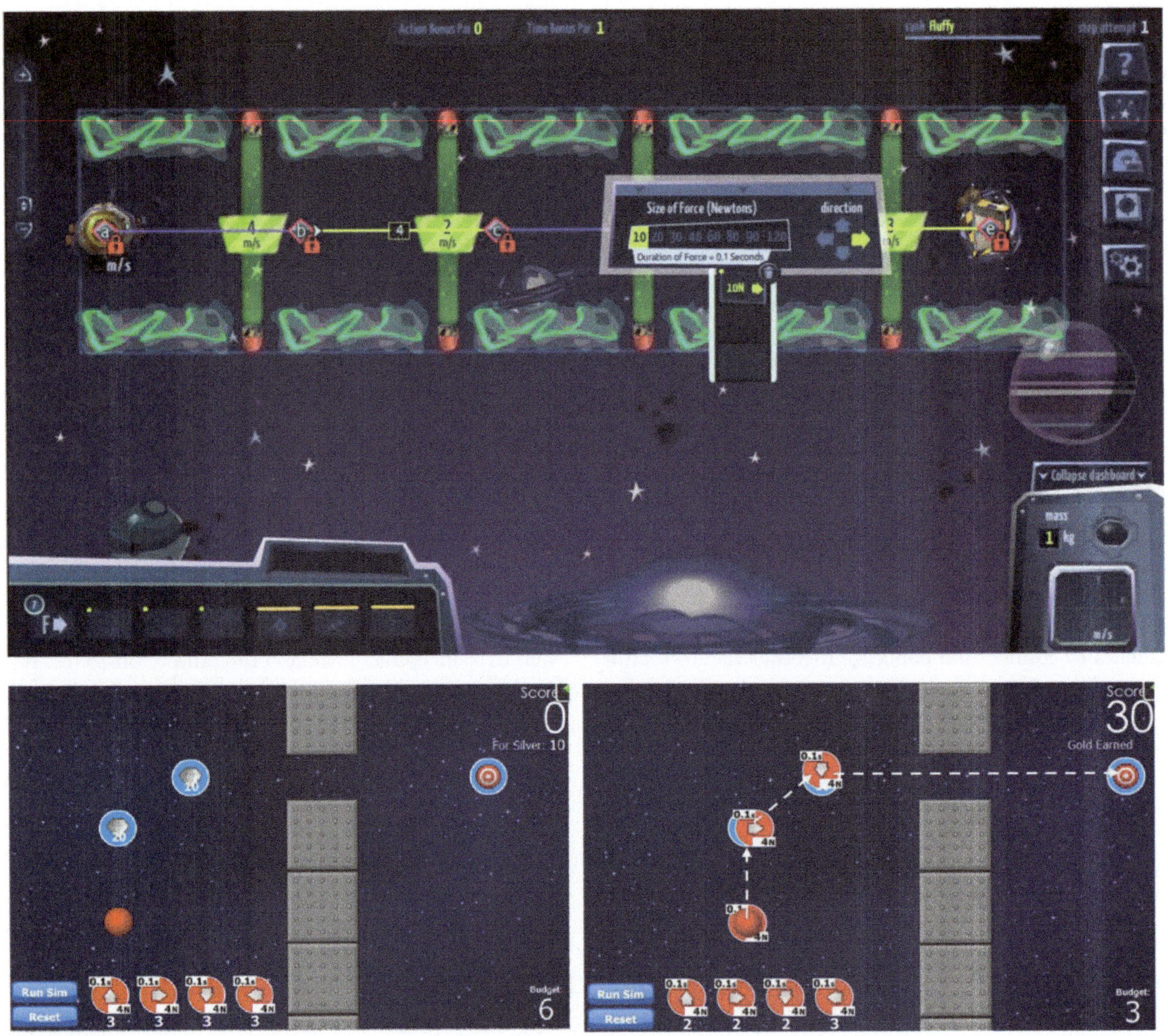

Figure 2 Simple example Fuzzy Chronicles level (top) and simple SURGE Next level and solution (bottom).

resource that was deeply entrenched in the minds of students and manifested itself in many ways throughout all of the students' game play.

As mentioned in our overview of KiP, shifting to correctly prioritizing the Force as Deflector p-prim is key to understanding formal Newtonian relationships underlying Newton's first law. diSessa explained the schematization of the Force as Deflector p-prim as follows: 'A force (e.g., shove) may act in concert with prior motion (momentum) to produce a compromise result, directionally between the two' (diSessa 1993, pp 218). From the perspective of canonical physics, while Force as Mover neglects the role of the momentum of an object, Force as Deflector takes that into consideration. Therefore, the latter enables us to correctly predict and explain situations in which application of two impulses on an object along two different directions may result in motion of the object along a 'compromise' direction.

In our study, the Force as Mover p-prim was initially the preferred resource among all students. Through the conceptually integrated nature of game play, however, students realized that their intuitive physics ideas did not hold true in all situations. If they wanted to successfully solve the levels, students were compelled to consider properties of forces that they may never have consciously considered. Each level in the game acted as a sandbox in which students could easily model and test their intuitive ideas about the relationships between force and motion and receive immediate feedback as to the appropriateness of those ideas. In this learning environment, we saw students discover that certain ideas were productive in certain situations, thus activating resources in a new situation and reorganizing knowledge elements into a more cohesive framework. These newly cued ideas were the intuitive foundations of Newton's first law, such as the notion that an object will continue to move in its original direction until another force acts on it.

During the initial levels, we observed that students tenaciously used the Force as Mover p-prim, even after it had proven unsuccessful in producing the target outcomes in similar situations in the immediately preceding levels. To be clear, Force as Mover is not a 'wrong' resource that students should never use. On the contrary, it can correctly explain commonplace situations in everyday life, as pointed out earlier. But it does not always work well as an explanatory resource in more complex situations that involve the combinations of forces along different directions. Levels in *SURGE Next* deliberately expose students to situations where Force as Mover is not productive, enabling students to iteratively revise and refine their reasoning through re-designing, re-deploying, and re-assessing their solutions. The nature of the solution process itself - i.e., the placement of impulses along the predicted path of Surge - made explicit students' underlying assumptions, and the ability to verify, revise, and refine their solutions offered them opportunities to reflect and consider other conceptual resources. Gradually, new resources such as Force as Deflector emerged and increased in cueing priority, but only after repeated attempts and failures to make the primary resource of Force as Mover work. Similar to Gee's argument, we found that modeling Surge's motion through the placement of impulses along their predicted paths allowed specific aspects of the players' interpreted experience to be interrogated and used for problem solving in ways that led from concreteness to abstraction.

Eventually, these resources were cued with a higher priority than Force as Mover, as students became more adept at recognizing scenarios in which these resources were appropriate. Students' intuitive thinking in *SURGE Next* evolved, showing productive growth toward expert-like reasoning during game play. Thus this work highlights conceptual change as a process of refining cueing priorities and conditions rather than conceptual replacement. Furthermore, this work demonstrates the importance of students' conscious awareness of the outcomes from individual navigation decisions for the conceptual change process.

Teacher thinking with *SURGE*: a case study

Around the same time as the microgenetic study, we conducted a case study of a teacher and his students using an early version of *Fuzzy Chronicles* (Van Eaton et al. 2013). The study explored how the teacher and students interacted with the representations in a version of *Fuzzy Chronicles* that included a timeline structure for placing navigation commands. The goal was to understand how the representations affected the teacher's and students' epistemologies of force. We had hoped that the teacher's and students' understanding of force and motion would become more nuanced and that they would connect their intuitive understanding of physics with formal, canonical understanding of Newton's laws. The study highlighted improvements in the teacher's and students' ability to make phenomenological predictions about what would happen next given a configuration of impulses and their ability to manipulate the representations in the game to successfully complete levels, but it also highlighted how the teacher and students ascribed subjective properties to the representations of forces in the game to reconcile phenomena and relationships in the game with their own intuitive understanding of Newton's laws.

The teacher's and students' thinking paralleled Aristotelian notions of force being 'used up' or 'spread out' over distance. Thus distance was foregrounded in student or teacher's intuitive thinking about force (i.e., force as a means to travel a set distance, not accelerate the object to travel at a specific velocity for a set time). The teacher and students reinterpreted structural features of the representations in the game to support these understandings and subsequently used these structural features to reconcile their intuitive understandings when discussing the game in terms of formal Newtonian definitions of relationships. In these discussions, the teacher and student were able to 'bend' formal statements of Newton's three laws in terms of the representations in the game to warrant their intuitive thinking in non-normative ways, such as interpreting forces applied against the direction of motion in terms of the wording Newton's third law.

We interpreted the case study findings as interactions between the representational nature of the game and the abstract concepts the game was intended to demonstrate (Van Eaton et al. 2013). As discussed earlier, Lehrer (2009) makes clear that students need to see and handle models of abstract concepts in order for meaningful conceptual change to happen; but the nature of the model is also key. Not only do representations capture essential dynamic features of the relationships they describe, but they also edit those relationships, foregrounding some elements and obscuring or omitting others (Lehrer and Schauble 2002; Lynch 1990), potentially both in desirable and undesirable ways. The representations we had designed in *Fuzzy Chronicles* scaffolded and refined the teacher and students' intuitive understanding of the relationships but are not sufficient to support a fundamental reinterpretation that the teacher and student could reconcile with normative interpretations of the relationships. Instead, the teacher and student reinterpreted structural features of the representation in ways to support their pre-existing non-normative interpretations. This case study thus explored the affordances of the representations and model they inscribed as well as the challenges of focusing teachers and students on the salient aspects of representations to support conceptual change. In other words, the case study highlights the intertwined relationship between focusing on representations, and the conceptual resources that are at play when teachers and students interact with the game.

Experimental outcomes and implications

In addition to the implications outlined above, our pilot studies with early versions of *SURGE Next* suggested that our approach to emphasizing prediction/anticipation rather than reaction was an improvement over our efforts in *SURGE Classic.* At the same time, however, these pilot studies showed how situation-dependent interaction design can be. Our intention was to incentivize predictive rather than reactive play. One key aspect of our approach involved requiring students to 'pre-place' the motion plan of their attempted solution, laying out impulses in space as opposed to enacting these impulses in real time. The other key aspect of our approach involved reducing the total number of navigational decisions/actions involved within individual game levels to increase the salience and consequence of each decision.

To explore the affordances of the first aspect of our design plan, we created two versions of *SURGE Next,* one requiring the player to pre-place navigational controls and the other requiring her to enact Surge's motion in real time. In line with the second aspect of our design plan, game levels in both the real-time and the pre-placed versions focused on applying a small number of impulses of the rather than the large number of rapid actions required by *SURGE Classic.* To our surprise, quantitative pilot studies comparing the two versions of *SURGE Next* showed that both approaches had advantages (Clark et al. 2013), suggesting that the critical benefit for both derives from focusing game-play on fewer more consequential decisions so that players anticipate and think carefully about decisions and actions (i.e., engage in prediction). The pre-placed approach encouraged extended prediction of a full level solution but allowed continual revision of the plan, while the real-time version allowed for planning but also incentivized careful attention and provided immediate feedback as an outcome for each choice.

Thus, both approaches supported prediction/anticipation in different ways. Interestingly, attentional cognitive covariates (Rueda et al. 2004) for individual students correlated with learning gains differentially across approaches in these studies (Clark et al. 2013). This has motivated an ongoing line of research in our project to better understand how cognitive and motivational factors of players interact with different approaches to structuring navigation to support prediction, reflection, and learning (e.g., Killingsworth, Adams, and Clark: Cognitive and Motivational Influences on Learning and Play in a Physics Game, submitted). We hope through this research to develop approaches to adapt navigation structures for students based on their profiles and game-play logs. In terms of the current manuscript, however, the findings from this research on *SURGE Next* underscore (1) the importance of incentivizing prediction/anticipation and (2) the emphasis of learning gains on intuitive understanding.

Research on *Fuzzy Chronicles* has simultaneously compared (1) pre-placed approaches that engage students in placing actions spatially on the level map with (2) pre-placed approaches where students pre-place actions in a *timeline* to emphasize the temporal relationships of motion rather than the positional relationships (Figure 3). As with the comparisons in *SURGE Next,* we are finding that different structures emphasize different affordances and cognitive demands by highlighting different relationships

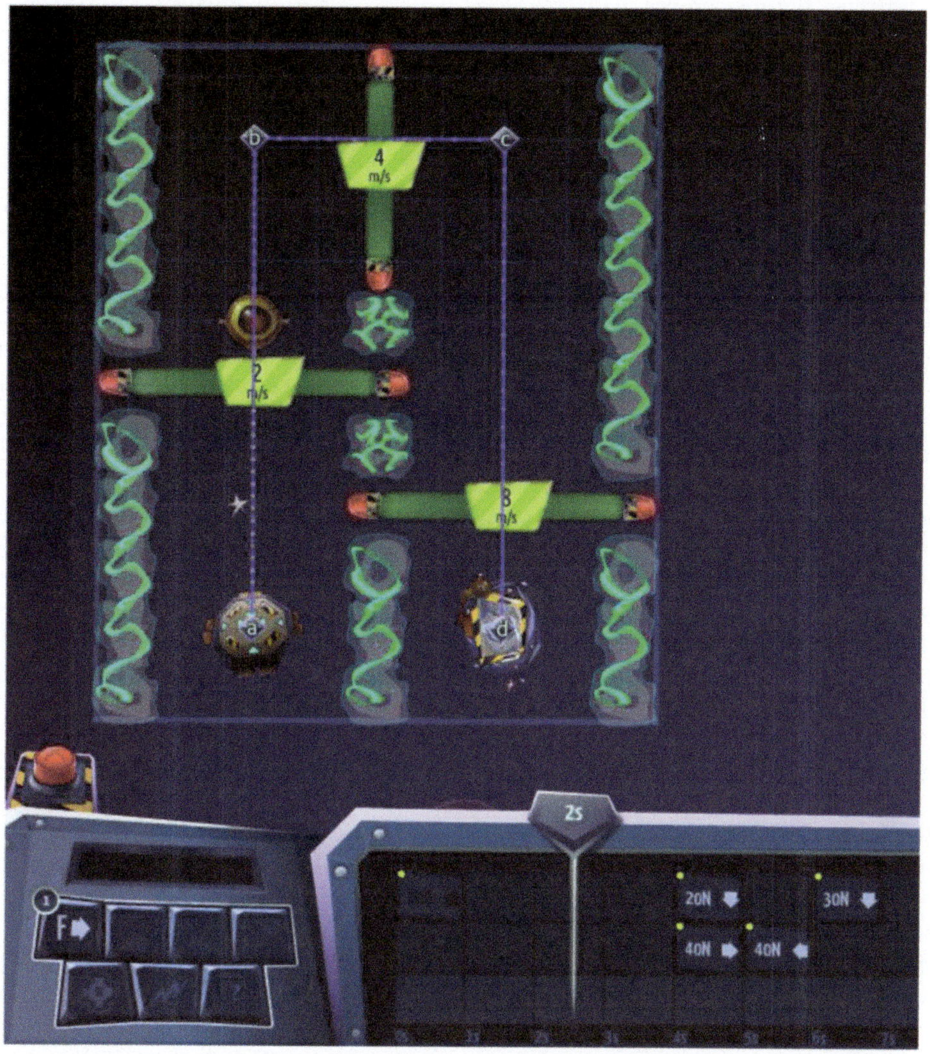

Figure 3 Simple Fuzzy Chronicles level with timeline placement of impulses to emphasize temporal relationships.

and aspects of the models structured by the students. The design challenges involve balancing these affordances and demands in a manner that allows students to focus on the core Newtonian relationships in a predictive, anticipatory, and conscious manner. The findings with *Fuzzy Chronicles* also parallel the findings from *SURGE Next* in their emphasis on the value of puzzle-like challenges with smaller numbers of high-salience decisions to support conceptually integrated designs and learning goals.

Self-explanation to scaffold articulation

To complement our increased emphasis on prediction in *Fuzzy Chronicles* and *SURGE Next,* we also began researching explanation functionality to scaffold students' articulation of the relationships they are exploring. Few games provide coherent structures for externalizing and reflecting on game play; more often, such articulation and reflection generally occur outside the game, through discussion among players or participation in online forums (Gee 2007b; Squire 2005; Steinkuehler and Duncan 2008). We are now working to develop supports for this articulation and reflection by encouraging explanation in the dialog between the players and computer characters.

Research on self-explanation by Chi and others provides insight into the value of explanation for learning (e.g., Chi et al. 1989; Roy and Chi 2005; Chi and VanLehn 1991). Encouragingly, research by Bielaczyc et al. (1995) shows that instruction that stresses generating explanations improves performance even after the prompts that drive the explanations are discontinued. Mayer and Johnson (2010) conducted preliminary work in embedding self-explanation in a game-like environment with encouraging results, including gains on transfer tasks. This emphasis on explanation is mirrored in research on science education. Work by White and Frederiksen (1998, 2000), for example, demonstrates the value of asking students to reflect on their learning during inquiry with physics simulations.

Interestingly, while many aspects of recreational game design are currently very sophisticated compared to most educational software, dialog in recreational games tends to involve relatively simple 'multiple-choice' dialog trees that are not difficult to create. Educational games can thus easily leverage this general approach and even improve upon it. After a player has completed a set of missions in *Fuzzy Chronicles*, a computer-controlled character in the game contacts the player and asks for help. The subsequent dialog prompts a player to select explanations to answer the computer character by explaining how the player's solution relates to more formal articulations of the relationships. Our goal is to present these invitations for dialog as puzzles that are engaging in their own right (Clark and Martinez-Garza 2012; Clark et al. 2012).

Adams and Clark (2014) conducted an experiment with an early prototype of the explanation functionality in *Fuzzy Chronicles* (Figure 4). The experiment compared three conditions. Students in the 'questions' version of the game chose explanations for key phenomena at specific moments in game play - before testing their solutions, after an incorrect solution, and upon successfully completing a stage (e.g., when asked why they needed to apply an impulse at the beginning of a level, students needed to choose 'according to Newton's first law the ship will not move unless an unbalanced force acts upon it'). Students in the 'tips' condition, by comparison, would receive a tip (i.e., be provided an explanation) at corresponding moments in play - when they started an attempt, after an unsuccessful attempt, and after completing the level. Finally, students in the control condition received feedback only about whether they succeeded on the level or not.

This first study taught us a great deal about the structure, timing, and placement of explanation functionality to manage cognitive load, engagement findings that have informed subsequent approaches. One take-home lesson involved managing the complexity of the dialogic interactions in the context of the game experience's overall complexity. In some prototype situations, adding the explanation questions increased the complexity of an already complex task, disrupting students' experience of *flow* (Csikszentmihalyi 1991; Kiili 2005). A challenge when designing games for learning is to balance flow with moments of conscious reflection for learning (Kiili and Lainema 2008; Mayer and Johnson 2010). Another take-home lesson involved the timing of the dialog episodes. In some instances, the explanation episodes worked against aspects of students' game play that served to 'segment' a level into smaller chunks to manage cognitive demands (c.f. Mayer 2009). Segmenting a level is useful metacognitive or 'epistemic action' (Kirsh and Maglio 1994) that facilitates cognition in challenging settings. We realized that future designs needed to balance complexity while still providing opportunities for students to articulate the relationships they are exploring.

These take-home lessons underscored the challenges in reengineering and applying the findings of research from one learning context to another, particularly to contexts as rich as digital games. We reengineered the dialog functionality based on these lessons (Figure 5) and are currently collecting data with the new design. The preliminary analyses suggest that these changes are substantial improvements and can scaffold students successfully in reflecting on their actions and improving learning gains (Clark et al. 2012). A repeated-measures ANOVA revealed that the full explanation condition

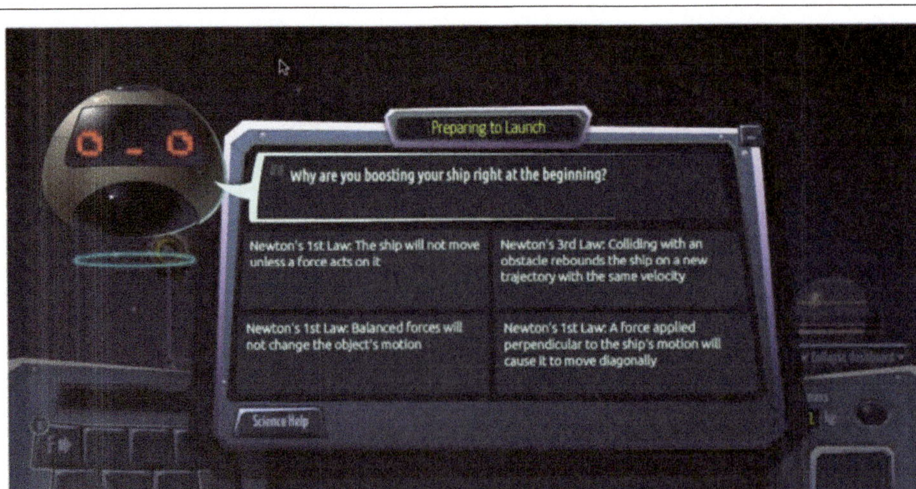

Figure 4 Early explanation functionality in *Fuzzy Chronicles*.

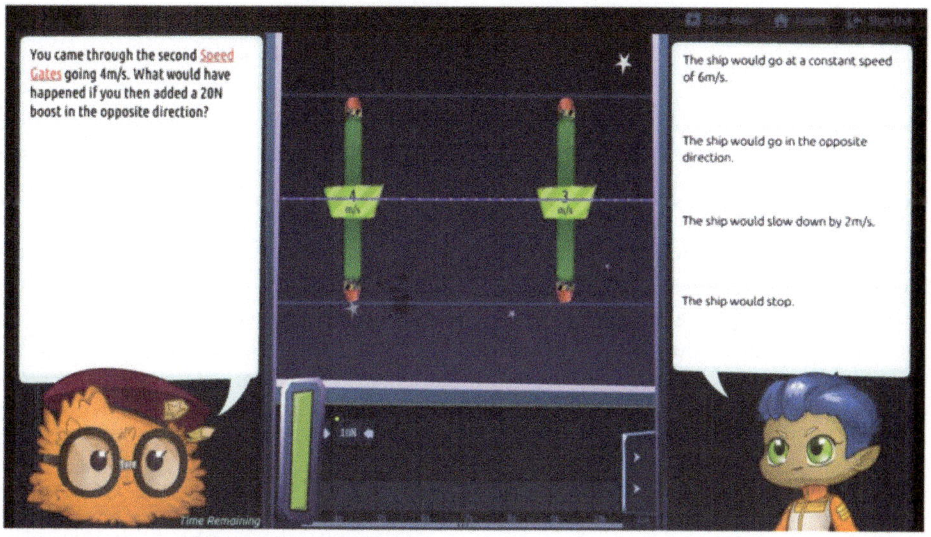

Figure 5 Revised explanation functionality in *Fuzzy Chronicles*.

outperformed the abbreviated explanation and tip conditions. Interestingly, although the full explanation condition required students to provide more answers and thus should have required more time, students in that condition actually completed slightly more levels in the game. This suggests that the full explanation conditions not only supported higher pre-post gains but also supported more efficient progress on the other parts of the game. We are currently conducting data-mining analyses of the data to explore these differences to better understand the mechanisms of learning supported through the full explanation condition.

Our results from this latest study have convinced us of the potential value of engaging students in the practices of explanation and articulation to enhance their understanding of the underlying relationships they are modeling in the game. We continue to refine and revise our design principles based on observations and data from the field clarifying synergistic approaches for integrating explanation and reflection into game play, as we will expand upon in a later section of this paper.

Toward disciplinary integration: integrating graphing with prediction and explanation

Through our work with integrating prediction and explanation into our designs, we have come to understand that conceptually integrated games need to create conditions for mathematizing situations and phenomena using domain-appropriate and task-appropriate symbolic representations. In this way, it is possible to engage students in modeling through game play. We developed this hypothesis in response to recurring patterns in findings across our studies. Nearly all students were able to develop productive intuitions about the underlying physical phenomena within the game as evident from the pre-post gains across studies, the microgenetic analysis (Krinks et al. 2013, Sengupta, Krinks, and Clark: Conceptual Change in Physics through Use of Digital Games, revised and resubmitted), the teacher case study (Van Eaton et al. 2013), and data mining analysis of log data from students' game play (Kinnebrew et al., in review). Students were generally not demonstrating strong abilities to connect that intuitive understanding across comparatively more formal, canonical representations of motion.

In order to address this issue, we set out to create additional opportunities in which students would engage in symbolizing salient aspects of motion phenomena and the underlying Newtonian dynamics. This symbolizing work was deeply integrated with the game experience so as to augment the effects of intuitive exploration and understandings achieved with prior designs. Our premise was that, as students progressed in our game, they should be able to *design* and *utilize* progressively more complex inscriptions of the kinematic phenomena they were exploring in the levels.

Designing these mathematical representations corresponds to *model development*, while utilizing them in order to accomplish a certain objective corresponds to *model deployment*, leading in turn to *refinement* of the model. Progressively increasing complexity involves generating and comparing multiple symbolic representations of the same phenomenon (e.g., dot traces and graphs of different types), as well as generating inscriptions of progressively more complex phenomena (e.g., situations involving constant speed, constant acceleration, and varying acceleration). We call this evolution of complexity *progressive symbolization*, appropriating Enyedy's (2005) use of the term. We envision progressive symbolization as a process of learning that can be supported *through* game play, by designing levels that progressively add symbolic depth and representational complexity to relevant game elements.

In our work, progressive symbolization within the game designs has proven valuable in several ways. First, the need for symbolization can be created within the narrative of the game; this enabled us to foster a deep *engagement* of the learners with the practice of modeling. Second, the symbolic representations generated by learners can be analogous to canonical representations that they will encounter in other contexts. This adds *authenticity* to learners' modeling work. Third, students have a meaningful experience of the relationship between work with representations on the one hand, and the development of knowledge and insights on the other hand - a recognition of the generative, constructive nature of working through representations to gain mastery of concepts and relationships. Fourth, students develop a deeper understanding of the underlying concepts and mathematical relationships. As argued earlier, this is also in tune with science and math education researchers' findings that engaging in modeling and progressively refining one's representation of some aspect of the world (e.g., a model or an inscription) can contribute to a deeper understanding of mathematical and scientific knowledge and practices (Gravemeijer et al. 2000; Hall and Stevens 1995; Lehrer and Pritchard 2002; Lehrer and Schauble, 2002).

To test these ideas, we extended *SURGE Next* to create *SURGE NextG. SURGE NextG* includes a graphing environment that enables real-time construction of mathematical representations based on periodic sampling of measures of Surge's motion (see Figure 6a,b,c). Students engage in modeling by generating, navigating between, interpreting, and reflecting upon both spatial records representing position in time (e.g., dot traces) and graphical representations of changes in features of motion over time (e.g., graphs).

Our goal with the design of *Surge NextG* was to further deepen the nature of students' modeling experiences by creating opportunities for students to engage in generating and reasoning about relations between multiple *genres* of inscriptions (e.g., dot traces and graphs of different features of motion, such as speed, displacement, and acceleration). This approach builds on a long history of having students match motion with graphs, control motion with graphs, or create graphs through motion with motion sensors. Some of the most detailed work to date in this area was conducted as part of the *SimCalc* projects, beginning with *MathCars* (Kaput 1994) and later *MathWorlds* (Rochelle and Kaput 1996; Hegedus and Roschelle 2013).

In *SURGE NextG*, students can generate multiple bar graphs, including an 'odometer' graph that shows total displacement as a function of time, graphs of signed x- and y-component displacements, and a 'speedometer' graph that shows total velocity as a function of time, and graphs of signed x- and y-component velocities. Each bar in the graph corresponds to a periodic measurement of distance traveled by Surge within successive time intervals - i.e., like the dot trace, each bar is the record of an instant, with the aggregate graphical representation emerging over time. Unlike with the dot trace, however, in the graphing environment, students can determine the frequency of measurements, either synchronizing them with the dot trace or making them more or less frequent. They can also alter several other features of the graph through provided controls. Finally, students can rewind and replay the completed level in order to examine temporal relationships between the graph and game motion more closely.

Incorporating graphing as a necessary interaction between the learner and the game (and thus shifting from conceptual integration toward disciplinary integration) has had additional implications and affordances for activity design. In particular, it has opened up opportunities for using graphical representations of plans, intentions, and predictions as mediators to connect virtual actions in the game with situations of physical motion in the real world. For example, in *SURGE NextG*, the students were asked to guide a ship through a nebula that was interfering with communication. Students watched a video of a ball first rolling down a ramp, then rolling up another ramp to reach its maximum height. Students were told this was a clue about how to guide the ship and asked to design a game level so that the ship's motion matched the motion of the rolling ball. Students were prompted to create and use graphs of the ship's motion when designing their level. Students were asked to draw a sketch of their solution and to explain how their design matched the video of the ball rolling on the ramp. Following the initial design, students were given 'updated information' from the captain in the form of a speed-time graph that the ship needed to generate and asked to redesign their solutions. Again, students were asked to sketch and to explain their designs.

We conducted a study with this version of *SURGE NextG* with four sections of seventh grade students taught by the same teacher (Sengupta et al. 2014; Learning Physics through Representational Translation in Video Games, in preparation). The study led to interesting results that highlight the benefit of symbolization as a gaming action. Each section was assigned to one of two graphing conditions (grapher vs. no grapher) and one of two collaboration conditions (collaborative vs. non-collaborative). We found that students in the grapher sections showed significantly greater pre-post test gains on key Newtonian relationships. Furthermore, the grapher students who

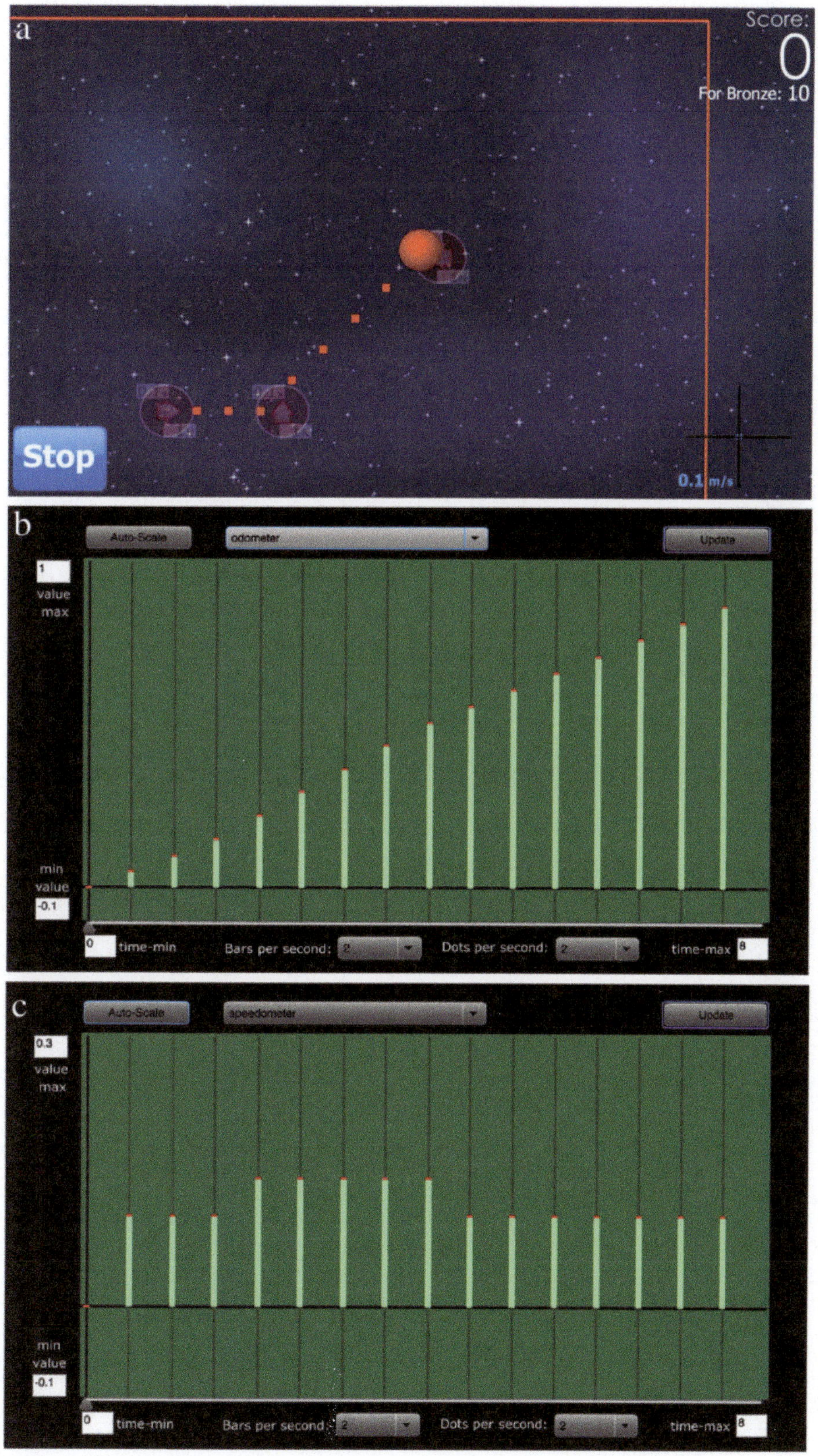

Figure 6 SURGE NextG. (a) A level depicting one-dimensional motion of Surge in *SURGE NextG*. **(b)** The displacement graph that accompanies the one-dimensional motion in *SURGE NextG*. **(c)** The corresponding velocity graph for that same motion in *SURGE NextG*.

framed their plan in a variable-focused way (e.g., thinking about the *meaning* of the relationships in the graph) rather than experientially (e.g., in terms of the *shape* of the graph) showed the highest gains of all.

These findings highlight the importance of progressive symbolization for developing deeper understandings of Newtonian relationships within the game. As students progressed through the levels of *SURGE NextG*, the game became a modeling tool for iteratively developing formal representations (graphs of motion) and connecting these representations to situations of motion in the real world. In the earlier levels, the game play was designed to familiarize students with the core computational representation of motion - dot traces - by engaging them in designing predictive trajectories of *SURGE*. In later levels, students iteratively designed inscriptions in *SURGE NextG* in order to further mathematize the dot-trace representations and use these two representations to model an example of constant acceleration in the real world. In doing so, students developed explanations (models) of motion, made predictions, and deployed their models to verify and further improve on them - and in the process, developed a deep understanding of conceptual relationships in kinematics. This relationship between meaningful symbolization and the development of conceptual understanding is central to disciplinary integration.

Deeper into disciplinary integration

We are currently developing a new game, *SURGE Symbolic* (Clark et al. 2014b), that carries the principles of disciplinary integration further, deepening the symbolization experiences of players while still attempting to stay true to the roots and conventions of recreational games (Figure 7). Specifically, *SURGE Symbolic* centers game play in manipulating and navigating across formal representations while simultaneously engaging players in dialog with computer characters to articulate the relationships inscribed within and across those representations.

Progressive symbolization

SURGE Symbolic engages students in a process of progressive symbolization with an emphasis on iteratively developing representational fluency and conceptual understanding. Play begins in the informal space without access to the Cartesian graphs. Initially, players only have the dot-trace representation and vector arrows for force and velocity. Cartesian representations of position, velocity, and force are gradually introduced to provide the player with tools to exert greater levels of control

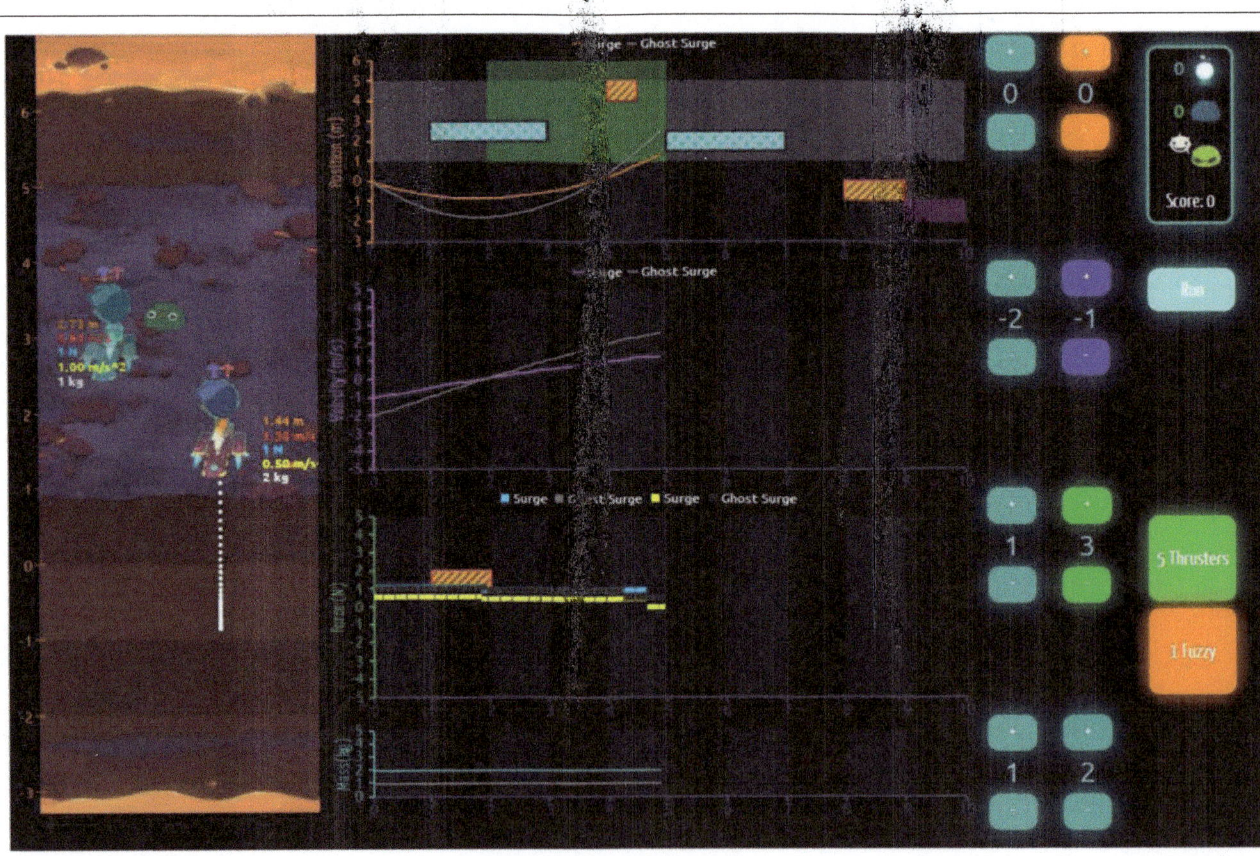

Figure 7 SURGE symbolic.

and prediction over what unfolds in the world space. Moreover, increasing focus is placed on coordination across multiple graphs. Thus play shifts from the informal space deeper and deeper into representational space. Successful game play depends on developing the ability to place multiple relationships in conversation with one another - gleaning the information that each can provide and understanding each as an important but partial perspective on the activity of the game.

Centering game play in the formal representations

Whereas earlier versions of *SURGE* focused more on layering formal representations over informal representations, *SURGE Symbolic* inverts this order, layering informal representations over formal representations while organizing game play explicitly around navigating and coordinating across representations. This provides multiple advantages compared to previous versions of *SURGE.* While earlier versions supported *reflection* on the results of game play through formal representations as a means to support strategy refinement (particularly in *SURGE NextG*), the formal representations were not the medium through which players *planned, implemented,* and *manipulated* their game strategies. In *SURGE Symbolic,* the Cartesian graphs of position, velocity, acceleration, force, and mass are where the puzzles are presented to players, where players plan and implement their actions and where players reflect on the outcomes of their plans. The informal space (which displays the Surge avatar and its physical surroundings) augments the formal representations, but the Cartesian graphs are the hub of all planning, action, and reflection. The graphs are the way that the player communicates with the game (i.e., controls the game) and the way that the game communicates the goals, challenges, events, and outcomes to the player. This is the opposite relationship from earlier versions of *SURGE,* where the informal space provided the hub of activity, while the formal spaces augmented reflection. Thus the Cartesian graphs now provide the language of control and planning as well as the language of description and reflection.

The emphasis on the Cartesian graphs also provides another key advantage. The navigation structures in earlier versions of *SURGE* preferentially foregrounded position, time, or motion. *SURGE Symbolic* emphasizes the *relationships* among all three by utilizing the formal Cartesian graphs as the navigation inscription. This focus on the unifying relationships and links between Cartesian graphs provides a more powerful foundation for exploring key Newtonian ideas, which themselves focus on these relationships.

Our approach extends prior work in using graphs as communications and control structures with 'representational expressivity,' (Hegedus and Moreno-Armella 2009) in two critical ways. First, concerning graph-bound representations as communication structures, our approach uses the Cartesian graphs for strategizing and acting, in which critical information about upcoming challenges is communicated to the player through the 'language' of the Cartesian graphs themselves. The position graph, for example, can present information about the specific regions of the game-world that will be affected by dangerous electrical storms at given times, as well as about locations where rewards or allies will appear to rendezvous with Surge. The velocity and acceleration graphs likewise indicate constraints on game-play, such as maximum or minimum speeds and maximum accelerations that must be observed by Surge or non-player characters during specific time periods, each of which can be tied to narrative elements in game scenarios. Thus again, while positive and negative events also unfold in the informal representations of the game, the hub of all prediction, action, and reflection about these events is integrated into the Cartesian graphs. As a result of this design approach, the Cartesian space emerges as a set of *scientific instruments* for the player, in the sense of providing access to data about the game world that are not available through other means. At the same time, the Cartesian graphs also play the role of an *instrument panel* or mission planner, offering fine-grained control over the movement of the Surge spacecraft.

Flexible dialog system to scaffold reflection and articulation

A key aspect of disciplinary integration focuses on supporting reflection and articulation about the progressive symbolization in which the player is engaging. Toward this end, players in *SURGE Symbolic* will engage in conversational exchanges with non-player characters, with the goal of supporting players in externalizing and articulating elements of their strategies. Thus, progress in coordinating representations and seeing representations as being in 'conversation' with one another is fostered and documented through dialog exchanges between players and non-player characters.

Toward this end, we have developed an adaptive branching structure for the dialog. At the most basic level, this allows students' choices in one frame of the dialog to change what the student encounters in the next frame of the dialog (Figure 8). This is standard functionality in games. What is more novel is that we can also integrate game levels into frames of the dialog so that students can (or even sometimes need to) work on navigation challenges as part of their response in a dialog frame. Furthermore, the response options provided to a student in a dialog frame can adapt depending on the student's actions in the navigation portion of that dialog frame.

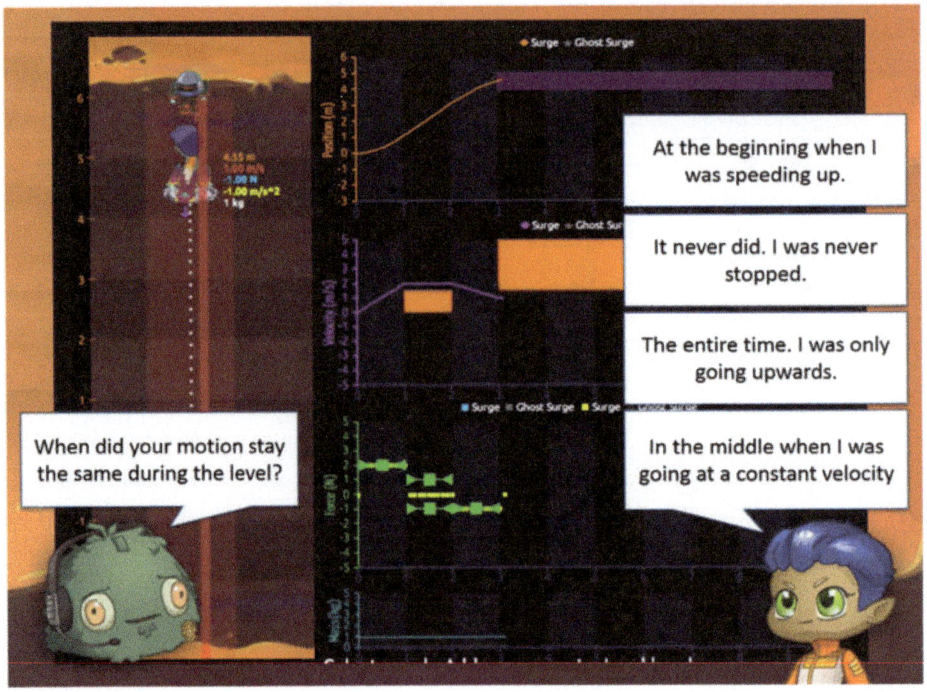

Figure 8 SURGE symbolic with integrated dialog.

Our goals for this functionality are threefold. First, we hope that providing more fluid and targeted responses to players' dialog choices will make the interaction feel more natural and engaging to players, thus increasing engagement and flow within the game.

Second, the new system allows us to develop adaptive scaffolding by adjusting students' experiences based on what they do in the game. If they struggle with a given challenge, they can be routed to additional experiences to make sense of that challenge. If they demonstrate mastery, their route can be expedited to more challenging encounters. If they make a dialog choice suggesting a misconception, the dialog can follow up with further dialog and exploration of those ideas. This functionality will allow us to build on our work with a hybrid p-prim/facet framework of student ideas (diSessa 1993; Krinks et al. 2013, Minstrell 2001; Sengupta, Krinks, and Clark: Conceptual Change in Physics through Use of Digital Games, revised and resubmitted) that can manifest within game play as a means of tracking students' progress and adjusting their experiences.

Third, the dialog system will allow us to more seamlessly integrate experiences from outside of the game into the game to support progressive symbolization. Similar to *SURGE NextG*, players will use *SURGE Symbolic* to develop models of examples of motion in the real world, in later levels in game play. In addition to supporting progressive symbolization, this will support preparation for future learning (Bransford and Schwartz 1999; Schwartz and Arena 2013), as it will allow students to connect the physics represented in the game with scenarios involving motion in the real world.

Generalizing disciplinary integration beyond Newtonian dynamics

Can disciplinary integration can be abstracted and generalized beyond Newtonian dynamics to other core topics? We argue that it can. A powerful framework for generalizing disciplinary integration is provided by Allan Collins and colleagues in their analyses of 'epistemic forms' and 'epistemic games' (Collins 2011; Collins, personal communication, June, 30, 2014; Collins and Ferguson 1993; Morrison and Collins 1995). More specifically, Collins and colleagues argue that the professional work of scientists can be understood in terms of epistemic forms (model types that are the target structures guiding scientific inquiry) and epistemic games (modeling strategies that are the sets of rules and strategies for creating, manipulating, and refining those model types). Collins and colleagues are considering shifting their terminology from 'epistemic forms and epistemic games' to 'model types and modeling strategies' to increase clarity of intent to a broader audience (Collins, personal communication, June 30, 2014), but we will use the original terminology of 'epistemic forms' and 'epistemic games' here to disambiguate from our own use of the terms models and modeling. Collins and colleagues new terminology of 'model types and modeling strategies,' however, underscores the tight fit with the focus of disciplinarily integrated games on models and modeling.

Collins and Ferguson (1993) argue that the advantages of focusing on models and modeling strategies as curricular goals are that they allow educators to move beyond a primary emphasis on 'teaching facts, concepts, and problem solving methods, along with particular theories and models' (Collins and Ferguson, 1993; p. 26), to 'some of the more important forms and games' to guide students' inquiries (p. 26). While Collins and Ferguson did not write with the intention of informing the design of actual digital games (they used the term 'game' as a metaphor), disciplinarily integrated games can be framed as building on the ideas of Collins and colleagues by structuring digital game play around epistemic games of designing and manipulating formal disciplinary representations (epistemic forms). More specifically, if we frame the puzzles in disciplinarily integrated games as distilling epistemic forms (model types) and the epistemic games (modeling strategies) for navigating and manipulating those forms, we open disciplinary integration well beyond our focus on Newtonian dynamics to span across disciplines.

Disciplinarily integrated games are inscriptional systems, and it is particularly important to consider the pedagogical value of the different symbolic systems deployed within a game, as well as the practices (i.e., actions or sets of actions, and the associated goals) that the players need to use in order to use these systems. For disciplinary integration, the forms and practices within the game need to be tied to representations and practices that are needed in order to develop professional scientific expertise. We posit that disciplinarily integrated games should support a key professional practice that cuts across scientific domains - modeling. This means that players' actions should involve the iterative development of inscriptions in the form of computational and mathematized representations of focal phenomenon in order to investigate key conceptual relationships in the domain, while also developing facility with the representations and inscriptions themselves. As mentioned earlier, this is at the heart of the 'Science as Practice' perspective: the history of science unambiguously shows that conceptual development in the sciences is deeply intertwined with the development of representational practices (Nersessian, 1998; Giere 1988; Pickering 1995; Lehrer and Schauble 2010).

Of note here is the use of multiple representational systems as tools for inscription. For example, in our work, dot traces and graphs are complementary representational systems, and when students used these systems *together* as part of their game play, they developed a deeper understanding of the target disciplinary ideas (i.e., concepts). Comparing how relevant aspects of important phenomenon can be represented using different inscriptional systems can support learners in developing a key characteristic of modeling expertise: communicativity (Lehrer, 2003; Lehrer and Schauble 2006b).

We therefore argue that disciplinarily integrated games engage students in playing epistemic games (leveraging modeling strategies) to manipulate and navigate challenges structured in epistemic forms (model types) as a means of (1) coming to understand those epistemic forms and epistemic games as important goals in their own right while (2) simultaneously coming to understand the disciplinary concepts driving the game. It is important to understand that this emphasis of disciplinary integration necessitates that we recognize that conceptual development and the development of representational practices (e.g., modeling) are deeply intertwined. This dual focus parallels the distinction in research on argumentation in the science classroom between 'learning to argue' and 'arguing to learn'. We assert that a joint focus on both is essential, because of their deeply intertwined nature. We therefore propose that disciplinary integration must target conceptual learning as well disciplinary learning in terms of the representational practices of the discipline.

One might then ask: how is designing for disciplinary integration different than designing a 3D virtual inquiry world (e.g., *Quest Atlantis, River City,* or *Crystal Island*)? We would argue that a key distinction in design involves the nature and breadth of focus. Virtual inquiry worlds generally engage students in the practices and Discourses (Gee 1990) of a discipline at the level of inquiry writ large. Much of the pedagogical power and engagement of 3D virtual inquiry worlds tends to focus heavily on their impressive affordances for role-playing, narrative, and identity-building (cf. Gee 2007a). While 3D virtual inquiry worlds are compelling and powerful, their scope and structure do involve tradeoffs in terms of the individual tasks or puzzles themselves, which are often themselves relatively mundane individually (e.g., click on a character to be told a piece of evidence, click on a location to get a reading on oxygen levels, or click on a location to bring up another mini-game to collect evidence).

Disciplinarily integrated games do not attempt the depth of immersion, identity-building, and role-playing of virtual inquiry worlds (and do not dispute their importance or value), but disciplinarily integrated games do afford potentially greater sophistication and refinement of the game-play surrounding the targeted epistemic forms and epistemic games by virtue of their tighter focus. Essentially, whereas 3D virtual inquiry worlds tend to cast students as scientists investigating a 'mystery' at the level of overarching inquiry, disciplinarily integrated games are more focused on specific epistemic games of manipulating specific epistemic forms. This focus allows for progressively deepening the puzzle at the heart of the game and all elements of the game, to emphasize the puzzle.

Disciplinary integration thus focuses foremost on aligning game play with modeling around a specific central set of disciplinary inscriptions rather than engaging in 'inquiry' more broadly. Disciplinary integration is fundamentally generative in that students develop, refine, and deploy models as actions that constitute game play. As students progress through curricular sequences, the game provides a sandbox for modeling phenomena in the real world. Thus, disciplinarily integrated games emphasize STEM practices, but in very focused ways, with any given disciplinarily integrated game focusing on a subset of epistemic forms, or even a single epistemic form, rather than on broader practices (e.g., 'inquiry' writ large).

In terms of examples beyond Newtonian dynamics, we would argue that *DragonBox* meets our criteria for disciplinary integration (http://dragonboxapp.com). *DragonBox* engages players in manipulating algebraic equations through the actual syntax, structures, and procedures of formal algebra. Players isolate boxes to grow their dragons. Players can transform and move and eliminate boxes in various ways. Everything gets introduced in a cartoony, pictorial, non-mathematical way, but gradually, the pictorial representations are pared back until players are moving through screens of more standard algebraic syntax. Another example is provided by *FoldIt*, which adopts molecular schematics as the target epistemic form and engages players in structuring proteins to fold into specific spatial configurations (http://fold.it). The puzzles and mechanics in these games are highly focused (e.g., *FoldIt*'s sequencing of molecules that will fold into specific shapes), providing clean, challenging, and engaging puzzles.

SURGE Symbolic, *DragonBox*, and *FoldIt* are but three possible examples for structuring disciplinary integration around epistemic forms and epistemic games. Framing disciplinary integration in terms of epistemic forms and games opens a vast trove of epistemic forms and epistemic games that span across disciplines (in fact well beyond STEM into the social sciences). Disciplinary integration of digital games thus provides a generalizable genre that holds promise as a vehicle for engaging students in key epistemic forms and games that cross multiple disciplines and respond to calls for greater emphasis on problem solving, 21st century skills, and engaging students in the practices of disciplines to develop deeper understanding.

Reflections and final thoughts

At the highest level, designing games for learning involves integrating learning goals, game design goals, and technology affordances. As with any design activity, game design is fundamentally a creative activity that is bounded not only culturally by the definitions, trajectories, and conventions of the genre it represents but also bounded materially by the economic and technological realities of producing the work itself. Unlike more historically established forms of design (e.g., architecture), game design has not fully explored the limits of its conventional boundaries. Cultural theorists like Berger (2002) advance the position that digital games are a 're-mediation' of earlier text forms, while game design experts stress the novel representational and interactive capacities of the medium (Crawford 1984).

A designer of educational games must attend not only to the conventional forms of the particular genre and subgenre of the game that is being created but also to whether or not the chosen forms are proper carriers of the concepts, systems, and relationships of the learning objectives. This is especially problematic in games for science learning because some of the most powerful ideas of science come in the form of systems, models, and relationships. It is not sufficient to design a compelling game that engages students. Games for science learning should also incorporate the models and structures that support the learning goals and optimize players' learning processes in light of those goals. In this regard, some game forms and concepts are likely more conducive to specific science learning processes and goals. Ultimately, the work of the designer of a game for science learning involves determining which specific conventions of game design support students' engagement with which specific science learning goals and processes.

This paper establishes learning theory as an essential guidepost for dealing with these design challenges and objectives. With KiP as an underlying theory, our early emphasis was on conceptual integration, as evident in the early versions of *SURGE Classic* and *SURGE Next*. Our design choices in these versions were driven by one key goal: to enable students to better articulate their intuitive understandings of the underlying physics. The iterative nature of game play provided students multiple opportunities of prediction and self-explanation, and in the process, supported students in productively reorganizing their understanding of the Newtonian relationships. In later versions of *SURGE*, we further emphasized practices central to modeling - both epistemic and representational - in order to support conceptual development. This was a result of our shift from KiP to SaP as the underlying theoretical framework. Game play now focuses on modeling through manipulation and navigation of formal disciplinary representations - a perspective that we have termed *disciplinary integration*.

Competing interests

The authors declare that they have no competing interests.

Authors' contributions

DC and PS are the equal lead authors and conceptualizers of the new thinking, designs, and writing in the manuscript. CB contributed to the authoring of the discussion about SURGE Symbolic and contributed by collaboratively implementing an early prototype of the SURGE Symbolic software and the graphing components of SURGE NextG. MM-G and SK contributed to the authoring of other specific sections. All authors read, edited, and approved the final manuscript.

Authors' information

The research reported here was supported by the National Science Foundation through grants 1019170 and 1119290 and the Institute of Education Sciences, U.S. Department of Education, through grant R305A110782. The opinions expressed are those of the authors and do not represent views of the Institute, the U.S. Department of Education, or the National Science Foundation.

Author details

[1]College of Education, Vanderbilt University, Box 230, 230 Appleton Place, Nashville, Tennessee 37203-5721, USA. [2]School of Education and Social Policy, Northwestern University, Annenberg Hall, 2120 Campus Drive, Evanston, Illinois 60208, USA.

References

Adams, DM, & Clark, DB. (2014). Integrating self-explanation functionality into a complex game environment: Keeping gaming in motion. *Computers and Education, 73*, 149–159.

Amin, TG. (2009). Conceptual metaphor meets conceptual change. *Human Development, 52*(3), 165–197.

Annetta, LA, Minogue, J, Holmes, SY, & Cheng, M. (2009). Investigating the impact of video games on high school students' engagement and learning about genetics. *Computers & Education, 53*(1), 74–85.

Berger, AA. (2002). *Video Games: A Popular Culture Phenomenon*. New Brunswick, NJ: Transaction Publishers.

Bielaczyc, K, Pirolli, P, & Brown, AL. (1995). Training in self-explanation and self-regulation strategies: Investigating the effects of knowledge acquisition activities on problem solving. *Cognition and Instruction, 13*(2), 221–252.

Bransford, JD, & Schwartz, DL. (1999). Rethinking transfer: A simple proposal with multiple implications. *Review of Research in Education, 24*, 61–100.

Champagne, AB, Klopfer, LE, & Gunstone, RF. (1982). Cognitive research and the design of science instruction. *Educational Psychologist, 17*(1), 31.

Chi, MTH, & VanLehn, KA. (1991). The content of physics self-explanations. *Journal of the Learning Sciences, 1*(1), 69–105.

Chi, MTH, Bassok, M, Lewis, MW, Reimann, P, & Glaser, R. (1989). Self-explanations: How students study and use examples in learning to solve problems. *Cognitive Science, 13*(2), 145–182.

Clark, DB. (2006). Longitudinal conceptual change in students' understanding of thermal equilibrium: An examination of the process of conceptual restructuring. *Cognition and Instruction, 24*(4), 467–563.

Clark, DB, & Martinez-Garza, M. (2012). Prediction and explanation as design mechanics in conceptually-integrated digital games to help players articulate the tacit understandings they build through gameplay. In C Steinkuhler, K Squire, & S Barab (Eds.), *Games, Learning, and Society: Learning and Meaning in the Digital Age* (pp. 279–305). Cambridge: Cambridge University Press.

Clark, DB, Nelson, B, Sengupta, P, & D'Angelo, CM. (2009). *Rethinking science learning through digital games and simulations: Genres, examples, and evidence*. Washington, DC: Paper commissioned for the National Research Council Workshop on Games and Simulations.

Clark, DB, Nelson, B, Chang, H, D'Angelo, CM, Slack, K, & Martinez-Garza, M. (2011). Exploring Newtonian mechanics in a conceptually-integrated digital game: Comparison of learning and affective outcomes for students in Taiwan and the United States. *Computers & Education, 57*(3), 2178–2195. doi:16/j.compedu.2011.05.007.

Clark, DB, Martinez-Garza, M, Biswas, G, Luecht, RM, & Sengupta, P. (2012). Driving assessment of students' explanations in game dialog using computer-adaptive testing and hidden Markov Modeling. In D Ifenthaler, D Eseryel, & G Xun (Eds.), *Game-based Learning: Foundations, Innovations, and Perspectives* (pp. 173–199). New York: Springer.

Clark, DB, Sengupta, P, Kinnebrew, J, Killingsworth, S, Krinks, K, Martinez-Garza, M, & Biswas, G. (2013). *Enhancing Games with Assessment and Metacognitive Emphases*. Washington, DC: Annual Report to the National Science Foundation.

Clark, DB, Brady, C, Sengupta, P, Martinez-Garza, M, Adams, D, Killingsworth, S, & Van Eaton, G. (2014a). *Evolving and balancing informal and formal representations. Proceedings of the Eleventh International Conference of the Learning Sciences*. Boulder, CO: ISLS.

Clark, DB, Tanner-Smith, E, & Killingsworth, S. (2014). Digital games, design, and learning: A systematic review and meta-analysis. Report to The Bill and Melinda Gates Foundation. Available at http://www.sri.com/work/projects/glasslab-research.

Collins, A. (2011). A study of expert theory formation: The role of model types and domain frameworks. In MS Khine & I Saleh (Eds.), *Models and Modeling: Cognitive Tools for Scientific Enquiry* (pp. 23–40). London: Springer.

Collins, A, & Ferguson, W. (1993). Epistemic forms and epistemic games. *Educational Psychologist, 28*, 25–42.

Council, NR. (2009). *National Research Council Workshop on Games and Simulations*. Washington, DC: National Academy Press.

Crawford, C. (1984). *The Art of Computer Game Design*. Berkeley, CA: Osborne/McGraw-Hill.

Csikszentmihalyi, M. (1991). *Flow: The Psychology of Optimal Experience*. New York: Harper Perennial.

D'Angelo, CM, Clark, DB, Nelson, BC, Slack, K, & Menekse, M. (2010). *Connecting tacit understanding from video games to formalized vector concepts*. Philadelphia, Pennsylvania: National Association of Research in Science Teaching (NARST) 2010 meeting.

Dickes, AC, & Sengupta, P. (2013). Learning natural selection in 4th grade with multi-agent-based computational models. *Research in Science Education, 43*(3), 921–953.

diSessa, AA. (1983). Phenomenology and the evolution of intuition. In D Gentner & AL Stevens (Eds.), *Mental Models* (pp. 15–33). Hillsdale, NJ: Lawrence Erlbaum Associates.

diSessa, AA. (1988). Knowledge in pieces. In G Forman & P Pufall (Eds.), *Constructivism in the Computer Age* (pp. 49–70). Hillsdale, NJ: Lawrence Erlbaum Associates.

diSessa, AA. (1993). Toward an epistemology of physics. *Cognition and Instruction, 10*(2 & 3), 105–225.

diSessa, AA, Gillespie, NM, & Esterly, JB. (2004). Coherence versus fragmentation in the development of the concept of force. *Cognitive Science, 28*(6), 843–900.

Duschl, RA, Schweingruber, HA, & Shouse, AW. (2007). *Taking Science to School: Learning and Teaching Science in Grades K-8 (National Research Council Board on Science Education, Center for Education, Division of Behavioral and Social Sciences and Education)*. Washington, DC: The National Academies Press.

Enyedy, N. (2005). Inventing mapping: creating cultural forms to solve collective problems. *Cognition and Instruction, 23*(4), 427–466.

Federation of American Scientists. (2006). *Report: Summit on Educational Games: Harnessing the Power of Video Games for Learning*. Washington, D.C: Federation of American Scientists.

Fox-Keller, E. (1983). *A Feeling for the Organism: The Life and Work of Barbara McClintock*. New York: W.H. Freeman.

Garris, R, Ahlers, R, & Driskell, JE. (2002). Games, motivation, and learning: A research and practice model. *Simulation & Gaming, 33*(4), 441–467. doi:10.1177/1046878102238607.

Gee, JP. (1990). *Social Linguistics and Literacies: Ideology in Discourses*. London: Falmer Press.

Gee, JP. (2007a). *Good Video Games and Good Learning: Collected Essays on Video Games, Learning, and Literacy (New Literacies and Digital Epistemologies)*. New York: Peter Lang Pub Inc.

Gee, JP. (2007b). *What Video Games Have to Teach us About Learning and Literacy. Second Edition: Revised and Updated Edition* (2nd ed.). New York: Palgrave Macmillan.

Gee, JP. (2008). Learning and games. In K Salen (Ed.), *The Ecology of Games: Connecting Youth, Games, and Learning. The John D. and Catherine T. MacArthur Foundation Series on Digital Media and Learning (pp. 21–40)*. Cambridge, MA: The MIT Press. doi:10.1162/dmal.9780262693646.021.

Giere, RN. (1988). *Explaining Science: A Cognitive Approach*. Chicago: University of Chicago Press.

Gravemeijer, K, Cobb, P, Bowers, J, & Whitenack, J. (2000). Symbolizing, modeling, and instructional design. In P Cobb, E Yackel, & K McClain (Eds.), *Symbolizing and Communicating in Mathematics Classrooms: Perspectives on Discourse, Tools, and Instructional Design*. Mahwah, NJ: Lawrence Erlbaum Associates.

Habgood, MPJ, & Ainsworth, SE. (2011). Motivating children to learn effectively: exploring the value of intrinsic integration in educational games. *The Journal of the Learning Sciences, 20,* 169–206.

Hall, R, & Stevens, R. (1995). Making space: A comparison of mathematical work in school and professional design practices. In SL Star (Ed.), *The Cultures of Computing* (pp. 118–145). London, UK: Basil Blackwell.

Hammer, D. (1996). Misconceptions or p-prims: How may alternative perspectives of cognitive structure influence instructional perceptions and intentions? *The Journal of the Learning Sciences, 5*(2), 97–127.

Hammer, D, Redish, EF, Elby, A, & Scherr, RE. (2005). Resources, framing, and transfer. In J Mestre (Ed.), *Transfer of Learning: Research and Perspectives* (pp. 89–120). Greenwich, CT: Information Age Publishing Inc.

Hegedus, SJ, & Moreno-Armella, L. (2009). Intersecting representation and communication infrastructures. *ZDM, 41*(4), 399–412.

Hegedus, S, & Roschelle, J (Eds.). (2013). *The SimCalc Vision and Contributions: Democratizing Access to Important Mathematics.* New York, NY: Springer.

Hesse, MB. (1974). *The Structure of Scientific Inference.* Berkeley, CA: University of California Press.

Hestenes, D. (1992). Modeling games in the Newtonian world. *American Journal of Physics, 60,* 732–748.

Hestenes, D. (1993). *MODELING is the Name of the Game.* Washington, DC: Presentation at the NSF Modeling Conference.

Hestenes, D, & Halloun, I. (1995). Interpreting the force concept inventory: A response to March 1995 critique by Huffman and Heller. *The Physics Teacher, 33*(8), 502–506.

Hestenes, D, Wells, M, & Swackhamer, G. (1992). Force concept inventory. *The Physics Teacher, 30*(3), 141–158.

Hines, PJ, Jasny, BR, & Merris, J. (2009). Adding a T to the three R's. *Science, 323,* 53.

Honey, MA, & Hilton, M (Eds.). (2010). *Learning Science through Computer Games and Simulations. National Research Council.* Washington, DC: National Academy Press.

Jeppsson, F, Haglund, J, Amin, TG, & Strömdahl, H. (2013). Exploring the use of conceptual metaphors in solving problems on entropy. *Journal of the Learning Sciences, 22*(1), 70–120.

Kaput, J. (1994). Democratizing access to calculus: New routes to old roots. In A Schoenfeld (Ed.), *Mathematical Thinking and Problem Solving* (pp. 77–156). Hillsdale, NJ: Lawrence Erlbaum Associates.

Kearney, M. (2004). Classroom use of multimedia-supported predict–observe–explain tasks in a social constructivist learning environment. *Research in Science Education, 34*(4), 427–453.

Kiili, K. (2005). *On Educational Game Design: Building Blocks of Flow Experience.* Tampere, Finland: Tampere University of Technology Press.

Kiili, K, & Lainema, T. (2008). Foundation for measuring engagement in education games. *Journal of Interactive Learning Research, 19*(3), 469–488.

Kirsh, D, & Maglio, P. (1994). On the distinguishing epistemic from pragmatic action. *Cognitive Science, 18,* 513–549.

Koster, R. (2004). *A Theory of Fun for Game Design.* Scottsdale, AZ: Paraglyph Press.

Krinks, KD, Sengupta, P, & Clark, DB. (2013). *Conceptual Change in Physics through use of Digital Games. Paper presented at annual conference of the National Association for Research in Science Teaching.* Puerto Rico: Rio Mar.

Latour, B. (1990). Drawing things together. In M Lynch & S Woolgar (Eds.), *Representation in Scientific Practice* (pp. 19–68). Cambridge, MA: MIT Press.

Lehrer, R. (2003). Developing understanding of measurement. In J Kilpatrick, WG Martin, & DE Schifter (Eds.), *A research companion to principles and standards for school mathematics* (pp. 179–192). Reston, VA: National Council of Teachers of Mathematics.

Lehrer, R. (2009). Designing to develop disciplinary dispositions: Modeling natural systems. *American Psychologist, 64*(8), 759–71. doi:10.1037/0003-066X.64.8.759.

Lehrer, R, & Pritchard, C. (2002). Symbolizing space into being. In K Gravemeijer, R Lehrer, B van Oers, & L Verschaffel (Eds.), *Symbolization, Modeling and Tool use in Mathematics Education* (pp. 59–86). Dordrecht, Netherlands: Kluwer Academic Press.

Lehrer, R, & Schauble, L. (2002). Symbolic communication in mathematics and science: Co-constituting inscription and thought. In E Amsel & J Byrnes (Eds.), *The development of symbolic communication.* Mahwah, NJ: Lawrence Erlbaum Associates.

Lehrer, R, & Schauble, L. (2006a). Cultivating model-based reasoning in science education. In RK Sawyer (Ed.), *The Cambridge Handbook of the Learning Sciences* (pp. 371–388). Cambridge, England: Cambridge University Press.

Lehrer, R, & Schauble, L. (2006b). Scientific thinking and science literacy: supporting development in learning in contexts. In W Damon, RM Lerner, KA Renninger, & IE Sigel (Eds.), *Handbook of Child Psychology* (6th ed., Vol. 4). Hoboken, NJ: John Wiley and Sons.

Lehrer, R, & Schauble, L. (2010). What kind of explanation is a model? In MK Stein (Ed.), *Instructional Explanations in the Disciplines* (pp. 9–22). New York: Springer.

Lehrer, R, Schauble, L, Carpenter, S, & Penner, D. (2000). The inter-related development of inscriptions and conceptual understanding. In P Cobb, E Yackel, & K McClain (Eds.), *Symbolizing and Communicating in Mathematics Classrooms: Perspectives on Discourse, Tools and Instructional Design* (pp. 325–360). Mahwah, NJ: Lawrence Erlbaum Associates.

Lynch, M. (1990). The externalized retina: Selection and mathematization in the visual documentation of objects in the life sciences. In M Lynch & S Woolgar (Eds.), *Representation in Scientific Practice* (pp. 153–186). Cambridge, MA: MIT Press.

Martinez-Garza, M, Clark, DB, & Nelson, B. (2013). Digital games and the US National Research Council's science proficiency goals. *Studies in Science Education, 49,* 170–208. doi:10.1080/03057267.2013.839372.

Mayer, RE. (2009). *Multimedia Learning* (2nd ed.). New York, NY: Cambridge University Press.

Mayer, RE, & Johnson, CI. (2010). Adding instructional features that promote learning in a game-like environment. *Journal of Educational Computing Research, 42*(3), 241–265.

McGonigal, J. (2011). *Reality is Broken: Why Games Make Us Better and How They Can Change the World.* New York: Penguin Press.

Minstrell, J. (2001). Facets of students' thinking: Designing to cross the gap from research to standards-based practice. In K Crowley, CD Schunn, & T Okada (Eds.), *Designing for Science: Implications for Professional, Instructional, and Everyday Science.* Mahwah: Lawrence Erlbaum Associates.

Morrison, D, & Collins, A. (1995). Epistemic fluency and constructivist learning environments. *Educational Technology, 35*(5), 39–45.

Munz, U, Schumm, P, Wiesebrock, A, & Allgower, F. (2007). Motivation and learning progress through educational games. *Industrial Electronics, IEEE Transactions on, 54*(6), 3141–3144. doi: 10.1109/TIE.2007.907030.

Nersessian, NJ. (1998). Modeling practices in conceptual change in science. In T Borsche, J Kreuzer, & C Strub (Eds.), *Cognition and Imagination* (pp. 149–168). Munich: Fink Verlag.

Nersessian, NJ. (2002). The cognitive basis of model-based reasoning in science. In P Carruthers, S Stich, & M Siegal (Eds.), *The Cognitive Basis of Science* (pp. 133–155). Cambridge: Cambridge University Press.

Nersessian, NJ. (2008). *Creating Scientific Concepts.* Cambridge, MA: MIT Press.

Pelletier, C. (2008). Gaming in context: How young people construct their gendered identities in playing and making games. In YB Kafai, C Heeter, J Denner, & JY Sun (Eds.), *Beyond Barbie and Mortal Kombat: New Perspectives on Gender and Gaming.* Cambridge, Mass: The MIT Press.

Pickering, A. (1995). *The Mangle of Practice: Time, Agency, and Science.* Chicago: University of Chicago Press.

Rapp, DN, & Sengupta, P. (2012). *Models and modeling in science learning. Encyclopedia of the Sciences of Learning (pp. 2320–2322).* New York: Springer.

Rochelle, J, & Kaput, J. (1996). Educational software architecture and systemic impact: The promise of component software. *Journal of Educational Computing Research, 14*(3), 217–228.

Roy, M, & Chi, MTH. (2005). The self-explanation principle in multimedia learning. In RE Mayer (Ed.), *The Cambridge Handbook of Multimedia Learning* (pp. 271–286). New York: Cambridge University Press.

Rueda, MR, Fan, J, McCandliss, BD, Halparin, JD, Gruber, DB, Lercari, LP, & Posner, MI. (2004). Development of attentional networks in childhood. *Neuropsychologia, 42*(8), 1029–1040. doi:10.1016/j.neuropsychologia.2003.12.012.

Salen, K, & Zimmerman, E. (2004). *Rules of Play: Game Design Fundamentals.* Cambridge: MIT Press.

Schwartz, D, & Arena, D. (2013). *Measuring What Matters Most: Choice-Based Assessments for the Digital Age.* Cambridge: MIT Press.

Scott, PH, Asoko, HM, & Driver, RH. (1992). Teaching for conceptual change: a review of strategies. In R Duit, F Goldberg, & H Niedderer (Eds.), *Research in Physics Learning: Theoretical Issues and Empirical Studies* (pp. 310–329). Kiel, Germany: Institute for Science Education at the University of Kiel.

Sengupta, P, Clark, D, Krinks, K, Killingsworth, S, & Brady, C. (2014). Integrating Modeling with Games for Learning Newtonian Mechanics. In N. Holbert & D. Weintrop (Org), N. Holbert (Chair), and Y. Kafai (Discussant), Combining Video Games and Constructionist Design to Support Deep Learning in Play. In J. Poleman, E. Kyza, I. Tabak & K. O'Neill (Eds.), Proceedings of "Learning and

Becoming in Practice," the 11th International Conference of the Learning Sciences (ICLS 2014), pp 1388 – 1395. University of Colorado at Boulder: ISLS.
Sherin, BL. (2001). How students understand physics equations. *Cognition and Instruction, 19*(4), 479–541.
Slack, K, Nelson, B, Clark, DB, & Martinez-Garza, M. (2010). *Influence of Visual Cues on Learning and In-Game Performance in an Educational Physics Game Environment.* Anaheim, California: Paper presented at the Association for Educational Communications and Technology (AECT) 2010 meeting.
Slack, K, Nelson, B, Clark, DB, & Martinez-Garza, M. (2011). *Model-Based Thinking in the Scaffolding Understanding by Redesigning Games for Education (SURGE) Project.* New Orleans, LA: Poster presented at the American Educational Research Association (AERA) 2011 meeting.
Smith, JP, diSessa, A, & Roschelle, J. (1993). Misconceptions reconceived: A constructivist analysis of knowledge in transition. *Journal of the Learning Sciences, 3*(2), 115–163.
Squire, K. (2005). Changing the game: What happens when video games enter the classroom. *Innovate, 1*(6), 25–49.
Squire, K. (2006). From content to context: Videogames as designed experience. *Educational Researcher, 35*(8), 19–29.
Squire, K. (2011). *Video Games and Learning: Teaching and Participatory Culture in the Digital age.* New York: Teachers College Press.
Steinkuehler, D, & Duncan, S. (2008). Scientific habits of mind in virtual worlds. *Journal of Science Education and Technology, 17*(6), 530–543.
Tao, P-K, & Gunstone, RF. (1999). The process of conceptual change in force and motion during computer-supported physics instruction. *Journal of Research in Science Teaching, 36*(7), 859–882.
Team, G-t-T. (2003). Design principles of next-generation digital gaming for education. *Educational Technology, 43*(5), 17–33.
Van Eaton, G, Clark, DB, & Beutel, D. (2013). *Designing Digital Objects to Scaffold Learning.* Memphis TN: Paper presented at the 16th International Conference on Artificial Intelligence in Education (AIED 2013).
White, B. (1984). Designing computer games to help physics students understand Newton's laws of motion. *Cognition and Instruction, 1*, 69–108.
White, B, & Frederiksen, J. (1998). Inquiry, modeling, and metacognition: Making science accessible to all students. *Cognition and Instruction, 16*(1), 3–118.
White, BY, & Frederiksen, JR. (2000). Metacognitive facilitation: An approach to making scientific inquiry accessible to all. In JA Minstrell & EH Van Zee (Eds.), *Inquiring into Inquiry Learning and Teaching in Science* (pp. 331–370). Washington, DC: American Association for the Advancement of Science.
Wilensky, U, & Reisman, K. (2006). Thinking like a wolf, a sheep, or a firefly: Learning biology through constructing and testing computational theories—an embodied modeling approach. *Cognition and Instruction, 24*(2), 171–209.
Wouters, P, van Nimwegen, C, van Oostendorp, H, & van der Spek, ED. (2013). A meta-analysis of the cognitive and motivational effects of serious games. *Journal of Educational Psychology, 105*, 249–265. Doi: 10.1037/a0031311.
Wright, W. (2006). Dream machines. *Wired, 14*(4), 110–112.

2

Exploring variation in measurement as a foundation for statistical thinking in the elementary school

Lyn D English[1*] and Jane M Watson[2]

Abstract

Background: This study was based on the premise that variation is the foundation of statistics and statistical investigations. The study followed the development of fourth-grade students' understanding of variation through participation in a sequence of two lessons based on measurement. In the first lesson all students measured the arm span of one student, revealing pathways students follow in developing understanding of variation and linear measurement (related to research question 1). In the second lesson each student's arm span was measured once, introducing a different aspect of variation for students to observe and contrast. From this second lesson, students' development of the ability to compare their representations for the two scenarios and explain differences in terms of variation was explored (research question 2). Students' documentation, in both workbook and software formats, enabled us to monitor their engagement and identify their increasing appreciation of the need to observe, represent, and contrast the variation in the data. Following the lessons, a written student assessment was used for judging retention of understanding of variation developed through the lessons and the degree of transfer of understanding to a different scenario (research question 3).

Results: The results were based either on the application of the hierarchical SOLO model or on non-hierarchical clustering of responses to individual questions in the student workbooks. Students' progress throughout the lessons displayed a wide range of explanations for the estimate of a single student's arm span, general surprise at the variation in measurements, and a large variety of hand-drawn representations based on the values or frequencies of measurements. Many different representations were also created in the software for the single student measurements and for the comparison of measurements for the two scenarios. Although the students' interpretations of their plots were generally more basic than sophisticated, the results of the assessment indicated that many students had developed the ability to transfer their appreciation of variation to another context and could clearly explain the meaning of variation.

Conclusions: The findings highlight the importance of an early focus on variation and distribution, with meaningful activities that motivate students to conduct and observe measurements, together with creating both hand-drawn and software representations to relate their experiences.

Keywords: Elementary school; Graphical representations; Measurement; Statistical thinking; Variation

Background

Since the introduction of statistics into school mathematics curricula about 25 years ago (e.g. Australian Education Council 1991; National Council of Teachers of Mathematics, 1989), there has been a growing awareness of the inadequacy of focusing solely on a procedural ability to calculate statistics. In particular, informal inference, a precursor to formal inference, has been highlighted as a foundational component that has not received the required attention especially in the elementary grades (Makar, in press). As described by Makar and Rubin (2009), informal inference is the process of using the evidence provided by data to answer questions beyond the data, acknowledging the uncertainty associated with the conclusion reached. Variation is the key to accepting a

* Correspondence: l.english@qut.edu.au
[1]Faculty of Education, Queensland University of Technology, Victoria Park Road, Kelvin Grove, Brisbane, Queensland, 4059, Australia
Full list of author information is available at the end of the article

conclusion with some degree of certainty (Franklin et al., 2007, p. 18).

Variation is in fact such a fundamental concept that generally in the literature it is taken as an undefined term, as does Moore (1990). Variation and its associated form variability, however, are complex words for fourth-grade students and need to be described in ways that allow students to develop an understanding of the concept. Variation emerges when young students collect data and all of the values are not the same or when they plot the data and *see* that there are changes in the shape of the plot with gaps between and clusters of points/values. At a basic level, statistical variation may be regarded as the difference in data values and spread seen in data representations. Once variation is acknowledged, however, the purpose of a statistical investigation is to understand it, represent it, summarise it and perhaps control it (Franklin et al., 2007; Moore, 1990).

Acknowledging the importance of variation in informal inference, this study sought to expose fourth-grade students to the concept of variation through a measurement activity that would reveal two different types of variation: variation as 'error' in the repeated measurement of a single student's arm span and variation as the difference observed in single measurements of arm spans of a class of students. In the first scenario, all students measured one student's arm span where the sources of variation did not lie in the entity itself (one arm span), rather in the measurers, the measurement processes and the instruments used. In the second scenario, variation arose from the entities being measured (all students' arm spans), together with the measurers, their measurement processes and instruments. Students' documentation of their measurements, their explanations of the variations they observed, and their hand-drawn and software representations displaying the variations formed the data for addressing our research questions.

In the first scenario, we primarily explored students' levels of development in detecting, representing (by hand and with technology) and explaining variation in linear measurement values. In the second scenario, our major research focus was on the plots students created with software and their ability to compare and explain differences between their representations in the two scenarios. Finally, to determine the success of the activity in terms of students' understanding of variation and their ability to apply this learning to a slightly different scenario, we administered an assessment 1 to 3 months after activity completion. Specifically, our research questions were:

1. What are students' levels of development in detecting, representing and explaining variation in linear measurement values?

2. How do students develop the ability to compare and explain differences between representations in the two scenarios?

3. Do students demonstrate understanding of variation and transfer of that understanding through delayed assessment questions?

In addressing the background literature for the study, we consider the variation component of statistical thinking and inference, including its presence in national curriculum documents. We then examine the role of variation in linear measurement and conclude with a review of the emergence of variation in statistical representation.

Variation

Variation lies at the heart of statistical reasoning - without it, statistics would not exist (Moore, 1990). Variation is linked to all aspects of statistical investigations (Cobb and Moore, 1997; Garfield and Ben-Zvi, 2007; Konold and Pollatsek 2002; Watson, 2006). Indeed, as Watson (2006) indicated, the reason data are collected, graphs are created and averages are computed is to 'manage variation and draw conclusions in relation to questions based on phenomena that vary' (p. 21). Variation as the foundation of statistics provides the basis from which inferences can be drawn during statistical decision making. The confidence with which one can make a decision, however, depends on creating a balance between variation and expectation (Watson, 2005). This balance is expressed in tests of significance or confidence intervals in senior secondary school courses, but learning to appreciate variation and its relationship to expectation (in this study prediction) needs to begin very early with appropriate hands-on experiences and student/teacher questioning.

The explicit recognition of variation in curriculum documents has been slow, but recent publications have begun to mention the concept. Most notable among these is the GAISE report (Franklin et al., 2007) prepared under the auspices of the American Statistical Association. The report presents a four-stage framework for carrying out statistical investigations, with every stage including a focus on variation. Formulating Questions *anticipates variation*, Collecting Data *designs for variation*, Analysing Data *accounts for variation in distributions* and Interpreting Results *allows for variation beyond the data*. Such an approach does not underpin national curriculum documents to the same extent. In Australia, the curriculum refers to variation in the general description for learning up to second grade, in terms of developing an awareness of variation in data but specific mention does not appear until third grade (Australian Curriculum, Assessment and Reporting Authority 2013b). In New Zealand, the curriculum notes 'acknowledging samples that vary' at level 3, and variables are introduced at level 4, with consideration of sources of variation as integral to planning a statistical investigation at level 5 (Ministry of Education, 2009). In the United States, the Common Core State Standards Initiative (CCSSI) (2010)) introduces variation in the sixth grade, the first year where a concentrated focus on Probability and Statistics is included in its curriculum. These curriculum recommendations are the result of earlier research and provide the motivation for further research.

There has been substantial research on older students' and adults' awareness of variation (e.g. Makar and Confrey, 2005; Reading, 2004; Wild and Pfannkuch, 1999) but less so on how this understanding can be developed with young children. As numerous researchers have lamented, this neglect is a major concern especially given that secondary school and university students are usually 'drilled' in the use of statistical techniques without appreciating or understanding why, when or how these are applied sensibly to a range of situations (Bakker, 2004; Garfield and Ben-Zvi, 2005; Reading, 2004). The sentiments of Pfannkuch (2005) encapsulate these concerns: 'Teaching has not focused on enculturating students into variation-type thinking and reasoning approaches. Much needs to be learnt about how to cultivate and develop this type of reasoning in students' (p. 84).

The studies on young learners' awareness of variation have indicated the presence of a primitive understanding that needs to be integrated, revisited and emphasised in statistics learning from the earliest grade levels (Garfield and Ben-Zvi, 2007; Lehrer and Kim, 2009; Lehrer et al., 2011; Watson and Kelly, 2002a, 2002b). The research-based classroom suggestions from these studies, however, are not being adopted in many classrooms because teachers lack the pedagogical content knowledge to make specific links to variation when they implement activities in data and chance (Watson, 2013). Explicit discussion of variation and its application across the curriculum is needed throughout the elementary school years, before students meet formal measures such as standard deviation in the secondary school years. Instructional approaches to developing an understanding of variation in the earlier grades have received limited attention. As Garfield and Ben-Zvi (2005) noted, designing a long-term program that will nurture this understanding is a complex and challenging endeavour. Their suggestions for intervention were considered in planning the present classroom activity.

Assessing the overall outcomes of instructional approaches has also received limited attention. Watson et al., (2003) developed a survey instrument in the context of a study involving lessons emphasising variation in grade levels 3, 5, 7, 9 (Watson and Kelly, 2002a, 2002b). The outcomes suggested four levels of increasing appreciation of variation: 'prerequisites,' including interpreting the context, simple graph reading and intuitive chance reasoning; 'partial recognition,' including putting ideas in context but focusing on single aspects and neglecting others; 'applications,' including consolidating ideas in context but inconsistency on the most salient features; and 'critical aspects,' employing complex justification or critical reasoning. Although assessment in the present study was more general than that of the Watson et al. survey, their research suggests levels of development that are useful for assessing learning outcomes.

Variation in linear measurement

In basic terms, linear measurement may be viewed as 'a comparative property of objects that embodies the amount of one-dimensional space between endpoints of the objects, which can be compared or quantified' (Szilagyi et al., 2013, p. 583). Drawing on the literature, Szilagyi et al. cited numerous competencies needed for length measurement, including awareness of attribute, unit-attribute relations, unit iteration, proportionality and the relation between number and measurement. Transitivity and conservation are also important features. Apart from Lehrer's research (e.g. Lehrer et al., 2011), which we subsequently address, the focus on the important role of statistical foundations in the development of understanding of length measurement has been largely neglected.

The lack of measurement connectivity across other strands of the mathematics curriculum has been lamented by Australian educators (Lowrie et al., 2012) with respect to the recently implemented curriculum, *The Australian Curriculum: Mathematics* (Australian Curriculum, Assessment and Reporting Authority 2013b). Their concerns reflect repeated calls for more links within and across topics and disciplines with similar conceptual underpinnings (e.g. Bobis et al., 2009). Although measurement understandings have been linked to the development of geometry, number and algebra (e.g. Booker and Windsor, 2010; Bragg and Outhred, 2004), few studies have addressed connections with statistical literacy. Lehrer's research (e.g. Lehrer, 2007; Lehrer and Kim, 2009; Lehrer et al., 2011), however, has used measurement in developing students' appreciation of measures of centre and of variability. As an initial step in developing statistical reasoning, Lehrer and his colleagues engaged students in generating variability through measurement error. The findings of their research highlighted the importance of student interactions, where they made visible their arguments for a measure's validity and considered situations where such measures might be insufficient.

Despite Lehrer's work, little attention has been given to variation in measurement in curriculum documents and professional mathematics teaching articles focusing on length (e.g. Clements and Bright, 2003). Although the word 'variation' appears in the Australian, New Zealand and United States mathematics curricula (Australian Curriculum, Assessment and Reporting Authority 2013b; Common Core State Standards Initiative CCSSI 2010;

Ministry of Education, 2009), it does not appear in relation to measurement. This is surprising given that variation is inherent in the entire measurement process - in the entity being measured, how the measurer undertakes the measuring process, the instruments used and how the measurements are interpreted. As a core understanding in the development of statistical literacy, variation includes interpreting and critically assessing various forms of measurement data. One of the goals of the present activity was the development of an appreciation of variation in measuring and measurements, and of the need for accuracy in measurement. Children need to understand what it means to make an accurate measurement, why accuracy is important, and the variation that can be expected in a measurement, especially if it is repeated (Lehrer, 2007; Watson and Wright, 2008).

The last understanding, of accuracy of measurement, is rarely addressed in the elementary curriculum yet as Konold and Pollatsek (2002) emphasised, it is an important context for various interpretations of average, an interpretation they refer to as 'signal in noise' (p. 268). From this perspective, each measurement is an estimate of an unknown yet specific value. We argue that connecting statistical and measurement topics can provide a powerful tool for targeting these currently neglected core understandings in the elementary curriculum and for addressing the long-standing concerns regarding students' difficulties with measurement (Smith et al., 2011).

Representing variation

Representing data in the elementary school years is typically limited to a few traditional graph types considered manageable by young students, such as picture graphs and simple column graphs, although recently using technology to produce these graphs has been suggested (see Australian Curriculum, Assessment and Reporting Authority 2013b, year 3). The focus has been largely on what types of graphs should be taught and when (e.g. Friel et al., 2001) and on appropriate scaling, labelling and directionality of plots (e.g. Leinhardt et al., 1990; Mevarech and Kramarsky, 1997). The ability of young students to create a wide range of representations of their own choosing is frequently underestimated (English, 2012, 2014; Russell, 1991). With a greater variety of graphs and other displays appearing in the media and elsewhere (e.g. Wall and Benson, 2009), students are being exposed more than ever to statistical representations that must be interpreted critically, where questions should be asked of the reliability of any claims made. This exposure is especially prevalent with the increased availability of technology, where students might create a range of representations without giving consideration to their appropriateness for the data being used (Konold, 2007).

Until recently, the explicit consideration of variation in relation to graphical representations has not been a feature of research. Yet, a key component of students' long-term development of statistical literacy is being able to interpret a message from a context with a distribution that displays variation, clustering, middles and unexpected values; this might not involve conventional textbook types of graphs (Lehrer, 2007; Wall and Benson, 2009; Watson et al., 2008). Early experiences with a range of representations that effectively display variation in data sets are important but have remained largely neglected in many elementary curricula until recently. Greater insights are needed into how young learners deal with variation in an immersive classroom environment including across disciplines (Watson, 2012), how they represent data in new ways of their own choosing, how they answer questions on comparing variation in different data sets and how they identify and justify the sources of variation they encounter.

In summary, this study addresses three underrepresented components of statistical development in the elementary grades. First, in integrating the strands of statistics and measurement in the curriculum, the study targets the neglected factor of variation in linear measurement. Second, the study highlights the importance of students' awareness, creation and understanding of variation in data representations, in contrast to traditional approaches where 'information' is simply read from a graph without being interpreted, analysed and questioned. Third, it focuses on an understanding and appreciation of informal inference, in this instance related to predicting a student's arm span length from data exhibiting variation, which is critical in interpreting data and distributions and making informed decisions.

Methods

Participants

Four year 4 (fourth grade) classes and one year 4/5 class from a large, middle socio-economic school participated during the first year of a 3-year longitudinal study (2012 to 2014). We focus only on the year 4 students ($N = 115$; mean age = 9.5 years) in the reporting of our findings, 43% of whom were classified as learners with English as their second language (ESL).

Design

The 3-year longitudinal study was conducted from 2012 to 2014. The study took a form of design research involving the three phases of (i) preparation and design of instructional materials, (ii) teaching experiments and (iii) retrospective analyses (Cobb et al., in press; Cobb et al., 2003). These phases were conducted in each year of the study, with subsequent years being informed by the outcomes of the previous. The teachers had input and took primary responsibility for implementing the instructional program within their own classrooms. In this article, we only consider one comprehensive activity from the first year of the study, although the learning progression we developed across the 3 years was informed by the outcomes of each successive activity in which the students were engaged.

Preparation phase: designing the activities

In the first year of the study we designed, in conjunction with the teachers' input, three sets of activities, namely, a preliminary benchmarking activity where the students created, implemented and analysed a playground survey (English and Watson, in press). The purpose of this benchmarking activity was to provide the research team with starting points for the main activities for the beginning year. This was followed by the measurement activity ('Measuring a Person's Arm Span'), which is the focus of this article. In the latter part of the first year, we implemented a multi-lesson probability activity that explored variation and expectation (English and Watson, in press).

In developing the activities, we drew upon a range of research but focused our attention primarily on the components of Garfield and Ben-Zvi's (2005) epistemological model for developing an in-depth understanding of variation, together with recommendations from the work of Lehrer and his colleagues (Lehrer, 2007; Lehrer et al., 2011), and previous positive outcomes with students in years 3 and 5 (Watson and Kelly, 2002a, 2002b). In particular, the suggestions of Garfield and Ben-Zvi were useful. Although their key ideas in each of the seven areas of knowledge of variability cover all years of schooling, the first three were especially relevant to our study, as was the last: (i) developing intuitive ideas of variation; (ii) describing and representing variability; (iii) using variability to make comparisons and (vii) considering variability as part of statistical thinking. These key ideas were the foundation of our planning for the activity conducted in year 4.

It was important in designing our program that it aligned with the school curriculum to ensure that the activities formed a core component rather than 'add-on' learning experiences. The teacher preparatory meetings conducted for each activity were thus vital in informing our design, as well as in enabling us to provide important professional development on the core statistical ideas to be developed. The present activity was designed in line with the *Australian Curriculum: Mathematics* (Australian Curriculum, Assessment and Reporting Authority 2013b), where the year 4 measurement strand states that students should 'Use scaled instruments to measure and compare lengths' (p. 43). For the data strand in year 4, the curriculum states that students should 'Select and trial methods for data collection ... Construct suitable data displays, with and without the use of digital technologies ... Include tables, column graphs ... Evaluate the effectiveness of different displays in illustrating data features including variability' (p. 45). Because one of the general capabilities of the Australian curriculum is Information and Communication Technology (ICT), which includes 'Investigation, Creating and Communicating with ICT' (Australian Curriculum, Assessment and Reporting Authority 2013a, p. 53), the software *TinkerPlots* (Konold and Miller, 2011) was introduced as the digital technology to 'construct suitable data displays'. The school was operating under this curriculum through the state education authority, where column graphs and picture graphs were specifically mentioned for year 4.

We targeted numerous learning objectives in designing the activity, not all of which are addressed in the research we report here. These objectives included developing students' appreciation of the need for accuracy in measurement and to pay careful attention to scale, competence in representing variation in measurement values and describing the shapes of data sets, confidence in predicting a representative measurement and skills in explaining variation in data sets. Learning to create various data displays in *TinkerPlots* and identify which displays best show the variation in a data set were also key objectives. An important learning feature was students' consideration of the most effective displays for showing the variation in the data sets, with the emerging understanding that there is very likely to be measurement error in the first scenario and, hence, the measurement in the second scenario is an approximation.

The creation of the activity involved several design iterations to ensure each component met our learning objectives and would generate adequate and appropriate data to gain insights into the students' learning. The authors and the senior research assistant worked on refining the activity, seeking teacher feedback as needed. Comprehensive teaching notes and corresponding student workbooks were developed, the latter serving as a core data source when completed by students.

Teaching experiment phase: implementing the activity

The 'Measuring a Person's Arm Span' activity comprised an initial teacher-led introduction to the activity, followed by student group work that was interspersed with whole class discussions on the groups' observations, their data representations and their findings. Implementation of the activity varied in time allocation per class, with an average duration of 5 h 10 min, spread across 3 days during 1 week for each class. Students worked in small groups (usually two or occasionally three), which were selected by the teachers based on students' ability to work collaboratively and communicate their thinking to others. The groups were of mixed achievement levels.

The teacher commenced the activity with a class discussion on how accurately 'we' can measure, different units of length we might use, and on ways length can be measured. The students were asked, 'If we all measure the same object will we get the same answer for its length?' On discussing issues of accuracy in this situation it was explained for the first scenario that, 'We are all going to measure the arm span of the same person and see if we get the same value. We will consider how to display and compare these values and see if we can make a "best guess" as to the person's arm span. We will then discuss how confident we feel about having exactly the right value.'

Once all the measurements had been recorded, the students were asked to suggest other methods of organising the data other than the list on the whiteboard. The students then completed three questions in their workbooks about the recorded measurement values, reflecting Garfield and Ben-Zvi's (2005) development of intuitive ideas of variability and describing variability (phase (i)):

1. Were all of the values the same? Why or why not?
2. Were you surprised at some of the values? Which ones? Why?
3. Write a summary of how accurate you think the measurements in the table are. What is your 'best guess' of the arm span of the person the class measured? How confident are you of this value?'

The language of the classroom often translated 'best guess' to prediction, a difficult word for some of the ESL students.

The students subsequently discussed in their groups different ways to create a representation that they considered 'best tells the story of the class measurements.' No direction was given as to what type of representation to construct. Each student, however, created his/her own representation in the workbook. The next question asked students to 'Write a summary statement about what your representation shows about the measurements your class made of the arm span of the person you measured'. The students were reminded to 'Think about the variation that is seen in your plot or picture,' reflecting Garfield and Ben-Zvi's (2005) ability to represent and describe variability (phase (ii)).

A whole-class stacked dot plot was then created on the white board. Students recorded their names and measured arm span values on PostIt notes and placed them in the correct positions on a horizontal axis drawn on the white board. The students were asked about the variation in values they observed and what they might expect if the arm spans of all students in the class were measured, as a prelude to the second measurement scenario. Prior to this second scenario, the students created their own dot plots of the single student's arm span measurements using the *TinkerPlots* software program. They were to include a textbox that explained the features of their graph, noting any clusters, gaps and outliers that might have occurred, again reinforcing the representing and describing of variation (Garfield and Ben-Zvi, 2005).

In the second scenario, the students were to measure and plot the arm span of all members of the class and record these measurements on the whiteboard. Due to time limitations, in most instances the researchers had to assist in taking these measurements. Prior to the measurements being taken, the students recorded their responses to two questions, namely:

1. Do you think all the values will be the same? Why/why not?
2. How accurate do you expect your results to be compared to our last lesson?

After recording their measurements on the white board, the student groups entered the data into a new data collection in their *TinkerPlots* files, which still contained their plots of the single student's arm span measurements. They were then to create a plot 'that best describes the [new] data set and tells the story.' This was to be accompanied by a text box containing a summary statement of what the plot shows and 'at least two sentences that describe the differences between this plot and the earlier one,' reflecting Garfield and Ben-Zvi's (2005) component of using variability to make comparisons (phase (iii)).

The activity concluded with a class discussion that highlighted the differences between the two scenarios and the variation in the two plots. The students were asked:

1. Why is there a difference in the spread/range for the two activities (scenarios)?
2. How confident are we of the values that we plotted in the second graph for each class member, having experienced the variation we found in the earlier plot for a single person?
3. Would it have been better to have made two or three or four measurements on each person and picked a 'typical' one?

These questions reflected Garfield and Ben-Zvi's (2005) last component of engendering consideration of variability in all parts of a statistical investigation (phase (vii)).

Retrospective analyses

The data to be used in the retrospective analyses were drawn from multiple sources. In each class, we selected two focus groups for in-depth analysis, where their work was video- and audio-recorded and subsequently transcribed. All whole class discussions were also recorded and transcribed, and all of the students' workbooks were scanned for analysis. Between 1 and 3 months after completion of the activity, an assessment was implemented in all classes except the year 4/5 class whose timetable prevented their completion of the assessment. Two of the classes had 30 students undertake the assessment a month after completing the activity. Of these students, many were classified as ESL and/or low-achieving. Of the other two classes, streamed as high achieving, 36 students completed the assessment after 3 months. Although some were classified as ESL, many of these had high levels of English. The teachers of the two classes with the longer delay did not review the activity with the students before completing the assessment. Although there was a difference in performance between the two groups of two classes, favouring the class with the longer delay, it was believed to be the result of streaming the classes, and the data were combined for analysis of all year 4 students. The work of any students without parental consent was not recorded and not included in the analysis.

The data addressed here are drawn from the students' completed workbooks, their *TinkerPlots* creations and accompanying textbox descriptions, the transcriptions of whole class and focus group discussions and the assessment. Codes were checked by each author and refined, with the senior research assistant undertaking a final overview; consensus was reached on all coding.

In analysing the responses of students in their workbooks and in creating plots in *TinkerPlots* with accompanying text in text boxes, two kinds of criteria were used. In one situation, students were providing descriptions or reasons associated with observations or conjectures. These differed somewhat between classes because of the data collected or the way the teacher handled the discussion. It was of interest to categorise these responses to gain an appreciation of the diversity of thinking in the measurement context, but the responses were not considered to be hierarchical in nature. For these data, we employed content analysis (Patton, 2002). A description of the categories and the percentages of responses in each are presented in tables in the 'Results' section. In other situations where students were constructing representations or more complex arguments, it was possible to suggest a hierarchical cognitive structure reflecting increasing use of the elements available for the response. The criteria for levels of response are reflective of levels of the SOLO model (Biggs and Collis, 1982) where code 1 generally is assigned to employing a single element or aspect from the context of the question (a unistructural response). At code 2, several elements may be used, usually presented in sequence (a multistructural response) and, at code 3, relationships are demonstrated among the elements (a relational response). The particular descriptions of these levels where applicable are presented in the tables in the Results section.

The assessment began with straightforward questions based on a screen dump from the software for two reasons. The first was to confirm the students had picked up the basics of interpreting the information in the *TinkerPlots* format, and the second was to provide easy questions at the start of the assessment. The coding values for the instrument are given in the Additional file 1 with the questions asked, along with the rubric provided to teachers. Of interest is the total score obtained as it reflects the overall understanding of students in adapting to *TinkerPlots* as a context for reaching the learning objectives of the measurement activity. Further, the responses to questions 10 to 15, including a request for the definition of variation, throw light on the degree of application of ideas associated with variation in the classroom scenarios, as well as in a related context.

Although this study was not accompanied by extensive surveying that could lead to the type of Rasch analysis reported by Watson et al. (2003), it is possible to consider descriptively whether the responses provided by students, first in their workbooks, second in class discussions, and later in a limited assessment situation, exhibited the type of thinking typical of the four levels of their developmental hierarchy of understanding variation. Because of the specific scenarios of the classroom activity and the interaction of the teacher and students, it is assumed that the students understood the measurement environment for the activity. Although some were classified as ESL students with little English, there was no indication from the video of the classroom that any student was unaware of the task of measuring one student's arm span. They had also created graphs through previous classroom experiences, and it was assumed that all students had reached level 1 of the developmental hierarchy, Prerequisites for Variation.

We report the results in terms of the three research questions cited previously, namely, (1) What are students' levels of development in detecting, representing and explaining variation in linear measurement values? (2) How do students develop the ability to compare and explain differences between representations in the two scenarios? (3) Do students demonstrate understanding of variation and transfer of that understanding through delayed assessment questions?

The first research question is based on variation in linear measurement of one student's arm span. This links directly to level 2 of the developmental hierarchy, Partial Recognition of Variation, which involves putting ideas in context and focusing on a single element. The context is the consideration of variation in length measurements, repeated for a single student. The second research question is related to students' understanding of comparing variation in the two scenarios and ability to represent it in a visual way and then explain the meaning. This is one of the types of consolidation of ideas expected at level 3 of the developmental hierarchy, Application of Variation, where perhaps not all significant features are recognised. The third research question is related to critically interpreting the variation seen within and between the data distributions and transferring this to another context. This is the sort of complex justification expected at level 4 of the developmental hierarchy, Critical Aspects of Variation.

Results

In reporting the results of the study in relation to the research questions, we first consider the outcomes from the classroom that are associated with the first two research questions. The third research question is addressed by the post-activity questions in the class assessment.

Research question 1: in the first scenario, what are students' levels of development in detecting, representing, and explaining variation in linear measurement values?

To determine the students' detection of variation and accuracy in their measurement values for the first scenario (measuring just one designated person in the class), we analysed their responses from the first three workbook questions (some of these responses were reported briefly in a conference paper of English and Watson, 2013). We identified different non-hierarchical categories of responses to each workbook question, with some students' responses encompassing more than one category, and some responses incomplete; hence the number of responses reported varies across the questions.

Workbook question 1: were all of the values the same? Why or why not?

Five main categories of responses were identified in the analysis of the first question. Although some responses were vague in presenting justifications for the different values, most students across the classes focused on the measuring tools and how they were used or their accuracy. Fewer students suggested measuring in different units, or the fact that the student being measured might have moved, as a reason for different values. The percentages for each category are given in Table 1.

Workbook question 2: were you surprised at some of the values? Which ones? Why?

Analysis of the children's responses ($N = 95$) to the question about surprising values yielded four categories (in addition to a category of four irrelevant or non-interpretable responses). Overwhelmingly, students identified an outlier or extreme/unusual value and included why it had occurred. Some students mentioned variation without focusing on a particular value, whereas others, especially in one class where there were no apparent outliers, noted the lack of variation, hence lack of surprise. The percentages are given in Table 2.

Workbook question 3: write a summary of how accurate you think the measurements in the table are. What is your 'best guess' of the arm span of the person the class measured? How confident are you of this value?

In analysing the students' assessment of the accuracy of their measurements, 101 responses were classified into eight groupings. The most frequently occurring category contained responses related to a modal idea, although the term mode was not used. Some other students focused on the idea of middle in choosing their prediction. Outside of these categories, students mentioned variation in the data, visual intuitions and reasons expressed for earlier questions. Outcomes are shown in Table 3.

Students' representations The students created representations in two ways for the data collected in the first

Table 1 Responses: were all of the values the same?

Description	Example	Percentage
Measuring tools/how tools used	No because some people used different measuring tools.	41
Tool not used accurately	No because the measuring tape can bend, same with string so the measurement could be wrong.	29
Different units of measurement	Some people used cm and some used m and cm.	8
Movement of person measured	No. Some are different because A might move his arms from recording to recording.	6
Nebulous differences	No, values came from different people.	15
Uninterpretable		1

Why or why not? ($n = 97$) (summarised from English and Watson, 2013).

Table 2 Responses: were you surprised at some of the values?

Description	Example	Percentage
Identifying extreme/ unusual value	I was surprised at the fact that somebody's value was 159 for it was much larger than the other values.	63
	I was surprised with 106 because it was too small and A is the largest person in the class.	
Variation in values	146 and 159 the differences is big, it is 13.	19
	Yes, I was surprised at the 146 measurement and the 150 measurement because of the veration [variation].	
Lack of surprise	I was not surprised because at the values because they looked like it was around where A's armspan would be.	13
	Nothing surprised me.	
Uninterpretable		4

Which ones? Why? ($n = 95$) (summarised from English and Watson, 2013).

scenario, namely, constructing a hand-drawn representation on a blank page in their workbooks and then later using the *TinkerPlots* software to represent their data. For both formats, the students were to record a summary statement about what their representations showed about the measurements, keeping in mind variation seen in the plot. First we consider the students' hand-drawn representations and the associated explanations.

Students' hand-drawn representations and summary statements For the hand-drawn representations, of the 84 students who completed this task, 6 students created two representations, making a total of 90. Of the 90 representations, 7% could not be interpreted, 36% focused on the actual measured values (V) and 58% focused on the frequency (F) with which the measured values occurred. Within these two types (measured values and frequency), it was possible to rank the representations based on their statistical appropriateness. For representations of value, it was considered that unordered lists were the most difficult to interpret, followed by unordered value plots with scales beginning at 0 or 10 (example V2 in Figure 1). Plots with scales beginning with a value of 80 or more (example V3 in Figure 1) were considered easier to interpret visually, whereas an ordered list was considered the most interpretable of representations of values.

For frequency representations, again order was considered more appropriate than non-ordered data as was a graphical presentation over tallies. Several of the plots appeared to represent frequency but were impossible to interpret (F0). Of the unordered representations, those based on tallies (example F1 in Figure 1) were considered more difficult to understand than those displaying frequency visually (example F2 in Figure 1). Of the representations that ordered the data, those based on tallies or totals (example F3 in Figure 1) were considered more difficult to interpret than those displaying frequency in plots. Further, the plots showing individual frequencies (example F5 in Figure 1), were thought more interpretable than those using intervals. Percentages of all levels are given in Table 4, with examples of some of the levels presented in Figure 1.

In writing a summary statement of what their hand-drawn representation conveyed about their data, of the 84 responses, some were not actually related to the data, such as mentioning colour or describing people. It was possible to employ a hierarchical coding of the responses

Table 3 Responses: summary, 'best guess,' and confidence ($n = 101$) (summarised from English and Watson, 2013)

Description	Example	Percentage
Mode/frequency	I believe J's armspan is between 150 cm to 155 cm. I am quite confident about this because most people chose those measurements.	35
	141, 141 is the most common of this table.	
Variation in relation to accuracy	The measurements were not very accurate because most of the measurements were different.	12
Average/central tendency	I think the value 154 cm is the most accurate value, for it is the average close to the middle values.	11
Visual approximation	I think the most accurate was M's with 1 m 50 cm because A's arms look about 1 m 50 cm. I am pretty confident it was M's.	9
Outlier	The real value was 140 and the fake one was 146 … because the number can't go up to 146.	4
Accuracy of tools	I think the best guess is 154 cm because the measuring tape was very straight.	4
Position of student	I thought the measurement are 50% accurate… Sometimes A's hand was down and up.	4
Nebulous statement	No, I don't think the measurement was that accurate. Around 134 cm. Confident.	23

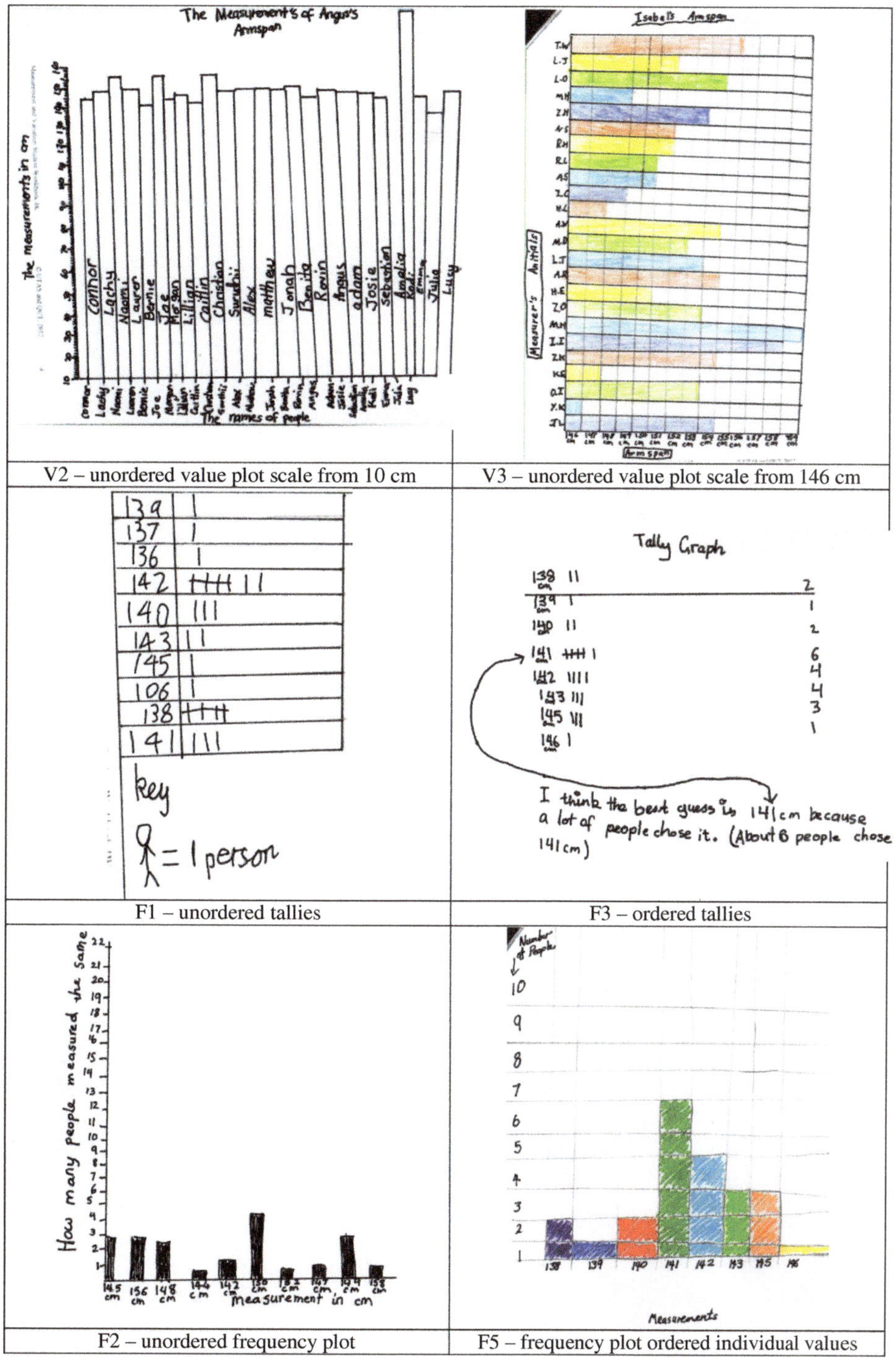

Figure 1 Examples of hand drawn representations of measurements of a single student.

linked to the SOLO model, with responses not related to the representation considered pre-structural and coded 0. A single acknowledgement of the graph as a focus was considered unistructural and coded 1. Putting together a description of either variation or expectation linked to the graph was considered multistructural (code 2), whereas linking both variation and expectation to the plot was considered relational (code 3) as this included the fundamental ingredients of a statistical analysis in making an 'informal inference' acknowledging variation. The most frequent response was to provide only a general description of the representation rather than its message. Table 5 reports the percentages of responses at each level with examples.

Table 4 Hand drawn representations of single student context (*n* = 90)

Type of plot	Level	Description	Percentage
V		Focus on measured *values*	36 (total)
	V1	Unordered list	6
	V2	Value plot - unordered, scale from 0 or 10 cm vertical (5) or horizontal (3)	9
	V3	Value plot - unordered, scale from ≥80 cm vertical (13) or horizontal (3)	18
	V4	Ordered list	3
F		Focus on *frequency* of measurements	58 (total)
	F0	Uninterpretable frequency	4
	F1	Tallies - unordered intervals (2) or individual frequencies (4)	7
	F2	Frequency plot - unordered intervals (2), individual frequencies (4) or pie in segments (1)	8
	F3	Tallies/totals - ordered individual totals (1) or individual frequencies (8)	10
	F4	Frequency plot - ordered intervals unequal width (2) or equal width (6)	9
	F5	Frequency plot - ordered individual frequencies unscaled ordered (1), bars (1), bars in squares (12), icons (3), or line (1)	20
0		Impossible to interpret	7 (total)

Students' TinkerPlots representations and summary statements Students worked in pairs to create *TinkerPlots* graphs for the measurement of a single student. Thirty-six groups created plots and text boxes for this task. The codes for levels of understanding displayed again reflected the SOLO hierarchy with some groups not providing interpretable text (code 0), some groups focusing on single isolated aspects of their plots (code 1), other groups describing sequentially several aspects of their plots appropriately (code 2) and one group going further to relate the information in an argument (code 3). Descriptions and the percentages of groups with each code are given in Table 6. One or two examples of each code are shown in Figure 2.

Research question 2: how do students develop the ability to compare and explain differences between representations in the two scenarios?

Rather than create hand-drawn graphs of class data, students were asked to use *TinkerPlots* to compare and contrast the two data sets for the single student and the class. Thirty-one pairs of students produced plots and text boxes for this part of the activity. The hierarchical coding levels are listed in Table 7, with code 0 files not addressing the question or including any further advance on the previous question. At code 1, groups gave evidence of considering the class data only, not comparing it to the individual student data, whereas at code 2, groups made basic statements comparing the plots for the two situations (individual student and class). At code 3, two or more of the comparison statements were linked to give reasons for the differences in the two plots. Examples for codes 1 to 3, including the plots and text, are shown in Figure 3.

Insights into the students' thinking in comparing the representations between scenarios were gleaned from the class and focus-group transcripts. For example, during a class discussion on the differences between the two plots, Neil explained, 'Shanna's was based on the same person and the other one was based on different [people], and it would be different measurement,' and 'Um, Shanna's arm span there's not like as much options

Table 5 Responses: interpreting the representations for the single student context (*n* = 84)

Code	Description	Example	Percentage
0	Description not related to the data	The way people measure.	8
	No response (although drew representation)		6
1	Strict description of graph (no summary of message)	I used a bar graph to show V's arm span.	35
2	Description of variation	My graph shows the amount of difference with different tools and their measurements, the variation: 26 people, 13 different answers.	27
	Description of expectation	The graph shows us that 141 cm is most likely to be S.	7
3	Description of both expectation and variation	In the variation of guesses their [there] were a lot of guesses around 1 m 50 cm so the answer would probably be around 1 m 50 cm. I also think this because it is not to[o] big or small.	17

Table 6 Responses: plots and text boxes in *TinkerPlots* for measurement of one student ($n = 36$)*

Code	Description	Percentage
0	Not interpretable; not addressing the question; no text box.	8
1	Literal reporting of aspects of the plot, for example, what variable the graph displays, labels on the axis, number of data values.	50
2	Description of explicit information read from the graph, for example, 1 or 2 of the following types of comment: specific measurements such as range, most frequent (popular) values, outlier.	39
3	Additional information beyond, but including, the types of comments in code 2, for example, at least 3 comments of the following type: specific measurements such as range, most frequent (popular) values, outlier, percent values in the plot, intervals, averages.	3

*If multiple plots and text were produced by a group, the highest code assessed is reported in the table.

in measurement, you can just do like one type cause it's her. Lots of people measure her and some people could get a not exact [measurement]'. In further discussion, another student explained why the two distributions differed, namely, 'Shanna's would be more squished because the numbers would be closer together cause it's the same person and in, at the class, we're all different so it's all further apart'.

Students' expectation of accuracy in the second scenario

In the second scenario, while collecting measurements of all class members, students were to respond to the workbook question, 'How accurate do you expect your results to be compared to our last lesson?' As the data from each class were genuine, two classes had values that would be classified as outliers, two classes showed a large degree of variation, but no 'certain' outliers, and one class had very consistent measurements.

Six levels of responses ($N = 85$) were identified for this question. Those with no reference to criteria were coded 0. Some responses made reference to the measurement task without further explanation (code 1), whereas most of the students drew connections with descriptions of events during the activity that could affect accuracy (code 2). The

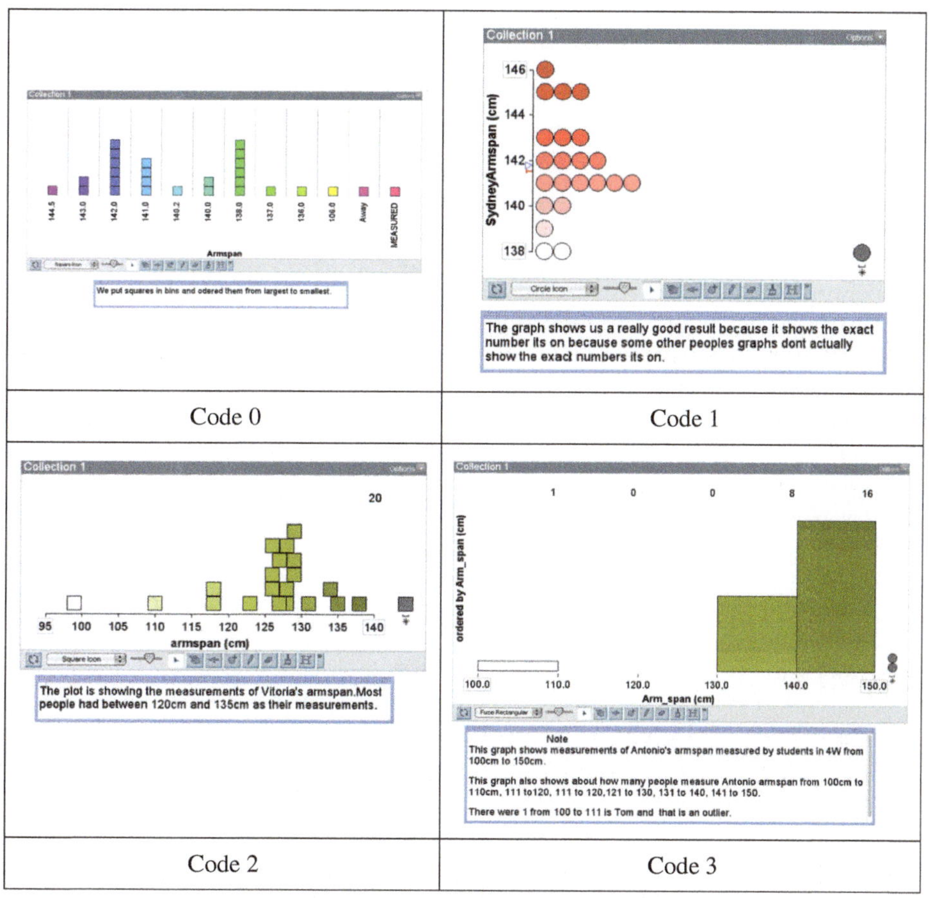

Figure 2 ***TinkerPlots*** **plots and text files for plots related to measuring a single student.**

Table 7 Responses: plots and text boxes in *TinkerPlots* comparing measurements for one student and class ($n = 31$)*

Code	Description	Percentage
0	Not an interpretable comparison; not addressing the question; no advance on the first part.	16
1	Discussion of class data only, usually in a similar fashion to the discussion of student data.	26
2	Basic statement on the difference between the two plots, for example, bumpy lines versus a triangle	39
3	Reason for difference in the arm span based on statistical information in the plot, for example, single student data bunched, class spread; most around 130 and 140, no outliers, not many same in class as single student.	19

*If multiple plots and text were produced by a group, the highest code assessed is reported in the table.

most frequent percentage of responses again mentioned the measuring tools and how they were used. Other responses featured the accuracy of the person measuring (because in several classes the researchers collected the data due to time constraints), the greater experience of the students, and rather nebulous comments on 'different' people measuring. There was only one response (code 3) that related the critical issue of the number of measurements made on the individual student compared to the single measurements on the class. Although this issue was discussed with the class before the class measurements occurred, and again in discussion following students' completion of their representations (as we illustrate next), there were other issues that attracted the attention of the students. The percentages for each level of response are given in Table 8.

Students' assessment of accuracy in second representation

Despite only one written response indicating an awareness of the role of repeated measurements in assessing accuracy between scenarios, there was evidence of this understanding in class discussion following students' completion of the two plots. Given the variation in values the students identified in the first representation, they were asked to consider their confidence level in the values displayed in their second representation. Viviane, for example, explained, 'I don't think they're exactly [accurate] because with S, in S's arm span we got lots of answers of the whole class and if, I think if we measured each of the person [second scenario] lots of times we would get different answers.' Inta added to this point by commenting that it 'would be better to do it three times because it would be like, once it could be 142, then the next one could be a different number and then the next one...' Another student further commented that, 'If you had three goes you could see, if you had 142 the first time, then 142 the next time, a different number the third time, you could estimate the 142 is the most popular, then you could do it again and see if it is the same.' Reference to this approach being 'a good idea' was emphasised by another student, explaining that, 'because ... the one that is the most [frequently occurring value] will be good and all the ones in the middle will be best and if one's too small and one's too high, you don't [use them], you'd usually use the bigger ones [more frequently occurring value/s].

Research question 3: do students demonstrate understanding of variation and transfer of that understanding through the assessment questions?

There were 26 marks possible on the assessment questions (Additional file 1). The distribution of scores for the 66 students who completed the questions is shown in Figure 4, where the median score is seen to be 18. The distribution is somewhat skewed, with a mean of 16.7 because of the three very low scores of students who spoke virtually no English. Without those three scores, the median becomes 19 and the mean becomes 17.5, which seems a reasonable reflection of the performance of the students. The teachers were pleased that half of their students had achieved scores of 69% or more.

In further evaluating the students' understanding of variation and distribution within and across data representations, we consider their responses to the assessment items Q10 through Q15 (Additional file 1).

In reviewing the results for Q10 (associated with the figure at the beginning of the Additional file 1), on describing the plot shown ('What it tells you about the people in the data set'), the maximum score was 4 for providing a meaningful and accurate account of the information in the plot. Although 20% of students did not score on Q10, 32% achieved a score of 4. The mean score across the students was 2.3 with 70% of the students achieving half marks or better.

Students scoring 1 provided very limited information on the plot, for example, 'The shape of the plot is like building in the path' and 'It tells me in the data set that the people are quite old.' Students scoring 2 gave some interpretation of the shape of the plot, with a sequence of observations: 'There are more in the middle and are kind of spreader (sic.) on the out sides' and 'There are seven people are taller than 170 cm, eight people who are shorter than 164 cm and there are nearly 50% of people in the centre'.

Scores of 3 reflected both the content and some limited comments on shape: 'It tells you 30 people heights. It shows a lot of option and goes from 146 cm to 188 cm.' 'It tells me about the people that their heights are all

Code	Text	Plot
Code 1	this plot shows directly how much everyones arm span is	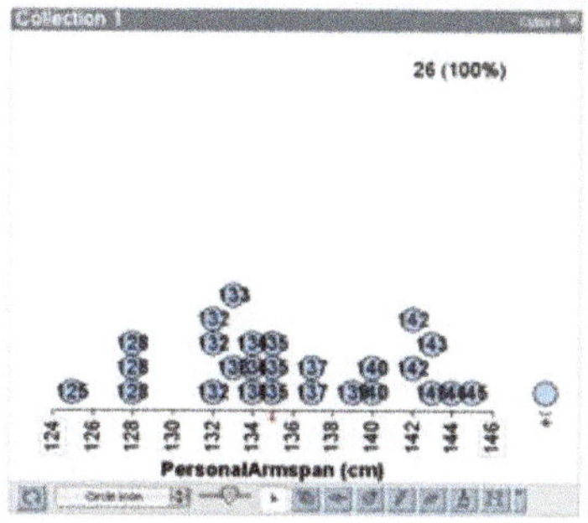
	this plot shows what the average is (140-150). And what percentage of the class guessed Antonio armspan was more than 140 and who guessed it was less.	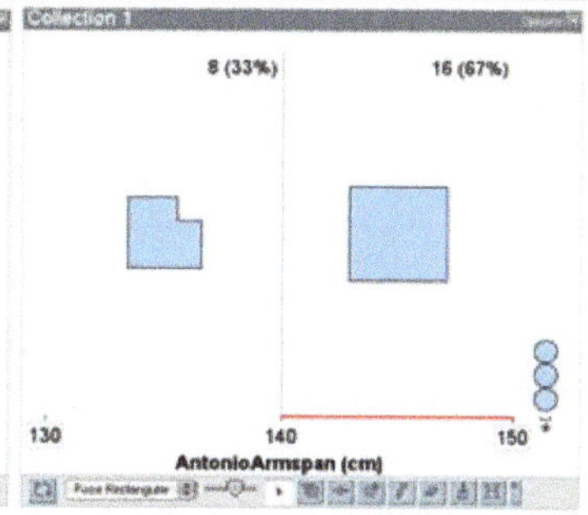
Code 2	We choose this plot because it is easy to read and understand. We think this plot is better than the pie graph we did for Isabel's armspan because it's easier to understand.	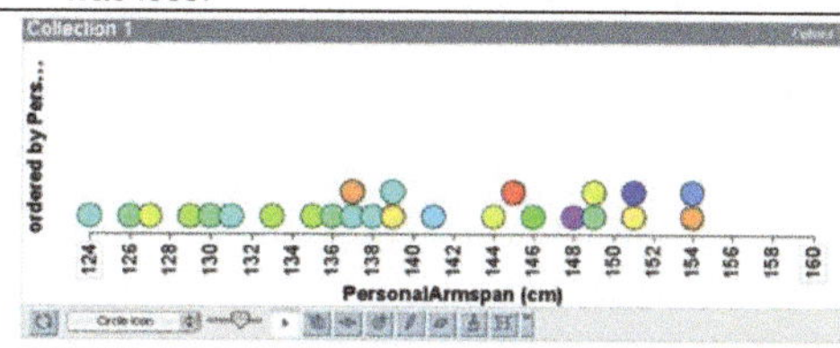
	When we compared the personal armspans graph and the Isabel's armspan graph, we found out that different people's armspans can have up to 30 cm difference.	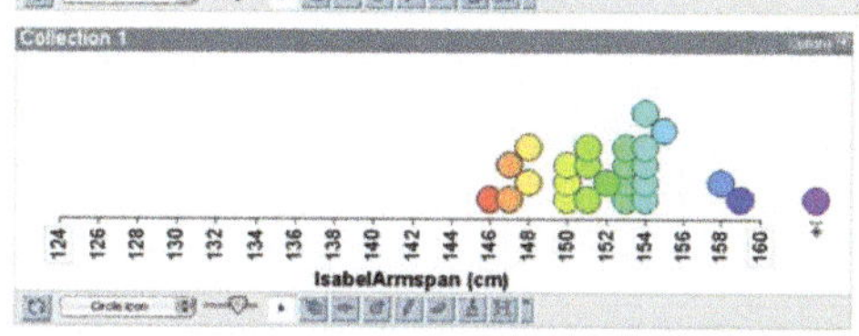
Code 3	This plot shows the names of my classmates and their measure of their proper armspan.	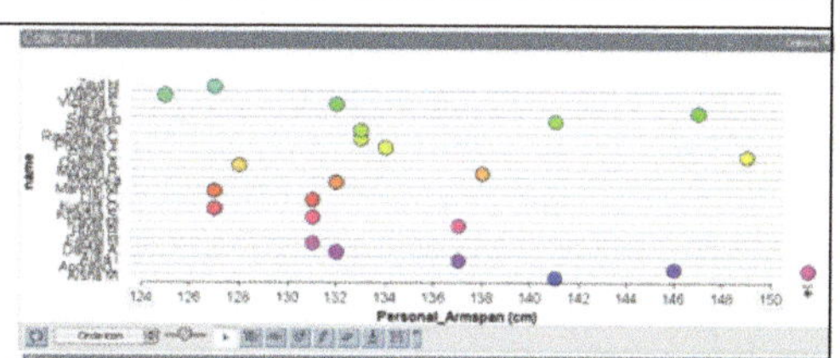
	The personal is more separedly because people always some are bigger and some smaller. The second graph is vitorias armspan and the persons balls are more squishi because it was just the measurement of 1 person and the first is different peoples armspan. That's why the first one is separate and the second one is more squishi.	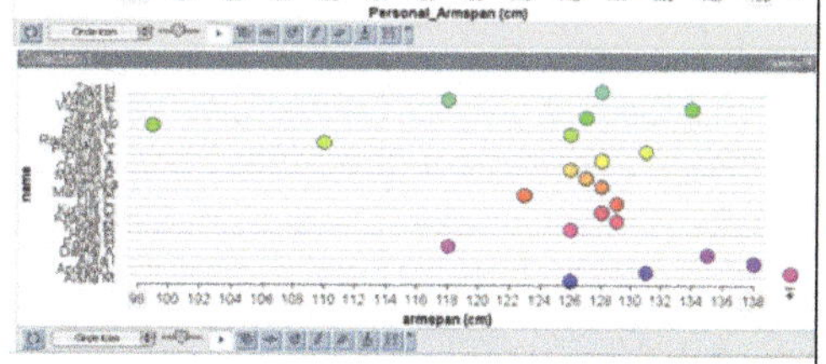

Figure 3 ***TinkerPlots*** **plots and text files for plots contrasting measurements for a single student and a class.**

different. Some people are small'. Students who scored 4 provided meaningful links to a summary of the data. These included 'It shows the average is about 164 to 170 cm which is in the middle and it is irregular with random bumps' and 'The shape is a bit of a triangle. This means it starts small on the edges and goes up to centre. Centre = 164 to 170 14 people are in the centre. There are eight people around the edges. The average person is about 167 cm'.

Q11 aligned with the classroom activity, asking students to distinguish between arm span measurements for a single student (lower plot) and a class (upper plot) (see Additional file 1), followed by the reason for being able to distinguish correctly. Seventy-seven percent of responses correctly distinguished the plots, 3% had labelling difficulties, and 20% either did not answer or did not use the labels provided. For Q12 where students explained how they decided which plot was which, 20% of students could not answer the question but 62% scored the maximum of 4, reflecting a good understanding of the classroom activity, as indicated in the sample responses below for a score of 4.

Table 8 Responses: accuracy between contexts (one student or class) (*n* = 85)

Code	Description	Example	Percentage
0	Uninterpretable	Good enough.	14
1	Nebulous comments on difference	No because people kept getting measured and it was different each time.	12
	Unexplained numerical values	At least 95%.	4
2	Measuring tools and how used	I think the [class] results are accurate because we were measuring on a flat surface and the tape was put in place accurat[e]ly.	33
	Reliability of person measuring	Yes they [the class] will be [more accurate] because the teachers measured it in the second lesson.	26
	Experience gained	Yes, I think they will be because now we have had practice at measuring we might be more accurate than last time.	10
		We have learnt more about measurement.	
3	Number of measurements*	I think it [class] wasn't really accurate because we measured S. a lot of times and for our class we only measured ourselfs [ourselves] 1 time.	1

*Most appropriate statistical response.

> The top one was the 19 students armspan because there was a lot of difference and the bottom one was Leo's armspan because it was all cramped up together. Leo's armspan didn't have a lot of variation because it is only one arm to measure and it should be nearly the same. While the 19 students one had alot of spread because its unlikely that one person could have a range of armspands [arm spans].
>
> If Leo's plot was the top one it would be impossible because Leo can't have that many armspans. If it was 19 people everyone would most likely have a different range. The top one has a bigger variation.

Responses that were scored 2 marks (11%) only considered one plot for the reasoning, for example, 'I know the second plot is Leo's Armspan because its bunch[ed] up in one place' and 'I think the bottom one is Leos (sic) because the scores are mostly the same and Leo only has one armspan.'

Q13 and Q14 were based on a plot that compared arm span measurements for two grades rather than one student and a class. Students were asked if there were an overall difference in the arm spans of these grade 6 and grade 7 students. The plot is shown above Q13 in the Additional file 1. Q13 asked for their answers and Q14 asked for two reasons for the decision. For Q13 (not scored), one student did not answer, 82% said 'Yes,' 12% said 'Not sure' and 5% said 'No'.

Two marks were possible for each reason in Q14, and there was an indication that students did slightly better for the first reason than the second. This is likely to have occurred because it is more difficult to think of two reasons than one. Overall, for both reasons, the mean score was 1.2. If a reason was repeated with little change, no mark was given for the second. The 'not sure' responses were generally followed by 'I don't know' or a blank. Some reasons for 'Yes' answers did not provide any specific information from the plot (score of 0), e.g. 'Yes, because you can see it' and 'People have differnet [different] heights in diff[e]rent age groups.' Scores of 1 generally only mentioned a single feature of the plot or a general recognition of the context: 'If you look at the top of the graph there is one dot in the very end' and 'Yes because normally Year

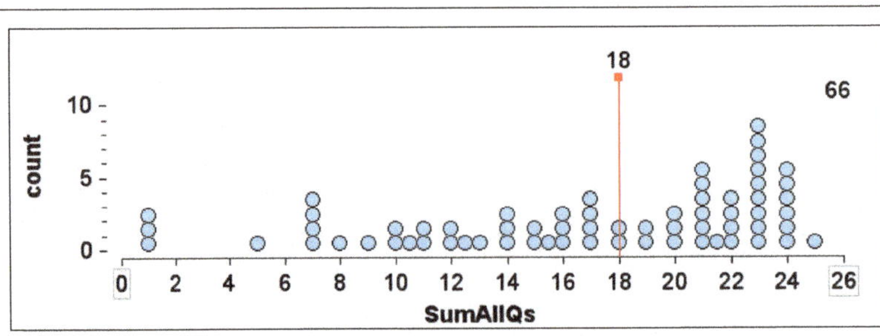

Figure 4 Distribution of marks on measurement assessment task.

7's have bigger armspans (sic.) and I've seen it.' Responses that scored 2 marks displayed a general recognition of difference in shape, as in, 'Because one is more to the right and one more to the left' and 'Because the graph shows that grade 6's are bunched up at the small end'. Two of the 'No' responses actually gave a reason for the classes to be different whereas the only valid reason supporting no difference was the following: 'I gave my answer no because the difference between the armspan (sic.) is not big (it is medium not big).'

For the final question, Q15, asking for the meaning of variation (worth 2 marks), the mean score was 1.4 with 64% of students achieving a score of 2. Many of the 26% of responses that were scored 0 were of the form, 'I don't know.' Others reflected an understanding of the context but not the nature of variation, such as, 'Long of armspan' or 'The number of people.' Responses with a score of 1 often used a word with the same root as variation, for example, 'I think it means varity [variety]' and 'Varying the amount by which something varies.' The concept of difference among some things being measured was reflected in score 2 responses: 'Variation means difference or many things, a variety for example, Sam's 131 cm and Jonah is 156 cm that's the variation'; 'It means how different things are (comparing);' and 'The diff[e] rences or similaritys [similarities] with something'.

The mean score (out of 16) for the scored items Q10 to Q15 was 10.3, with a median of 12, suggesting that the students had developed a reasonable understanding of the core concepts that were targeted in the activity. In particular, the students appeared to have developed a basic understanding of variation (Q15), scoring a mean of 1.4 out of 2. This understanding was borne out in students' responses to Q10 where well over half the class could describe and interpret the shape of the plot of heights. Likewise, for Q11 and Q12, the majority of students could identify the correct labels for the two arm span plots and could explain why this was the case.

Discussion

In reflecting on our findings, we address each research question in turn, beginning with the students' developments in detecting, representing and explaining variation in linear measurement values. We next consider their learning as they compared and explained differences between representations in the two measurement scenarios, including identifying variation and distributions, judging measurement accuracy and appreciating the role of repeated measurements. Finally, we review the students' retention and transfer of variation and distribution, including describing plots and their shape and identifying value clusters and outliers. In reflecting on our findings we touch upon the issue of how students conceive of variation and distribution, in terms of whether the former is seen as generating the latter or vice versa.

Detecting, representing and explaining variation in linear measurement values

With respect to the first research question (measuring one designated class member), the students recognised that the use of different measuring tools and how accurately they were used led to variation in values obtained and difficulty in predicting the student's actual arm span. Any outliers that occurred were readily detected and, if no such values existed, the students considered their cluster of values to predict the approximate arm span of the student. This reference to a modal notion was evident in the students' reflections on their accuracy, with recognition of the 'most popular' value/s as the likely arm span measurement. Variation in values, however, was considered by some to indicate less accuracy, as was the way in which the measuring tools were used. Although the language of informal inference was not used at this grade level, the students' best guesses or predictions were made with implicit acknowledgement of the uncertainty associated with the presence of variation.

The use of a real-world measurement activity, in which variation is a naturally occurring feature, provided a rich context for students' appreciation of phenomena that vary. As Lehrer's research has indicated (e.g. Lehrer et al., 2011), engaging young students in creating variability through measurement error is a powerful way of making visible the impreciseness in measuring - from the tools chosen, how they are manipulated and how measurements are recorded and interpreted. Experiences in undertaking repeated measurements are especially important here as they reveal the inherent variation more explicitly and convincingly. Furthermore, as observed by Lehrer et al. (2011), as students attempt to take repeated measures they became more aware of the phenomenon being measured and how any changes in that phenomenon would impact on the measurements generated. What the present activity provided was a hands-on experience of variation in a context designed to build beginning recognition of variation. In terms of the Watson et al. (2003) developmental hierarchy, this early identification of variation represents at least the second level of development for nearly all students, whereas many students reached the third level for this component of informal inference.

An awareness of the 'affordances and constraints of measures in light of characteristics of distribution' (Lehrer et al., 2011, p. 275) was becoming apparent as the students proceeded to represent and interpret their data by generating a range of representations, both hand-drawn and using the *TinkerPlots* software. Recognition of clusters of values was evident in their hand-drawn representations, with over half of the students focusing on the frequency with which the measured values occurred. Students' representations enabled them to gain a sense of the 'signal in noise' (Konold and Pollatsek, 2002, p. 268) in their data, that is, an indication of what the actual arm span measurement of the designated person might be.

Although the ordering of values and the creation of frequency plots with meaningful scales were prevalent in these hand-drawn representations, many (approximately one third) featured less sophisticated displays of actual measured values. Although our analysis focused on the statistical sophistication of the students' data displays rather than the type of representation, it is worth noting that a wide range of representations was produced. There was the use of lists, tally marks, bar graphs, circle graphs, dot plots, and histograms, with some students creating more than one representational form.

In contrast to this representational diversity were the somewhat limited descriptions of what the representations conveyed about the data. Nearly half of the responses provided only a general description of the representation rather than its message, typical of partial recognition of variation (level 2). Nevertheless, approximately a third of responses made reference to the variation and expectation that their hand-drawn representation revealed.

The students displayed similar responses in their text box explanations of their software representations, with a simple reporting of the plot features prevalent. Although there was some reference to data distribution features such as the range and most frequent values, it appeared that interpreting representations beyond a literal reading (cf. Curcio, 2010) was a new experience for the students and that more attention is required here, especially given young students' competence in generating a range of representational types (English, 2013).

Comparing and explaining differences between representations in two scenarios

The comparison of data from the two scenarios provided the opportunity for students to develop and display a consolidation of ideas related to variation in a realistic context. Identifying variation across these data sets represented development at level 3 of the Watson et al. (2003) hierarchy, although there were some inconsistencies in the presentation of arguments as evident in the students' written responses on accuracy. The class discussion transcripts, however, indicated some students could express in colloquial language ideas that they found difficult to express in written language in their workbooks.

The observed outcomes in the classroom suggested that a focus on developing students' 'metarepresentational competence' is needed, a term that diSessa and his colleagues (e.g. diSessa, 2004; diSessa et al., 1991) proposed to indicate the range of students' capabilities in constructing and using external representations prior to direct instruction - and even independently of it. This metarepresentational competence, however, needs to be accompanied by the development of conceptual competence (diSessa, 2004); specifically, students should be able to interpret and explain the statistical features displayed by their representations. As diSessa noted, research is limited here, and the role of student-created representations in conceptual development is complex. Further investigation is needed on how certain strengths or limits of metarepresentational competence might advance or hinder conceptual competence, especially as students move from non-software to software-generated representations. At the same time, it is necessary to address whether metarepresentational competence and conceptual competence grow together as students develop the statistical competencies we have explored here (English, 2013).

Although we cannot answer these questions directly from our results, students' comparisons of their software generated representations for the two measurement scenarios appeared to indicate concurrent conceptual and metarepresentational development. Over half of the student pairs could detect distribution differences, with some responses more sophisticated than others. Drawing analogies between familiar shapes (e.g. triangle) and the data distribution display was common, but reference to specific statistical information (e.g. clusters of values, variation) was not as prevalent.

In terms of judging measurement accuracy between the two scenarios, the majority of students recognised variation in the tools used and the reliability with which they were used. A few commented on the learning they had gained from the first scenario as a reason for improved accuracy in the second, suggesting a metacognitive awareness of the knowledge they had developed. This awareness has not received the attention it warrants, as both Lester (2013) and Schoenfeld (2013) have emphasised. Indeed, very little is known about how to develop students' metacognitive abilities even though they play a critical role in mathematical problem solving and learning in general.

The role of repeated measurements, the most appropriate statistical response to the question regarding measurement accuracy in the second scenario, was only mentioned once in the students' workbook responses. Follow-up class discussion, however, suggested some appreciation and understanding of the impact of repeated measurements. Very little attention has been given to this important component, which is critical to the development of long-term statistical reasoning (Cobb and Moore, 1997; Lehrer et al., 2011; Noll and Shaughnessy, 2012; Thompson et al., 2007). For elementary students to develop competency with measurement, they need to be exposed to experiences in which they witness, first-hand, the impact of repeated measurements and hence the variation that is inherent in processes of measurement.

Retention and transfer of variation and distribution

Students' understanding of variation and distribution within and across data representations was further gauged from the assessment items (third research question). In general, the students were able to describe the plots of the type they had created, noting the plot shape and identifying value clusters and outliers. On the one hand, the extent to which they provided meaningful links to a summary of the data, such as reference to centre or average or most, was not prevalent; however, we did not specifically introduce the formal notions of mean, median and mode, because these are not part of their fourth-grade curriculum. On the other hand, the majority of the students were able to distinguish between plots displaying measurements for a single student and for all students, indicating a sound understanding of the core ideas of the classroom activity.

For the assessment item that asked students to distinguish between two groups (a more general comparison than they had considered in class), 77% of students achieved a score of 1 or 2 for their first reason. This dropped to 68% for the second reason. Because the students had not seen a comparison like this before, it was felt that the performance indicated an encouraging degree of transfer of understanding of variation and the ability to think critically in a similar but non-identical context. Furthermore, well over half of the students could clearly explain the meaning of variation, demonstrating that this core concept had been absorbed meaningfully for these students.

Students' application of critical reasoning, typical of level 4 in the developmental hierarchy of Watson et al. (2003), was not as prevalent in their workbooks as we would have liked. This could have been due partially to the time constraints necessitating the researchers to assist in the measurements of the class arm spans. The class discussion, however, helped students make the desired connection with accuracy of measurement. Further, on the post-activity assessment questions, many students were able to define variation and demonstrate justifications typical of the level 4 developmental hierarchy.

These findings raise the issue of how students viewed variation and distribution. It could be that variation was seen as generating distribution, which Prodromou and Pratt (2006) considered to be half of the desired understanding. That is, this 'data centric' perspective needs to be complemented by a 'modelling perspective' where distribution is perceived as variation from an ideal model (pp. 70-71). Yet, as Noll and Shaughnessy (2012) noted, coordinating both perspectives can be challenging for young students especially when school curricula focus on one at the expense of the other. Watson's (2009) research on developing awareness of distribution, for example, suggested that students' natural intuition about variation could be overshadowed when curricula emphasise expectation. We thus argue that attention needs to be focused on both perspectives in order to sow the seeds for strong statistical reasoning. Clearly more research is warranted here including how students think about data distributions in different contexts (Noll and Shaughnessy, 2012). Because data are the basic building blocks for the study of distributions and their variation tells the stories therein, it is essential that students develop a meaningful appreciation that is deeper than numbers on a page or dots on a line. Although the language of distribution may be very complex for students to absorb in fourth grade alongside variation, slowly students should develop the notion suggested by Wild (2006) that distribution is 'the lens through which statisticians look at the variation in data' (p. 10).

Conclusions

Variation is the foundation of all of statistics and an underlying feature of all measurement. It is thus paramount that an early start is made in providing meaningful activities that are motivating both in their intrinsic interest for the students in carrying out and observing the measurements and in the challenge of creating representations to tell the story of their experiences. In terms of the mathematics curriculum (at least in Australia), the study demonstrates the advantage of linking internal sections of the curriculum in meaningful ways. As noted earlier, the measurement part of the mathematics curriculum has generally received diminished attention in recent years, and activities such as this can regenerate interest in measurement as well as contributing to the development of essential understandings in statistics. In terms of variation itself, the study reinforces the importance of the GAISE approach (Franklin et al., 2007) to variation in all stages of a statistical investigation. It is to be hoped that future versions of mathematics curricula reflect this way of thinking in setting the foundations for the statistics component of the curricula.

We have highlighted a number of issues in need of further research and ultimately inclusion in school curricula. These issues include more studies that utilise real-world situations where variation is a naturally occurring feature. In the present case, the creation of variability through measurement error provides a powerful means of making visible the impreciseness in measuring, an understanding that needs greater attention in the elementary school. More opportunities for students to make data comparisons, to create and interpret data representations and recognise their core distributional features and to read critically 'beyond the data' (cf. Curcio, 2010) are also in need of research and curriculum development. Part of this research is the underrepresented component of metarepresentational competence (e.g. diSessa 2004), which we have argued is particularly important in students' software generated representations. Finally, the issue raised earlier regarding coordinating the two perspectives on variation and distribution, that is, variation as generating distribution and distribution as variation from a desired 'model' (Prodromou and Pratt, 2006), warrants increased curriculum and research consideration.

In concluding, the limitations of the study warrant noting. Given that the study was conducted in a regular classroom setting, a number of usual obstacles were faced. These included the limited time available, the overcrowding of computer labs, last-minute timetable changes and unexpected events or changes of direction in classroom discussions. In follow-up feedback, however, all teachers were positive about their participation in the study and expressed surprise at the achievements of some students whom they did not consider would meet the expectations of the activity.

Additional file

Additional file 1: Post-activity assessment including example responses. Coding values for the instrument.

Competing interests
The authors declare that they have no competing interests.

Authors' contributions
The authors shared equally in all parts of the study. Both authors read and approved the final manuscript.

Author details
[1]Faculty of Education, Queensland University of Technology, Victoria Park Road, Kelvin Grove, Brisbane, Queensland, 4059, Australia. [2]Faculty of Education, University of Tasmania, Private Bag 66, Hobart, Tasmania 7001, Australia.

References

Australian Curriculum, Assessment and Reporting Authority. (2013a). *General capabilities in the Australian Curriculum, January, 2013*. Sydney, NSW: ACARA.
Australian Curriculum, Assessment and Reporting Authority. (2013b). *The Australian curriculum: mathematics, version 5.0, 20 May 2013*. Sydney: NSW: ACARA.
Australian Education Council. (1991). *A national statement on mathematics for Australian schools*. Melbourne: Author.
Bakker, A. (2004). Reasoning about shape as a pattern in variability. *Statistics Education Research Journal, 3*(2), 64–83.
Biggs, JB, & Collis, KF. (1982). *Evaluating the quality of learning: the SOLO taxonomy*. New York: Academic Press.
Bobis, J, Mulligan, J, & Lowrie, T. (2009). *Mathematics for children: challenging children to think mathematically* (3rd ed.). Frenchs Forest, NSW: Pearson Education.
Booker, G, & Windsor, W. (2010). Developing algebraic thinking: using problem solving to build from number and geometry in the elementary school to the ideas that underpin algebra in high school and beyond. *Procedia – Social and Behavioral Sciences, 8*, 411–419.
Bragg, P, & Outhred, L. (2004). A measure of rulers – the importance of units in a measure. In MJ Horne & AB Fuglestad (Eds.), *Proceedings of the 28th International Conference of the International Group for the Psychology of Mathematics Education (PME)* (Vol. 2, pp. 159–166). Bergen: PME.
Clements, DC, & Bright, G. (2003). *Learning and teaching measurement: 2003 yearbook*. Reston, VA: National Council of Teachers of Mathematics.
Cobb, GW, & Moore, DS. (1997). Mathematics, statistics, and teaching. *American Mathematical Monthly, 104*, 801–823.
Cobb, P, Confrey, J, diSessa, A, Lehrer, R, & Schauble, L. (2003). Design experiments in educational research. *Educational Researcher, 32*(1), 9–13.
Cobb, P, Jackson, K, & Munoz, C (in press). Design research: A critical analysis. In LD English & D Kirshner (Eds.), *Handbook of international research in mathematics education* (3rd ed.). New York: Routledge.
Common Core State Standards Initiative (CCSSI). (2010). *Common core state standards for mathematics*. Washington, DC: National Governors Association for Best Practices and the Council of Chief State School Officers. Available at: http://www.corestandards.org/assets/CCSSI_Math%20Standards.pdf.
Curcio, FR. (2010). *Developing data-graph comprehension in Grades K-8* (3rd ed.). Reston, VA: National Council of Teachers of Mathematics.
diSessa, AA. (2004). Metarepresentation: native competence and targets for instruction. *Cognition and Instruction, 22*(3), 291–292.
diSessa, AA, Hammer, D, Sherin, B, & Kolpakowski, T. (1991). Inventing graphing: metarepresentational expertise in children. *Journal of Mathematical Behavior, 10*, 117–160.
English, LD. (2012). Young children's metarepresentational competence in data modelling. In J Dindyal, L Pien Cheng, & S Fong Ng (Eds.), *Mathematics education: expanding horizons (Proceedings of the 35th annual conference of the Mathematics Education Research Group of Australasia, eBook* (pp. 266–273). Singapore: MERGA.
English, LD. (2013). Reconceptualising statistical learning in the early years. In LD English & J Mulligan (Eds.), *Reconceptualising early mathematics learning* (pp. 67–82). Dordrecht: Springer.
English, LD. (2014). Promoting statistical literacy through data modelling in the early school years. In E Chernoff & B Sriraman (Eds.), *Probabilistic thinking: presenting plural perspectives* (pp. 441–457). Dordrecht: Springer.
English, LD, & Watson, J. (2013). Beginning inference in fourth grade: Exploring variation in measurement. In V Steinle, L Ball, & C Bardini (Eds.), *Mathematics education: yesterday, today and tomorrow (Proceedings of the 36th annual conference of the Mathematics Education Research Group of Australasia)* (pp. 274–281). Melbourne: MERGA.
English, LD, & Watson, JM. (in press). The development of probabilistic understanding in fourth grade. *Journal for Research in Mathematics Education*.
English, LD, & Watson, JM. (in press). Statistical literacy in the elementary school: Opportunities for problem posing. In F Singer, N Ellerton, & J Cai (Eds.), *Problem posing: From research to effective practice*. Dordrecht: Springer.
Franklin, C, Kader, G, Mewborn, D, Moreno, J, Peck, R, Perry, M, & Scheaffer, R. (2007). *Guidelines for assessment and instruction in statistics education (GAISE) report: A preK-12 curriculum framework*. Alexandria, VA: American Statistical Association. Retrieved July 3, 2009 from http://www.amstat.org/education/gaise/.
Friel, SN, Curcio, FR, & Bright, GW. (2001). Making sense of graphs: critical factors influencing comprehension and instructional implications. *Journal for Research in Mathematics Education, 32*, 124–158.
Garfield, J, & Ben-Zvi, D. (2005). A framework for teaching and assessing reasoning about variability. *Statistics Education Research Journal, 4*(1), 92–99.
Garfield, J, & Ben-Zvi, D. (2007). How students learn statistics revisited: a current review of research on teaching and learning statistics. *International Statistical Review, 75*(3), 372–396.
Konold, C. (2007). Designing a data analysis tool for learners. In MC Lovett & P Shah (Eds.), *Thinking with data* (pp. 267–291). New York: Lawrence Erlbaum.
Konold, C, & Miller, CD. (2011). *TinkerPlots: dynamic data exploration [computer software, Version 2.0]*. Emeryville, CA: Key Curriculum Press.
Konold, C, & Pollatsek, A. (2002). Data analysis as the search for signals in noisy processes. *Journal for Research in Mathematics Education, 33*(4), 259–289.
Lehrer, R. (2007). Introducing students to data representation and statistics. In J Watson & K Beswick (Eds.), *Mathematics: essential research essential practice (Proceedings of the 30th Annual Conference of the Mathematics Education Research Group of Australasia)* (Vol. 1, pp. 22–41). Adelaide: MERGA.
Lehrer, R, & Kim, M. (2009). Structuring variability by negotiating its measure. *Mathematics Education Research Journal, 21*(2), 116–133.

Lehrer, R, Kim, M, & Jones, RS. (2011). Developing conceptions of statistics by designing measures of distribution. *ZDM Mathematics Education, 43*, 723–736.
Leinhardt, G, Zaslavsky, O, & Stein, MK. (1990). Functions, graphs and graphing: tasks, learning and teaching. *Review of Educational Research, 60*(1), 1–64.
Lester, FK. (2013). Thoughts about research on mathematical problem-solving instruction. *The Mathematics Enthusiast, 10*(1&2), 245–278.
Lowrie, T, Logan, T, & Scriven, B. (2012). Perspectives in geometry and measurement in the Australian Curriculum: Mathematics. In B Atweh, M Goos, R Jorgensen, & D Siemon (Eds.), *Engaging the Australian National Curriculum: Mathematics—Perspectives from the field* (pp. 71–88). Online Publication: Mathematics Education Research Group of Australasia.
Makar, K (in press). Developing young children's emergent inferential practices in statistics. *Mathematical Thinking and Learning.*
Makar, K, & Confrey, J. (2005). Using distributions as statistical evidence in well-structured and ill-structured problems. In K Makar (Ed.), *Proceedings of the Fourth International Research Forum on Statistical Reasoning, Thinking and Literacy (SRTL-4). SRTL4 - 2005: Fourth International Research Forum on Statistical Reasoning, Thinking and Literacy.* New Zealand: University of Auckland.
Makar, K, & Rubin, A. (2009). A framework for thinking about informal statistical inference. *Statistics Education Research Journal, 8*(1), 82–105. www.iase-web.org/documents/SERJ/SERJ8(1)_Makar_Rubin.pdf.
Mevarech, ZR, & Kramarsky, B. (1997). From verbal descriptions to graphic representations: stability and change in students' alternative conceptions. *Educational Studies in Mathematics, 32*, 229–263.
Ministry of Education. (2009). *The New Zealand curriculum: mathematics standards for years 1–8.* Wellington, NZ: Author. Available at http://nzcurriculum.tki.org.nz/The-New-Zealand-Curriculum/Learning-areas/Mathematics-and-statistics.
Moore, DS. (1990). Uncertainty. In LS Steen (Ed.), *On the shoulders of giants: new approaches to numeracy* (pp. 95–137). Washington, DC: National Academy Press.
National Council of Teachers of Mathematics. (1989). *Curriculum and evaluation standards for school mathematics.* Reston, VA: Author.
Noll, J, & Shaughnessy, JM. (2012). Aspects of students' reasoning about variation in empirical sampling distributions. *Journal for Research in Mathematics Education, 43*, 509–556.
Patton, MQ. (2002). *Qualitative research and evaluation methods* (3rd ed.). Thousand Oaks, CA: Sage Publications Inc.
Pfannkuch, M. (2005). Thinking tools and variation. *Statistics Education Research Journal, 4*(1), 83–91.
Prodromou, T, & Pratt, D. (2006). The role of causality in the co-ordination of the two perspectives on distribution within a virtual simulation. *Statistics Education Research Journal, 5*(2), 69–88. http://iase-web.org/documents/SERJ/SERJ5%282%29_Prod_Pratt.pdf.
Reading, C. (2004). Student description of variation while working with weather data. *Statistics Education Research Journal, 3*(2), 84–105.
Russell, SJ. (1991). Counting noses and scary things: children construct their ideas about data. In D Vere-Jones (Ed.), *Proceedings of the Third International Conference on the Teaching of Statistics* (pp. 158–164). Dunedin, NZ: University of Otago.
Schoenfeld, AH. (2013). Reflections on problem solving theory and practice. *The Mathematics Enthusiast, 10*(1&2), 9–34.
Smith, JP, van den Heuvel-Panhuizen, M, & Teppo, A. (2011). Learning, teaching, and using measurement: introduction to the issue. *ZDM Mathematics Education, 43*, 617–620.
Szilagyi, J, Clements, DH, & Samara, J. (2013). Young children's understanding of measurement: evaluating a learning trajectory. *Journal for Research in Mathematics Education, 44*, 3.
Thompson, PW, Liu, Y, & Saldanha, LA. (2007). Intricacies of statistical inference and teachers' understanding of them. In MC Lovett & P Shah (Eds.), *Thinking with data* (pp. 207–231). New York: Lawrence Erlbaum.
Wall, JJ, & Benson, CC. (2009). So many graphs, so little time. *Mathematics Teaching in the Middle School, 15*, 82–91.
Watson, JM. (2005). Variation and expectation as foundations for the chance and data curriculum. In P Clarkson, A Downton, D Gronn, M Horne, A McDonough, R Pierce, & A Roche (Eds.), *Building connections: theory, research and practice (Proceedings of the 28th annual conference of the Mathematics Education Research Group of Australasia, Melbourne* (pp. 35–42). Sydney: MERGA.
Watson, JM. (2006). *Statistical literacy at school: growth and goals.* Mahwah, NJ: Lawrence Erlbaum.
Watson, JM. (2009). The influence of variation and expectation on the developing awareness of distribution. *Statistics Education Research Journal, 8*(1), 32–61.
Watson, JM. (2012). History and statistics: connections across the curriculum. *AGORA, 47*(3), 58–64.
Watson, JM. (2013). Statistical literacy, a statistics curriculum for school students, the pedagogical content needs of teachers, and the Australian Curriculum. *Curriculum Perspectives, 33*(3), 58–69.
Watson, JM, & Kelly, BA. (2002a). Can grade 3 students learn about variation? In B Phillips (Ed.), *Proceedings of the Sixth International Conference on Teaching Statistics: developing a statistically literate society, Cape Town, South Africa.* Voorburg, The Netherlands: International Statistical Institute. Retrieved from http://iase-web.org/documents/papers/icots6/2a1_wats.pdf.
Watson, JM, & Kelly, BA. (2002b). Grade 5 students' appreciation of variation. In A Cockburn & E Nardi (Eds.), *Proceedings of the 26th Conference of the International Group for the Psychology of Mathematics Education* (Vol. 4, pp. 385–392). Norwich, UK: University of East Anglia.
Watson, J, & Wright, S. (2008). Building informal inference with *TinkerPlots* in a measurement context. *Australian Mathematics Teacher, 64*(4), 31–40.
Watson, JM, Kelly, BA, Callingham, RA, & Shaughnessy, JM. (2003). The measurement of school students' understanding of statistical variation. *International Journal of Mathematical Education in Science and Technology, 34*, 1–29.
Watson, JM, Fitzallen, NE, Wilson, KG, & Creed, JF. (2008). The representational value of hats. *Mathematics Teaching in the Middle School, 14*, 4–10.
Wild, CJ. (2006). The concept of distribution. *Statistics Education Research Journal, 5*(2), 10–26.
Wild, CJ, & Pfannkuch, M. (1999). Statistical thinking in empirical enquiry (with discussion). *International Statistical Review, 67*(3), 223–265.

3

An exploratory study of informed engineering design behaviors associated with scientific explanations

Şenay Purzer[1*], Molly Hathaway Goldstein[2], Robin S Adams[2], Charles Xie[3] and Saeid Nourian[3]

Abstract

Background: Design and science inquiry are intertwined during engineering practice. In this study, we examined the relationship between design behaviors and scientific explanations. Data on student design processes were collected as students engaged in a project on designing energy-efficient buildings on a blank square city block surrounded by existing buildings using a computer-aided design program, Energy3D, with built-in solar energy simulation capabilities. We used criterion sampling to select two highly reflective students among 63 high school students.

Results: The main data sources were design replays (automatic playback of student design sequences within the CAD software) and electronic notes taken by the students. We identified evidence of informed design such as problem framing, idea fluency, and balancing benefits and trade-offs. Opportunities for meaningful science learning through engineering design occurred when students attempted to balance design benefits and trade-offs.

Conclusions: The results suggest that design projects used in classrooms should emphasize trade-off analysis and include time and resources for supporting trade-off decisions through experimentation and reflection. Future research should explore ways to visualize patterns of design behavior based on large samples of students.

Keywords: Computer-aided design; Engineering design; Informed design; Scientific inquiry; Trade-offs

Background

Engineering and technological design has been considered to be a component of K-12 education curricula and standards in a number of countries since the 1970s. Many industrialized countries such as Australia, Great Britain, New Zealand, and the US have implemented reforms for engineering education in K-12 schools to promote technological literacy as well as competencies to create and evaluate design solutions (Cajas 2001; Lachapelle and Cunningham 2014). While engineering design has been a part of the National Science Education Standards in the US (National Research Council 1996), it has gained a new sense of importance worldwide with the increased number of studies examining engineering in association with science learning, twenty-first century skill development, and academic motivation (Brophy et al. 2008; Penner et al. 1997; Sadler et al. 2000; Purzer et al. 2014) and with the publication of a number of reports such as *A Framework for K-12 Science Education* (National Research Council 2012), the *Next Generation Science Standards* (Achieve 2013), and *STEM Integration in K-12 Education* (National Academy of Engineering and National Research Council 2014).

Scientific inquiry vs. engineering design

Given that engineering is a relatively new subject as compared to science for many educators, curriculum developers, and policy makers, there are many attempts to understand features of scientific inquiry and engineering design and how they might relate or interact with each other (Lewis 2006; National Research Council 2012; Schunn et al. 2012). Lewis (2006) provides a brief history on the push for inquiry in educational standards and identifies key differences and similarities between inquiry and design. He notes that inquiry was first viewed as an intellectual process - the attitudes and activities associated with discovery (Bruner 1961). Over time, definitions of inquiry focused on the intellectual processes peculiar

* Correspondence: spurzer@purdue.edu
[1]School of Engineering Education, Purdue University, Wang Hall 4545, 516 Northwestern Avenue, West Lafayette, IN 47906, USA
Full list of author information is available at the end of the article

to particular aspects of science that were crucial to understanding the nature of science. As such, scientific inquiry became to be understood as more than a technique (i.e., a process or inquisitive stance) but as the content and practices of science (i.e., the role of scientific theory in generating new lines of investigation and how science is done). Scientific inquiry represents the diverse ways in which scientists study the natural world and develop explanations based on the evidence derived from research (National Research Council 1996, p. 23). While scientific inquiry involves observations, posing questions, and examining various sources of information to see what is already known, there is no single scientific method (Penner et al. 1997), and while scientific investigations may share a common set of deductive or inductive reasoning activities, there is 'no fixed sequence of steps that all scientific investigations follow' (National Research Council 1996, p. 3). Instead, inquiry is characterized as a fluid process in which the outcomes are not absolute, but rather tentative.

Similar to scientific inquiry, design is understood to be a complex cognitive activity (Cross 2001; Lawson and Dorst 2009) where there is no one generalized design method (Dubberly 2004) although variations of methods share many elements such as posing, generating, evaluating, and choosing solutions (Lawson and Dorst 2009). Designers tackle and resolve ill-defined or wicked problems in which solutions are neither right nor wrong but rather sufficient (Cross 2006; Goel and Pirolli 1992). This uncertainty requires that designers construct or frame problems, which involves taking into account the problem context and the needs of diverse stakeholders. This occurs through identifying constraints or boundaries on the space in which the designer searches for a solution. Constraints cover a large and often under-determined space from objective parameters (governed by natural or mathematical principles) to subjective values (Goel and Pirolli 1992; Jonassen 2000). As such, designers need to consider trade-offs to select among a set of plausible solutions and may need to revisit early problem formulations or backtrack on design decisions as needed.

Since design problems are often not amenable to exhaustive analysis, the designer uses abductive reasoning to impose conjectures to manage ambiguity and make solutions possible (Dorst 2011; Kolko 2010). They also rely on other cognitive reasoning tools such as analogical reasoning to search for solutions and manage ambiguity (Ball and Christensen 2009; Paletz et al. 2013; Daugherty and Mentzer 2008), visual thinking to amplify the inventive uses of mental imagery (Fish and Scrivener 1990; Goldschmidt 1991; Goldschmidt and Smolkov 2006), and representational thinking to translate abstract requirements into concrete ideas and communicate these ideas to others (Bucciarelli 1996; Cross 2006). Overall, the design process may be characterized as a goal-directed and iterative activity where the mode of problem solving is described as solution-focused (as compared to problem-focused) since a designer learns about the problem through proposing solutions and synthesizing ideas.

As Lewis (2006) describes, notable divergences between engineering design and scientific inquiry include purpose (starting points that emphasize pure versus applied dimensions), the role of constraints (constraints in design are intrinsically woven into design reasoning), the role of trade-offs (science has no parallel to this form of reasoning), and the role of context (design problems are shaped by context whereas science problems seek to transcend context). Two central ways design converges with Scientific inquiry include (a) reasoning processes such as analogical reasoning as navigational devices to bridge the gap between problem and solution and (b) uncertainty as a starting condition that demands expenditure of cognitive resources in the form of search strategies, mental models and visual representations to rehearse and communicate thought, and decision-making via testing and evaluation (Lewis 2006). As stated earlier, both design and inquiry are often referred to as procedures, although no generic procedure exists, and are taught as content in their own right, although they must draw upon a base of knowledge to formulate and solve problems.

Another key point of commonality between engineering design and scientific inquiry is that both emphasize learning by doing. For example, a key performance dimension of design is learning while designing (Crismond and Adams 2012). This includes learning by doing and reflecting, from brainstorming and prototyping, through iteration and feedback from failure, by noticing and troubleshooting, as well as drawing and dialoging with ideas, materials, and people (Adams et al. 2003; Crismond and Adams 2012; Lawson and Dorst 2009; Schön 1993). Similarly, scientific inquiry is characterized as a process of transformative learning that allows expression of both teacher and student voices (Lewis 2006).

While much has been written about comparing design and scientific inquiry, there are limited studies focusing on how K-12 students engage in engineering design and scientific inquiry simultaneously while solving complex and ill-defined problems (Svihla and Petrosino 2008; National Research Council 2009). In this study, we used a computer-aided design software that captured student design activities allowing us access to fine-grained data on students' explanations and actions. More specifically, we asked:

How are secondary school students' design behaviors associated with scientific explanations in informing design decisions?

Conceptual framework

Engineering and science manifest and interact to support learning

Learning one (e.g., engineering) through the other (e.g., science) represents an underlying philosophy integrating scientific inquiry and design in K-12 education. Previous research suggests that engineering design is an effective approach to supporting science learning (Apedoe et al. 2008; Hmelo et al. 2000; Kolodner 2002; Kolodner et al. 2003; Doppelt et al. 2008; Schnittka and Bell 2011). Well-documented and effective approaches for which design provides a vehicle for learning science include Learning By Design (LBD) (Kolodner 2002), Model Eliciting Activities (MEA) (Zubrowski 2002), and Knowledge and Skill Builders (Burghardt and Hacker 2004). As an example, the LBD model of constructing and testing real devices provides students with opportunities to test their conceptions and discover the holes in their own knowledge as well as predict the performance of their designs (Kolodner 2002).

Parallel to accounts of design approaches to enhance science learning are those that use science as a vehicle for prompting design. For example, Lewis (2006) describes two activities that ask students to develop design ideas by applying science concepts they learned previously. The first activity by Snetsinger et al. (1999) involves application of electrical and mechanical energy concepts to the design of wind turbines. The second activity by Subramanian (1999) applies thermal expansion principles into the design of bimetallic household products. Despite these examples, there are concerns about the so-called 'design-science gap' (Vattam and Kolodner 2008). A challenge is that such learning is not easily amenable to traditional assessment methods. In classroom practice, critical aspects of science learning tend to be set aside (Apedoe and Schunn 2013) as students focus on aesthetic features or on building and construction as opposed to experimentation, analysis, and justification of design decisions.

Using a conceptual framework that characterizes the interaction between scientific inquiry and design, this study offers an emergent theory of how secondary students learn and apply science concepts through engineering design. The study also offers tools for understanding how engineering and science manifest and interact and the kinds of learning associated with this interaction. As shown in Figure 1, this framework is situated in a shared space of convergence - learning while designing. This space includes learning science through design (where design is the vehicle for learning science), learning design through science (where science serves as vehicle for prompting a design task), and learning design. For this study, learning science focuses on specific concepts that are relevant to the design task. Both learning science and learning design goals are essential and in alignment with the NGSS (Achieve 2013).

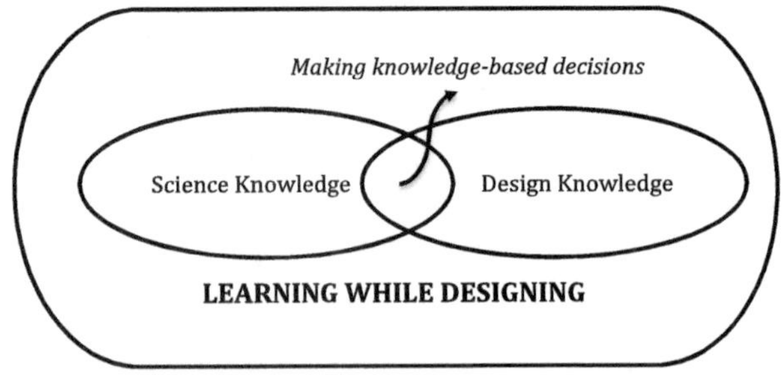

Figure 1 Science and design knowledge informing design decisions.

The intersection of science and design knowledge marks the nature of the interaction between science inquiry and design, making and explaining knowledge-based decisions. Crismond and Adams (2012) describe this as using knowledge of physical laws, how things work, methods of construction, everyday knowledge, application of known cases, and knowledge gained from design revisions and experiments. The framing illustrates the ways science inquiry and design occur concurrently feeding one another. For example, simulation data collected through experimentation can inform the design of specific features. Similarly, the design of multiple prototypes with comparable features can guide scientific inquiry with the goal of evaluating the performance of these alternatives. Together, these activities guide the explanation of relationships among design criteria as well as help inform decisions about making trade-offs among these criteria.

Informed design behaviors

To qualitatively characterize patterns of student design behaviors, we used Crismond and Adams (2012) *Informed Design Learning and Teaching Matrix*. The design of this matrix was based on a meta-literature review of more than 50 studies and synthesized key performance dimensions of informed designing and behaviors that distinguish novice and expert designers. Our goal was to explore how these behaviors manifest at the interactions between science and engineering. One of these key performance dimensions is 'using design strategies effectively'. This is defined as knowing when and how to use a range of design practices and strategies, and being open to altering a design approach or decision to accommodate new information and time constraints. These key performance dimensions were translated into nine observable design strategies that were further translated into nine 'contrasting set' statements that could act as a guide for noticing how beginning vs. informed designers do the selected strategies.

As shown in Table 1, the matrix describes a two-step learning trajectory from 'beginning designer' (that depicts assumptions about prior knowledge and skills of learners as they enter a learning progression) to 'informed designer' (that depicts what learners are expected to know and do by the end of the progression). Here, an informed designer is one whose level of experience includes some formal training in design, and level of competence lies somewhere between that of the novice and expert designer. Collectively, the nine statements represent key elements of design learning that make up effective practice, and each statement describes the signs of beginning designers' less effective design approaches as compared to how informed designers would more effectively perform the same strategy. For example, for the pattern of *ignore* vs. *balance benefits and trade-offs*, beginning designers are prone to ignore complexity and trade-offs and make design decisions without weighing all options or attend only to pros of favored ideas or cons of lesser approaches. In contrast, informed designers use words and graphics to display and weigh both benefits and trade-offs before selecting a solution. For the pattern, *haphazard or linear* vs. *managed and iterative designing*, beginners design in haphazard ways or do design steps once and in a linear manner. Informed designers do design in a managed way, improving on ideas iteratively through feedback and using strategies multiple times as needed, in any order.

Methods

Research participants and classroom context

This exploratory study was conducted at a large public high school located in the Northeast United States. Sixty-three students were enrolled in the engineering track during the spring 2013 semester in five courses that comprised the engineering track. Our intent was to target the students with the richest reflective notes from all students in the sample. We reviewed notes from students who completed at least two unique designs. In reviewing each student's designs, we looked at richness of reflection notes over their three designs. These reflective

Table 1 Informed design patterns (Crismond and Adams 2012)

Beginning vs. informed design patterns	Description
Pattern A. Problem solving vs. problem framing	Beginning designers feel that understanding the design task is straightforward, a matter of comprehending the challenge as a well-structured problem, which they prematurely and immediately attempt to solve. Informed designers seek initially to explore and comprehend the challenge as the best they can, delaying decisions to frame the problem effectively.
Pattern B. Skipping vs. doing research	Beginning designers skip doing research in favor of generating solutions immediately. Informed designers do research to build knowledge broadly about the problem and potential solutions.
Pattern C. Idea scarcity vs. idea fluency	Beginning designers can start a design project with very few or even just one idea, which they may not want to discard, add to, or revise. Informed designers want to design with an abundance of ideas and practice idea fluency to explore the design space and initially seek to avoid favoring any single solution.
Pattern D. Surface vs. deep drawing and modeling	Beginning designers propose and sketch ideas that superficially resemble viable solutions but do not support deep inquiry into how (and if) a solution might function or behave. Informed designers use multiple representations (gestures, words, text, simulations, prototypes) to explore and investigate design ideas in ways that support deep inquiry into how a system works.
Pattern E. Ignore vs. balance benefits and trade-offs	Beginning designers ignore or pay too little attention to design criteria and constraints, make design decisions without weighing options and trade-offs, or attend only to pros of favored ideas and cons of lesser approaches. Informed designers balance systems of benefits and trade-offs, using words and graphics, when they consider plans or make and justify decisions.
Pattern F. Confounded vs. valid tests and experiments	Beginning designers run few tests on their design prototypes, and when they run tests, they can confound experiments that cannot provide useful information about potential solutions and their performance. Informed designers conduct valid tests as part of their investigations that help them learn quickly about key variables, materials, users, and ways to optimize performance of prototypes.
Pattern G. Unfocused vs. diagnostic troubleshooting	Beginning designers use unfocused, non-analytical ways to view prototypes during testing and troubleshooting ideas. Informed designers focus their attention on problematic areas and subsystems when troubleshooting devices and proposing ways to fix them.
Pattern H. Haphazard or linear vs. managed and iterative designing	Beginning designers design in haphazard ways, working at random on whatever problems emerge or they treat design as a set of strategies to be done once in linear order. Informed designers design as an iterative process, improving ideas and prototypes based on feedback and cycling back to upgrade their understanding of the problem, managing time and resources strategically, and using design strategies multiple times as needed, in any order.
Pattern I. Tacit vs. reflective design thinking	Beginning designers do tacit designing when they think and act with little self-reflection and do little monitoring of their own or others' actions either in the moment or after the work is done. Informed designers practice reflective thinking in a metacognitive way by reviewing and keeping tabs on design strategies and thinking while working and after work is finished.

Note: For full matrix, see Crismond and Adams (2012).

notes included scientific explanations and provided information on students' actions and the reasoning associated with these actions.

For this exploratory study, we were purposeful in our selection of the cases. We wanted to select students from the same section to account for a similar course experience. The subsample that met all selection criteria ultimately included two senior high school students with the richest reflective notes from a course, named capstone design. Such reflectivity suggests that these students were at a place more than average in the beginning-informed designer spectrum. Each student, given the pseudonyms of Andrew and Brent, generated two design solutions addressing a design challenge described in the following section.

Design challenge

The design problem, the solar urban design challenge (Xie et al. 2014b), asked students to design energy-efficient, passive solar buildings on a blank square city block surrounded by existing buildings of different heights (see Figure 2).

The design challenge, described in Figure 3, involves the use of design practices to consider solar radiation as it varies over a day and over seasons, analyze simulation data, consider constraints, make trade-offs, and optimize solutions (e.g., minimize the energy required to heat a building in the winter and minimize the energy required to cool a building in the summer). The Energy3D environment allows verification or testing of design performance within the software (Xie et al. 2014a).

Students used a computer-aided design (CAD) software, Energy3D, to design solutions for the built environment based on solar energy and heat transfer concepts (i.e., science knowledge) addressing the following engineering principles (i.e., design knowledge) outlined in the NGSS (Achieve 2013).

- HS-PS3-3. Design, build, and refine a device that works within given constraints to convert one form of energy into another form of energy.
- HS-ETS1-1. Analyze a major global challenge to specify qualitative and quantitative criteria and constraints for solutions that account for societal needs and wants.
- HS-ETS1-3. Evaluate a solution to a complex real-world problem based on prioritized criteria and trade-offs that account for a range of constraints, including cost, safety, reliability, and esthetics as well as possible social, cultural, and environmental impacts.
- HS-ETS1-4. Use a computer simulation to model the impact of proposed solutions to a complex real-world problem with numerous criteria and constraints on interactions within and between systems relevant to the problem.

Data sources

Design replays

The Energy3D software collected logs of student design actions in the background as students were sketching buildings, conducting experiments, collecting data using simulations, and taking reflective notes. These learner data were used to reconstruct the entire design process with all important actions restored for analysis. The snapshots (computer models, *not* images) were played back just like running a slide show. Student notes (text

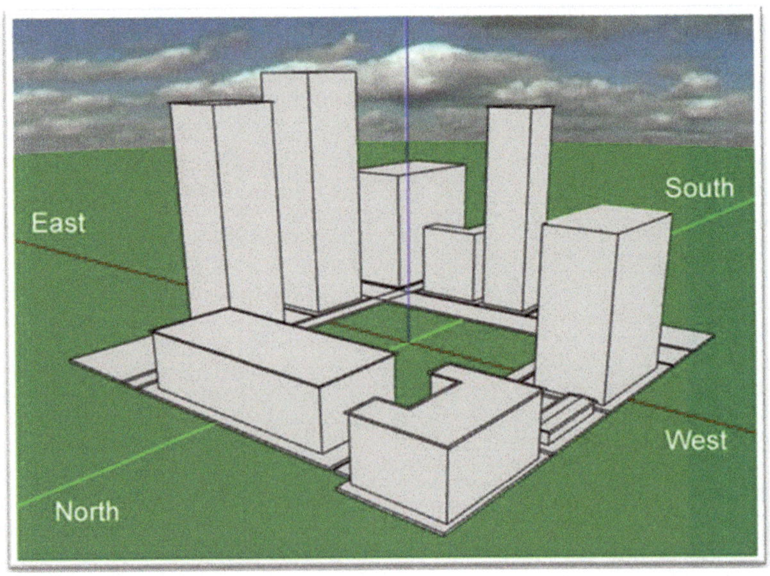

Figure 2 Solar urban design challenge.

City Block Design Challenge – Goals and Constraints

Build at least two high-rise buildings: These are for residence and offices. No new construction, however, is allowed to be taller than the highest existing buildings in the neighborhood.

Build at least two low-rise buildings: These are for shops or services such as restaurants, book stores, or pharmacies. They should not be taller than 20 meters.

Build with a balance of built and open space: Approximately ⅓ of the block must be constructed with high-rises and ⅓ with low-rises. The remaining ⅓ must be open space. The proportions do not need to be exact, however.

Build at most eight new buildings (including high- and low-rises): in total are allowed in the block.

Don't add windows: We assume that windows will be added proportionally to the total surface areas of each building later.

Parking areas, subway, or bus stations need not be considered.

Optimize solar gains of the high-rise buildings in the winter and summer: The locations and shapes of the high-rise buildings should be chosen such that they receive **as much total solar energy on December 31st as possible** to lower the heating costs in the winter ***AND*** **as little total solar energy on June 30th as possible** to lower the cooling costs in the summer.

No need to consider the solar gains of the low-rise buildings: They do not need a lot of sunlight because they accommodate business facilities that usually do not have many windows.

Figure 3 City block design challenge.

strings) to explain or reflect on their designs were replayed synchronously to their design actions such that we can coordinate the analyses of *what they did* and *what they thought.*

The computer recorded every action of the students. The datasets collected were large in that each design challenge required 5 to 7 h of classroom time to complete and summed up to approximately 20 megabytes at the end of a design project for a single active student. The replay of students' design actions can be sped up to provide a compressed view of the full design process, similar to time-lapse photography. In addition, these design replays can be stopped and restarted with one keystroke to better analyze each design action when needed.

Figure 4 presents the simulation of solar path (also called virtual heliodon), which students use to view the path of the sun. Another simulation allows viewing of the daily radiation heat map on all building surfaces. These features are helpful in understanding shadows related to both heating and cooling and enable students to visualize warmer and cooler parts of the building in multiple seasons. Figure 4 shows system capabilities in assisting students in balancing benefits and trade-offs from both a heating and cooling perspective as well as taking different seasons into account.

Electronic notes

The Energy3D system includes a note tool that allows students to enter electronic notes while designing. During the classroom implementation, students were encouraged to note their design process, decisions, and thinking and were instructed to take notes 'like an engineer' such as reasons for creating or selecting design features, describing tests to conduct about the performance of the current design, documenting performance and interpreting test results, and making plans for next steps. The student design rationales, collected through electronic notes within the system, were used in conjunction with the process data to gain a much clearer picture of student actions, learning, and reflection.

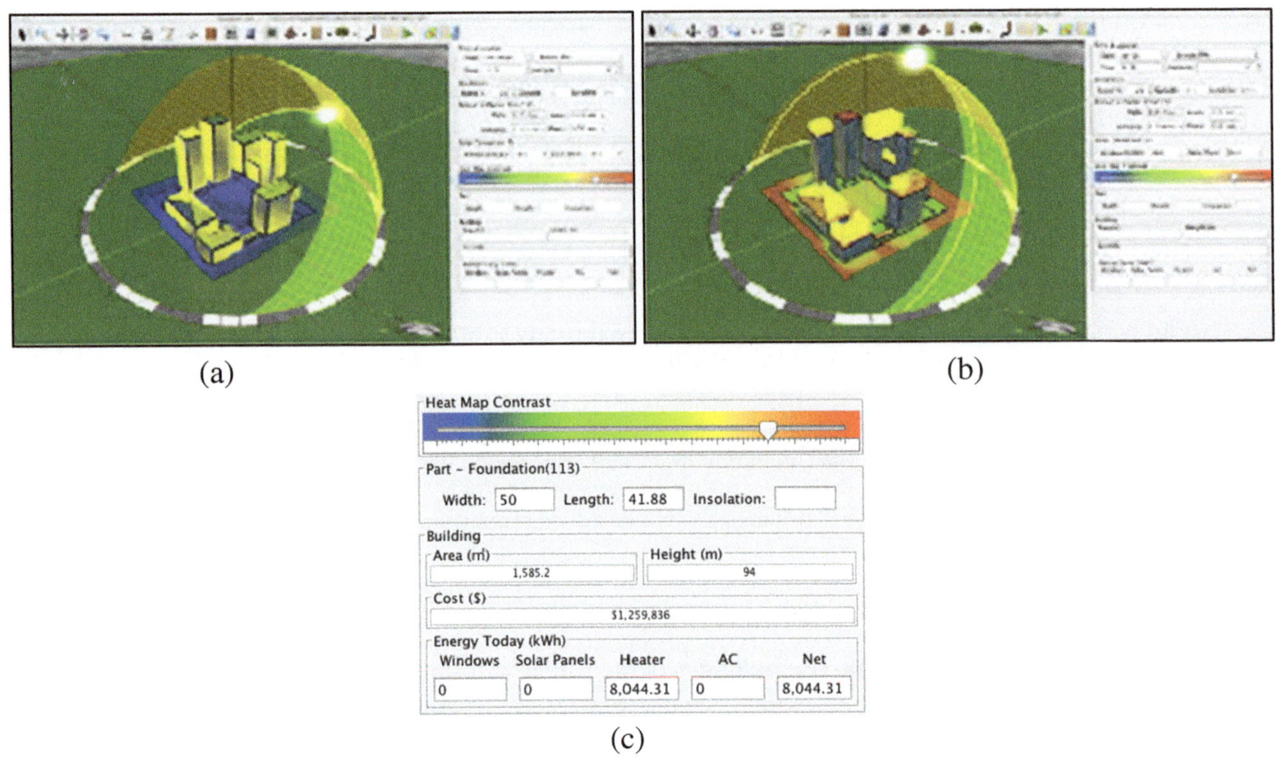

Figure 4 Energy3D simulations **(a)** analysis for December **(b)** analysis for July **(c)** detailed view of the quantitative analysis for December.

Data analysis

Because we were interested in the interaction between science inquiry and design, which was defined as making and explaining knowledge-based decisions in Figure 1, design decisions were our unit of analysis. To characterize observable patterns of student design behaviors within the video playbacks and student notes, we developed and used the informed design coding protocol based on the *Informed Design Learning and Teaching Matrix* (Crismond and Adams 2012). Finally, we used Valkenburg's (1998) representational system to visually display students' decision-making over time in terms of observable student design patterns. This also provided a mechanism for connecting macro-level iterations that addressed system-wide performance to micro-level iterations that addressed local issues.

Development of the informed design coding protocol

Each set of design decisions (moves), with student notes as further evidence when available, was mapped against the *Informed Design Learning and Teaching Matrix* (Crismond and Adams 2012). Table 2 includes examples of these behaviors as exhibited by Andrew and Brent. We did not consider pattern d, deep drawing, and modeling, from the *Informed Design Learning and Teaching Matrix*, due to the fact that the given project uses a CAD system without the explicit use of other forms of representations.

Each student's design replays were reviewed in 10-s increments, which corresponded to 6 to 7 min of the actual class time, similar to time-lapse photography. Prior studies show data from such low-fidelity approaches are compatible with high-fidelity approaches where the observer is physically co-located with the student observed (Baker et al. 2006; Zhang et al. 2014). In addition, this approach allowed researchers to see subtle actions that are not obvious to the human eye. While designing, students typically made CAD design moves at a pace that allows these steps to be accelerated for analysis.

Within each 10-s increment, student design actions (moves) were reviewed and coded using the action categorization scheme presented in Figure 5. This categorization was used in combination with student notes to understand design episodes when the student was working within one goal or frame of the problem (see Figure 6). For example, within a frame, a student may write notes in which he reflects upon or considers the actions he has been taking in relation to a goal such as revising the roof while reflecting about increasing shade and decreasing the energy profile in the summer. Next, these chunks of time with similar goals served as input for characterization and visualization of the intersection of scientific explanation and design processes. Together, these actions formed a coherent design episode.

Valkenburg's (1998) representational system was then used to visually display students' decision-making over time in terms of observable student design patterns. This also provided a mechanism for connecting macro-level iterations. Figure 5 shows the symbols that were used to create visual representations of the design episodes based on the informed design coding protocol. Each design episode started with a goal, represented with an oval. The triangles are representative of moves or student actions such as making, editing, or changing roof shape. When a connection to a science concept is made, this was indicated with a blue dot. Student reflections are shown with a diamond.

Results and discussion

The analysis of Andrew's and Brent's design notes and design actions, resulted in a series of coherent activities reflecting informed design behaviors. Brent's full design process is used for this illustrative example to show how he made connections to science concepts. Andrew exhibited similar patterns in his design process as well. In Figure 6, all design episodes for Brent are represented in sequential order, composed of six episodes. All seven patterns of informed design behaviors were evident in both Andrew and Brent's design processes: problem framing, doing background research, idea fluency, balancing benefits and trade-offs, diagnostic troubleshooting, managed and iterative designing, and reflective design thinking.

As illustrated in Figure 6, the use of science concepts appeared in four episodes (episodes 1, 2, 3, and 5) along with trade-off analysis he engaged in. Where there was no trade-off analysis, there were no explicit connections to science. Reflective design thinking was also evident in these episodes. Episodes 4 and 6 were the only two instances where Brent did not make a science connection. These episodes also did not include any written reflections or evidence of an explicit trade-off analysis. During idea fluency, when Brent affluently generated and tested a large number of ideas, there was no evidence of reflective thinking and consequently no scientific explanations.

Throughout his design process, Brent made connections to two science concepts: heat transfer and seasonal solar path. As illustrated in Episode 1 in Figure 6, he conducted experiments that resulted in scientific explanations on the relationship between building geometry (more specifically surface area) and the solar energy gains. In

Table 2 Informed design coding protocol

Informed design patterns	Data description
Problem framing (understand the challenge)	Student spent time reviewing the criteria and constraints and specifically mentioned these elements in the student notes
Doing background research (build knowledge)	Student tested design features early in the episode (i.e., designed a basic building to get a sense of its baseline performance)
Idea fluency (generate ideas)	Student worked with a large variety of ideas (i.e., building height, width, roof characteristics, or location). Student was able to work with one idea element at a time (i.e., building height) or several elements at a time.
Balance benefits and trade-offs through experimentation (weigh options and make decisions through conducting experiments)	Student made design moves (adjust building height, width, roof characteristics, location) and performed the solar path analysis to determine the performance associated with the move. Sometimes notes regarding the experimental nature of the move were explicit. Student ran the solar analysis in two different seasons, weighing design options based on performance in summer and winter and making a decision. Student might change these building characteristics based on the analysis or might explicitly mention the positives and negatives about their design within a particular season.
Diagnostic troubleshooting (troubleshoot)	Student made a move to resolve a specific perceived issue in the design (e.g., 'In the summer the building's roof puts a shadow almost all the way to the bottom of the building making the sunlight on that area be very cold (dark blue color) while the other sides such as the back and etc. still received a substantial amount of heat…')
Managed and iterative designing (revise/iterate)	Student started with a good working solution but explored ways to make it better. This differs from fluency; in that, this is a micro-level improvement on a solution. Small revision or 'tweak' to one characteristic of a design that usually occurs later in an episode. Could be accompanied by reflection if other elements of the Informed Design Matrix are involved.
Reflective design thinking (reflect on process)	Student made electronic notes in the system that are more than recordkeeping of values but show consideration for how their design efforts affect performance

Framework	Description	Source of evidence	'Symbol' in representation system
Design goal	The goal of a sequence of activities or the frame of actions	Student notes	⬭
Design moves	The activities students can do within the system (e.g., make, edit, delete, change shape, change orientation, simulation, etc.)	Design replays from log file	▽
Self-reflection	Reflection or thinking about the actions in relation to the goal or frame	Student notes - explanations that link goals to actions	◇
Science concept	Denotes existence of or reference to a science concept	Student notes - explanations	●

Figure 5 Action visualization protocol.

episodes 1 and 2, he recognized that the larger the surface area the greater the heat gain was. He also associated surface area with specific geometric shapes. For example, he justified building a parabola-shaped building (i.e., a U-shaped building) to increase the amount of solar heat energy transferred to the building. As his reflective notes in episodes 3 and 4 show, Brent made explicit efforts to establish a trade-off between heating in winter and cooling in summer.

Hence, it appears that exhibiting design behaviors of balancing benefits and trade-offs through experimentation was more conducive to students making connections to science concept during engineering design. According to Jonassen (2012), the trade-off analysis is a rational model of decision-making and an avenue for metacognitive awareness that opens opportunities for learning (Jonassen 2012). In our study, we similarly found evidence of systematic experimenting, scientific explanations, and decision-making at times when trade-off was to be made. Moreover, in authentic engineering design practice, reasoning through benefits and trade-offs of different design alternatives is an important component of decision-making (National Research Council 2012). In balancing benefits and trade-offs, students practice weighing options from experimentation and making decisions rather than focusing solely on the features of their design solutions.

The actions associated with trade-off analysis did not occur in a continual form. In fact, there was evidence of macro iterations in Brent's full design processes starting from episode 1 leading to episode 6. These macro iterations occurred between idea fluency and trade-off analysis and exposed managed and iterative designing. In episodes 1, 2, and 3, Brent's focus was on trade-off analysis with some evidence of knowledge building, he engaged in idea fluency in episode 4. In episode 5, he went back to trade-off analysis and then moved back to idea fluency in episode 6. In the informed design coding protocol, idea fluency represents the student working with a large variety of ideas (i.e., building height, width, roof characteristics, or location) with the ability to work with one idea element at a time (i.e., building height) or several elements at a time. Idea fluency represents exploration of design alternatives in greater breadth and/or depth. In the exploratory cases of Andrew and Brent, there were no explicit evidence for science connections during idea generation and testing; however, macro iterations were evident between generating multiple designs through idea fluency and balancing benefits and trade-offs. It is possible that idea fluency allowed students to apply their new understandings into designs or gain information about their designs that are later tested more systematically through trade-off analysis. The visualization of the design episodes of Brent allowed us to better understand students' design goals through their design processes and reflective notes.

This exploratory study concludes that students explicitly explore and develop scientific explanations when balancing design benefits and trade-offs. Such decision-making through trade-off leads to opportunities for meaningful science learning. There are two critical variables that are likely to influence this phenomenon. First, learning becomes apparent through reflective design and reflective notes that illustrate the negotiation of benefits and trade-offs. Hence, without the reflective thought process or structures that reinforce the expressing of such thinking, learning may not be possible.

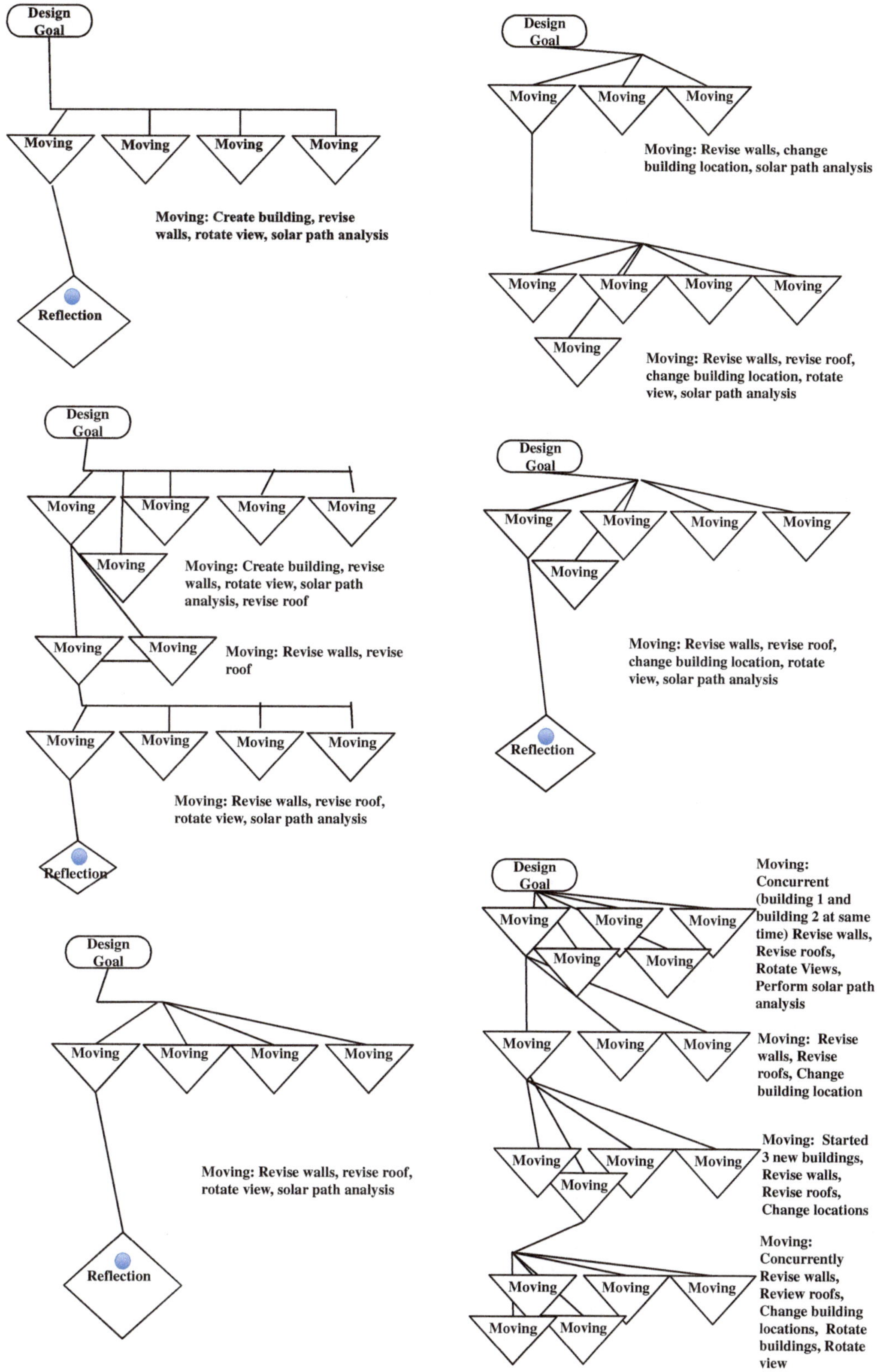

Figure 6 Brent's full design process.

Second, people in general, not just students, struggle with evaluating trade-offs (Scholten and Sherman 2006), demonstrating that such decision-making is not necessarily a naturally easy process (Papadouris 2012). Without well-constructed design problems, most students cannot consider or fully engage with the complexity of weighing trade-offs in making design decisions.

Conclusions

As noted in the introduction, while engineering design has been considered to be a component of K-12 education curricula and standards for decades, there is little research on how the students learn to apply science through design. In this study, we attempted to untangle and deconstruct two high school students' engineering practices as intertwined activities between engineering design and scientific explanations. Analyzing design behaviors as a series of design episodes provided ways to visualize student design processes, which was facilitated by the Energy3D system. Student design replays and reflective notes provided evidence that characterized engineering and scientific practices. As a result, we present a framework for explaining this intersection and an emergent theory of engineering-science integration.

This exploratory study included two highly reflective high school students who were able to engage in divergent and convergent behaviors. Future research should explore patterns for a more diverse group of students and ways to visualize these patterns with large samples of students. In conclusion, the results suggest that for science learning to occur, design projects used in classrooms should allow and emphasize trade-off analysis and include time and resources for supporting trade-off decisions through experimenting, data gathering, and reflection. Abilities to conduct trade-off analysis should be a desired learning objective in its own right and should be appropriately scaffolded for students.

Competing interests

The authors declare that they have no competing interests.

Authors' contributions

SP, MG and RA co-designed the informed design coding protocol, outlined data analysis procedures, and finalized the manuscript. MG carried out the data analysis and drafted the manuscript. CX and SN are the lead software developers of Energy3D, developed the solar urban design challenge model, and collected all data. All authors read and approved the final manuscript.

Acknowledgements

This work presented in this manuscript is based upon work supported by the National Science Foundation under Grant DUE #1348547 and DUE #1348530. Any opinions, findings, and conclusions or recommendations expressed in this paper, however, are those of the authors and do not necessarily reflect the views of the NSF. We thank Anthony Iarrapino, William Jumper, and Roger Morneau of Lowell High School, Massachusetts, for pilot-testing our software and materials in their classes.

Disclaimer

We, the authors, feel obliged to clarify that inquiry is not limited to natural sciences but serves many other disciplines such as history. Design as a set of strategies is itself an inquiry and serves a number of disciplines such as architecture, choreography, education, and engineering. However, these two terms (design and inquiry) have specific meanings in K-12 STEM education. Hence, in this manuscript when we use the term inquiry, we are referring to scientific inquiry and when we use the term design we are referring to design inquiry.

Author details

[1]School of Engineering Education, Purdue University, Wang Hall 4545, 516 Northwestern Avenue, West Lafayette, IN 47906, USA. [2]School of Engineering Education, Purdue University, Armstrong Hall, 701 West Stadium Avenue, West Lafayette, IN 47906, USA. [3]The Intelligent Learning Environments Laboratory, The Concord Consortium, 25 Love Lane, Concord, MA 01742, USA.

References

Adams, RS, Turns, J, & Atman, CJ. (2003). Educating effective engineering designers: the role of reflective practice. *Design Studies, 24*(3), 275–294.

Apedoe, XS, Reynolds, B, Ellefson, MR, & Schunn, CD. (2008). Bringing engineering design into high school science classrooms: the heating/cooling unit. *Journal of Science Education and Technology, 17*(5), 454–465.

Apedoe, XS, & Schunn, CD. (2013). Strategies for success: uncovering what makes students successful in design and learning. *Instructional Science, 41*(4), 773–791.

Ball, LJ, & Christensen, BT. (2009). Analogical reasoning and mental simulation in design: two strategies linked to uncertainty resolution. *Design Studies, 30*(2), 169–186.

Baker, RS, Corbett, AT, & Wagner, AZ. (2006). Human classification of low-fidelity replays of student actions. In *Proceedings of the Educational Data Mining Workshop at the 8th International Conference on Intelligent Tutoring Systems.*

Brophy, S, Klein, S, Portsmore, M, & Rogers, C. (2008). Advancing engineering education in P-12 classrooms. *Journal of Engineering Education, 97*(3), 369–387.

Bruner, JS. (1961). The act of discovery. *Harvard Educational Review, 31*, 21–32.

Bucciarelli, LL. (1996). *Designing engineers*. Cambridge: MIT Press. Chapter 1–2, 6.

Burghardt, MD, & Hacker, M. (2004). Informed design: a contemporary approach to design pedagogy as the core process in technology. *The Technology Teacher, 64*(1), 6–8.

Cajas, F. (2001). The science/technology interaction: implications for science literacy. *Journal of Research in Science Teaching, 38*(7), 715–729.

Crismond, DP, & Adams, RS. (2012). The informed design teaching and learning matrix. *Journal of Engineering Education, 101*(4), 738–797.

Cross, N. (2001). Design cognition: results from protocol and other empirical studies of design activity. In CM Eastman, WM McCracken, & W Newstetter (Eds.), *Design Learning and Knowing: Cognition in Design Education.* New York: Elsevier Press.

Cross, N. (2006). *Designerly ways of knowing*. London: Springer. Chapter 1–2.

Daugherty, J, & Mentzer, N. (2008). Analogical reasoning in the engineering design process and technology education applications. *Journal of Technology Education, 19*(2), 7–21.

Doppelt, Y, Mehalik, MM, Schunn, CD, Silk, E, & Krysinski, D. (2008). Engagement and achievements: a case study of design-based learning in a science context. *Journal of Technology Education, 19*(2), 22–39.

Dorst, K. (2011). The core of 'design thinking' and its application. *Design Studies, 32*(6), 521–532.

Dubberly, H. (2004). How do you design? A compendium of models. Dubberly Design Office, San Francisco CA. [–Retrieved from http://www.dubberly.com/wp-content/uploads/2008/06/ddo_designprocess.pdf]

Fish, J, & Scrivener, SA. (1990). Amplifying the mind's eye: sketching and visual cognition. *Leonardo, 23*(1), 117–126.

Goel, V, & Pirolli, P. (1992). The Structure of design problem spaces. *Cognitive Science, 16*(3), 395–429.

Goldschmidt, G. (1991). The dialectics of sketching. *Creativity Research Journal, 4*(2), 123–143.

Goldschmidt, G, & Smolkov, M. (2006). Variances in the impact of visual stimuli on design problem solving performance. *Design Studies, 27*(5), 549–569.

Hmelo, CE, Holton, DL, & Kolodner, JL. (2000). Designing to learn about complex systems. *The Journal of the Learning Sciences, 9*(3), 247–298.
Jonassen, DH. (2000). Toward a design theory of problem solving. *Educational Technology Research and Development, 48*(4), 63–85.
Jonassen, DH. (2012). Designing for decision making. *Educational Technology Research and Development, 60*(2), 341–359.
Kolko, J. (2010). Abductive thinking and sensemaking: the drivers of design synthesis. *Design Issues, 26*(1), 5–28.
Kolodner, JL. (2002). Facilitating the learning of design practices: lessons from an inquiry into science education. *Journal of Industrial Teacher Education, 39*(3), 9–40.
Kolodner, JL, Crismond, D, Fasse, BB, Gray, JT, Holbrook, J, Ryan, M, et al. (2003). Problem-based learning meets case-based reasoning in the middle-school science classroom: putting a learning-by-design curriculum into practice. *Journal of the Learning Sciences, 12*(4), 495–548.
Lachapelle, CP, & Cunningham, CM. (2014). Engineering in elementary schools. In S Purzer, J Strobel, & ME Cardella (Eds.), *Engineering in pre-college settings: synthesizing research, policy, and practices*. West Lafayette, IN: Purdue University Press.
Lawson, B, & Dorst, K. (2009). *Design expertise*. Oxford, UK: Architectural Press (Elsevier).
Lewis, T. (2006). Design and inquiry: bases for an accommodation between science and technology education in the curriculum? *Journal of Research in Science Teaching, 43*(3), 255–281.
National Academy of Engineering and National Research Council. (2014). *STEM integration in K-12 education: status, prospects, and an agenda for research*. Washington, DC: The National Academies Press.
National Research Council. (1996). *National science education standards*. Washington, DC: National Academies Press.
National Research Council. (2009). *Engineering in K-12 education: understanding the status and improving the prospects*. Washington, DC: National Academies Press.
National Research Council. (2012). *A framework for K-12 science education: practices, crosscutting concepts, and core ideas*. Washington, DC: National Academies Press.
Achieve. (2013). *Next generation science standards: for states, by states*. Washington, DC: National Academies Press.
Paletz, S, Schunn, CD, & Kim, KH. (2013). The interplay of conflict and analogy in multidisciplinary teams. *Cognition, 126*(1), 1–19.
Papadouris, N. (2012). Optimization as a reasoning strategy for dealing with socioscientific decision-making situations. *Science Education, 96*(4), 600–630.
Penner, DE, Giles, ND, Lehrer, R, & Schauble, L. (1997). Building functional models: designing an elbow. *Journal of Research in Science Teaching, 34*(2), 125–143.
Purzer, Ş, Strobel, J, & Cardella, ME. (2014). *Engineering in pre-college settings: synthesizing research, policy, and practices*. West Lafayette, IN: Purdue University Press.
Sadler, PM, Coyle, HP, & Schwartz, M. (2000). Engineering competitions in the middle school classroom: key elements in developing effective design challenges. *The Journal of the Learning Sciences, 9*(3), 299–327.
Scholten, M, & Sherman, SJ. (2006). Tradeoffs and theory: the double-mediation model. *Journal of Experimental Psychology, 135*, 237–261 and 552.
Schön, DA. (1993). *The reflective practitioner: How professionals think in action*. New York: Basic Books.
Schnittka, C, & Bell, R. (2011). Engineering design and conceptual change in science: addressing thermal energy and heat transfer in eighth grade. *International Journal of Science Education, 33*(13), 1861–1887.
Schunn, CD, Silk, EM, & Apedoe, XS. (2012). Engineering in and for science education. In J Shrager & S Carver (Eds.), *The journey from child to scientist: Integrating cognitive development and the education sciences* (pp. 207–225). Washington, DC: American Psychological Association.
Snetsinger, C, Brewer, C, & Brown, F. (1999). Capture the wind: students get a charge from wind energy. *The Science Teacher, 66*, 38–42.
Subramanian, K. (1999). Practical physics. *The Science Teacher, 66*, 37–39.
Svihla, V, & Petrosino, AJ. (2008). *Improving our understanding of K-12 engineering education. Paper presented at the International Conference on Engineering Education*. Greece: Heraklion.
Valkenburg's, R. (1998). The reflective practice of design teams. *Design Studies, 19*(3), 249–271.
Vattam, SS, & Kolodner, JL. (2008). On foundations of technological support for addressing challenges facing design-based science learning. *Pragmatics & Cognition, 16*(2), 406–437.
Xie, C, Zhang, H, Nourian, S, Pallant, A, & Bailey, S. (2014a). A study of the instructional sensitivity of CAD logs based on time series analysis. *International Journal of Engineering Education, 30*(4), 760–778.
Xie, C, Zhang, H, Nourian, S, Pallant, A, & Hazzard, E. (2014b). A time series analysis method for assessing engineering design processes using a CAD tool. *International Journal of Engineering Education, 30*(1), 218–230.
Zhang, Z, Xie, C, & Nourian, S. (2014). *Detecting iterative cycles of engineering design from student digital footprints in computer-aided design software. Poster presented at the 2014 International Conference of the Learning Sciences*. Boulder CO: International Society of the Learning Sciences.
Zubrowski, B. (2002). Integrating science into design technology projects: using a standard model in the design process. *Journal of Technology Education, 13*(2), 47–65.

4

The landscape of PreK-12 engineering online resources for teachers: global trends

Aikaterini Bagiati[1*], So Yoon Yoon[2], Demetra Evangelou[3], Alejandra Magana[4], Garene Kaloustian[5] and Jiabin Zhu[6]

Abstract

Background: The newly formed discipline of engineering education is addressing the need to (a) enhance STEM education for precollege students and (b) identify optimum ways to introduce engineering content starting, perhaps, from the early ages. Introducing engineering at the Prekindergarten through 12th grade (PreK-12) education level requires significant changes in teacher preparation and support. It highlights the need for developing developmentally appropriate content knowledge and pedagogical methods, thus revealing the challenges of preparing teachers to incorporate this type of knowledge base into their practice. Although professional development offered by universities, school districts, and other educational entities provides the primary source of formal learning tools for teachers, an increasing number of teachers also utilize other informal web-based resources regularly. This paper examines available PreK-12 engineering web resources offered by entities formally related to education in seven different languages, namely Arabic, Chinese (Mandarin), English, French, Greek, Korean, and Spanish.

Results: Findings showed how different educational systems designated different attention to the entry level ages when introducing engineering content. Differences in the terminology used to identify STEM resources for introducing these topics also became apparent. Similarities suggest that a large number of resources available on the web were originating in all researched languages. However, the developmental appropriateness and content validity of many of these resources remained questionable in many cases. In general, there was a plethora of isolated activities and lesson plans but significantly fewer complete engineering curricula available to teachers on the web.

Conclusions: This study presents a comparative analysis of the international landscape of PreK-12 engineering education and provides guidelines and samples of state-of-the art resources in each language for teachers interested in introducing their students to engineering as a reliable starting point towards PreK-12 engineering information gathering.

Keywords: PreK-12 STEM; PreK-12 engineering; Open web resources; Open educational resources teacher preparation; International comparison; Early engineering

Background

The technological challenges of our world affect every aspect of our social, cultural, and economic structures (Campos et al. 2000; Punie 2012) while modern governance adopts the position that 'science, technology, engineering, and math (STEM) disciplines are the drivers of technological advancement, innovation and foundational infrastructure that leads to secure economic future' (Watt et al. 2007, p. 759). Understanding that STEM, technology and engineering in particular, can be critical to a country's welfare (Sanders 2009), the development of human capital in the STEM fields presents a major challenge as recent trends point to a diminishing interest in these fields (Kuenzi 2008; Becker 2010; Dimopoulos et al. 2011). Success will be measured by our ability to reverse the trend, through the transformation of the educational processes in fundamental ways (Campos et al. 2000; Punie 2012).

A head start for the advancement of STEM education has lead scholars to the study of curricular ideas prior to college (Bagiati and Evangelou 2008; Brophy et al. 2008; Bagiati 2011) not only because of the long preparation necessary for success in the STEM fields but also to address student motivation in a timely manner. Student motivation, which needs to be fostered in the early childhood years, has emerged as an important influencing factor for attracting students to engineering domains

* Correspondence: abagiati@mit.edu
[1]MIT-SUTD Collaboration Office, Massachusetts Institute of Technology, Cambridge, MA, 02139, USA
Full list of author information is available at the end of the article

(Graziano et al. 2012). Given these trends, many institutions are now providing open educational resources (OER) specifically tied to STEM, and sometimes to engineering in particular.

This drive for open access web resources comes at a time of generalized interest in Prekindergarten through 12th grade (PreK-12) STEM education in many countries aiding the development of the new content. Scholars now seek to understand and enhance the ways PreK-12 teachers are advancing their education and identifying optimum ways to introduce engineering in their classrooms (Brophy et al. 2008; Katehi et al. 2009; National Research Council 2009; Moore 2010; Bagiati 2011; Wang et al. 2011; Bagiati and Evangelou (in press(a); Bagiati and Evangelou (in press (b)). Introducing engineering at the PreK-12 level, however, reveals a need for a deep understanding of the content and methods that are also developmentally appropriate at each grade level (Bagiati and Evangelou 2008; Bagiati 2011; Bybee 2011). To complement this effort, scholars are seeking to understand how teachers prepare to incorporate this new content into practice (Shulman 1986; Bagiati and Evangelou 2008; Wang et al. 2011; Bagiati and Evangelou (in press (a)).

In many countries, ministries of education, universities, school districts, and various other educational entities responsible for offering formal teacher education and on-going professional development support teachers in remaining current in their expertise. Teachers now also utilize a variety of other ways to stay current and informed as professionals (Bagiati et.al. 2010), including peer-to-peer (Lock 2006; Borko et al. 2009) or individual efforts to (a) enhance their skills by investigating new content and to (b) access, comprehend, incorporate, and adopt new practices. Teachers use the Internet more than books or journals in order to understand new concepts and to find curricula or small-scale activities to incorporate into their teaching (Hedtke et al. 2001; Recker 2006).

This approach is gaining popularity with teachers worldwide irrespective of the diversity of educational systems, norms, and practices, as it allows teachers to balance preparation with job and family commitments (Borko et al. 2009; American Association of Colleges for Teacher Education 2013). Information and communication technologies appear to 'provide more flexible and effective ways' for teachers to prepare and remain updated (Jung 2005, p. 94) while at the same time allowing them the opportunity to expand and connect to the global teacher community. In this new context, the access to open web-based educational resources is despite the challenge of searching and verifying online learning resources ascertaining the quality and validity of the material. Many educators limit their information seeking primarily within search engines and do not take full advantage of educational-related digital libraries (Perrault 2007). Teachers' expectations in screening educational resources include quality of the resource, as well as additional contextual information beyond that resource (Recker et al. 2004); specifically characteristics, such as age-appropriateness, accuracy, and contemporariness (Recker et al. 2004). Accessing and screening open web resources on PreK-12 engineering education present additional barriers including factors, such as content validity, accessibility, and language.

Content validity

In recent years, 'teaching is becoming one of the most challenging professions in our society where knowledge is expanding rapidly' (Jung 2005, p.94). Having extensive experience with in-service PreK-12 teachers, we are aware of the difficulties when attempting to identify valid engineering-related curricula online. Teachers, especially at the early education level, usually do not receive formal exposure or preparation for the implementation of engineering in class (Bagiati and Evangelou (in press (a)). STEM content, particularly engineering content, is considered a very challenging topic for teachers to conceive and successfully implement in class. For STEM education in particular, concepts, such as *engineering, technology*, and *design*, are easily misunderstood and misrepresented in class (Yaşar et al. 2006; Hsu et al. 2011; Bairaktarova et al. 2012). This makes it even harder for them to understand the need and become able to identify and evaluate the appropriateness of resources among the uncategorized plethora of information to be found on the web.

Prior small-scale research studies on the topic (Bagiati et al. 2010, 2011) have shown an adequate number of resources on PreK-12 engineering curricula, lesson plans, and activities available on the web. However, these studies have shown that the pedagogical and content reliability of such resources are limited. Elementary and early engineering education is still at its infancy (Bagiati et al. 2010; Bagiati 2011), and content validation is difficult to distinguish within the currently available content, even to engineering education specialists. The existing content is either addressed directly as engineering or gets introduced within an integrated STEM context. However, when discussing the educational level that the PreK-12 websites are targeting, things appear so far to be uneven. The majority of websites only offer educational resources for older grade level audiences, such as high school or middle school students.

Accessibility

Open educational resources (OER) are supported by UNESCO, and many countries support this idea (Johnstone 2005) by offering a wide variety of OER. However, the Internet governance and Internet freedom policies set by individual governments, are sometimes causing access to these resources to be limited or making OER completely unavailable within a country. Restrictions on accessibility might not always be applied to the content of the resources per se but they may apply to the software platform that the developers have chosen in order to share content. Furthermore, educational entities developing educational content suggest user regulations that may cause accessibility issues as well. Additional challenges to accessing OER may be encountered as a direct result of insufficient technology infrastructure.

Language barrier

Up to date, the vast majority of the Internet content is in English (Gounari 2009, p. 170; Pimienta et al. 2009), and even though the development of web content in languages other than English is rising, 'the dominance of the English language unavoidably affects access for non-English speakers. At the same time, those non-English sites are mostly limited to speakers of the specific language—a linguistic reality that compromises the "globality of the medium"' (Gounari 2009, p. 170).

Advancement in the development of online translation software has partially addressed this challenge and will continue to do so to virtually eliminating the linguistic barrier among users. However, a more persistent issue of access comes from the variety of disciplinary terms used in local education nomenclature (e.g., engineering vs. technology, design, or STEM).

In the English context, in certain European countries as well as in the United States, the English acronym STEM is popularly used to describe courses or educational content integrating science, technology, engineering, and mathematics within a PreK-12 educational curriculum (Sanders 2009). In recent years, there are additional efforts to highlight the *E* in PreK-12 ST*E*M education (Sanders 2009). The term *engineering education* was found to also be widely used, however, mainly at the college level in order to describe the wider concept of undergraduate or graduate studies within a school of engineering, and not so much, if at all, to describe PreK-12 content or practices. Furthermore, terminology, such as *STEM education* or *engineering education*, is not the norm in many educational systems around the world (e.g., in European countries, such as Spain, France, and Greece, in Arab-speaking countries, and in Asian countries, such as China and South Korea), where terms, such as *invention education*, *creativity education*, or *technology education*, are used in a broader sense to describe the same content. As an example, the education system of France is going through a transformation on how to perceive PreK-12 science, math, and technology education with implications on how material and resources are provided for the public - schools, teachers, and other professionals. The emphasis has shifted from teaching content per se to *skills* that children should acquire at each grade level. Thus, the terms '*investigation*' and '*inquiry*' are critical within the web search for more specific content, namely science. Within a contemporary transformation of terminology in the field of *Science*, incorporating skill-based terminology, such as *inquiry* and *investigation* with its many variations and epistemological, psychological, and/or educational meaning, has led to a more hands-on approach to the field as a whole (Giordan 2010). Lebeaume (2011) highlights that the proposed amendments of the French education system (content-based teaching/learning to skill-based teaching/learning) 'breaks down barriers between strictly disciplinary teachings since this deems unproductive for investment of educational achievements as a whole' (p. 2).

Our short exposure to the variations of approaches, regulations, and nomenclature shows how the global landscape of PreK-12 engineering web resources is considerably uneven for teachers to explore.

Purpose of the study

A scientific discipline is characterized by shared terminology negotiated and established in order to facilitate communication among scholars. In the newly formed discipline of engineering education, this process is on-going and acknowledges and respects existing nomenclatures across different cultures and educational systems. This paper aims to compare the international landscape on PreK-12 engineering education. We identified engineering educational websites constructed by credible organizations formally related to education, examined types of engineering education resources by grade level, and explored differences in the terminology to search engineering-related educational resources across seven languages; namely, Arabic, Chinese (Mandarin), English, French, Greek, Korean, and Spanish.

Additionally, we have placed a particular interest in identifying resources targeting early education. Resources targeting early education have a value of developmental nature attached to them. Moreover, they have a particular strategic significance, as the existence and quality of such resources reveal how soon different countries approach introduction to engineering and the importance that they place on this first introduction. Existing infant and toddler curricula designed to date follow a comprehensive approach to assist children development, and more specifically, to assist development of approaches to learning, social, emotional, and physical development, communication, and development of gross and fine motor skills (Copple and Bredekamp 2009). Although development in all aforementioned areas is essential for the child to be able to then successfully develop STEM thinking and learning, and while children play at this age can be considered precursor to engineering thinking and acting (Brophy and Evangelou 2007, Bagiati and Evangelou (in press (b)), the infant and toddler curricula are not designed to target STEM or engineering in particular. To date, the first curricula designed to specifically target STEM, design, and engineering are starting at the PreK level. Therefore, in order for our study to follow the most holistic approach while investigating engineering curricula, we chose to start our investigation at the Prekindergarten level.

The research questions guiding this study are as follows:

(a) What is the number of websites containing resources related to PreK-12 engineering-relevant content developed by entities formally related to education?
(b) Which percentage of the identified websites addresses early education?
(c) What is the curricular scope of the resources developed?
(d) What terminology in each of the represented languages is used to identify PreK-12 engineering related content?
(e) Are the resources identified openly accessible to teachers?

We believe that this study will (a) help future engineering content developers better understand their global audience and (b) help PreK-12 teachers in their attempt to self-educate and introduce engineering education in their schools. Furthermore, we expect research findings to enhance global discourse in regards to adaptation and implementation of the PreK-12 engineering content.

Methods

Cross-cultural collaboration

Researchers participating in this study had to comply with three fundamental criteria: (a) be native speakers of one language examined in the study, (b) be familiar with the discipline of engineering education and educational research, and (c) have personal experiences of a PreK-12 educational system of the language under examination. These criteria were adopted based on our understanding that 'among different educational systems, and according to different educational/technological cultures, similar content might be presented using varied terminology' (Lock 2006, p.2). All researchers but one were involved with the discipline of engineering education in the United States and all are graduates of different schooling systems located in Asia, Europe, Latin America, and the Middle East. Furthermore, two researchers are experts in the field of early education and child development.

The seven languages examined in this study cover a large portion of the Internet users. Figure 1 presents the countries around the globe where the seven languages are being used in the formal education system.

As of 2011, as presented in Table 1, all languages, except Greek, were listed among the top languages used on the Internet. More than 67.1% of the world Internet users and 55.8% of the world population use the seven languages that were explored. Approximately, 30.3% of the world population has access to the Internet. Among the seven languages, Korean speakers had the most Internet users (55.2%) of the language population, followed by English (43.4%) and Spanish (39.0%).

Taking a look at the languages spoken around the world, we see that in the United States where the predominant language is English, a big segment of the population is also fluent in Spanish or another language. English is also used in many Caribbean, Asian, and African countries. In Canada, in addition to English, French is also used. Around the world, there are more than 30 francophone countries, while Spanish is the official language in 20 countries and spoken in many more. In the case of Europe, the European Union (EU) strongly encourages mobility among people of different EU countries, and in many countries, people speak more than their native language. On the same time, Chinese has attracted a lot of interest in recent decade and the number of people learning one of the major dialects is expanding. In conclusion, more and more people are now able to explore resources developed in languages other than their own, so teachers residing in countries other than the ones highlighted in Figure 1 may also use the languages explored.

Procedures

Each researcher collected and analyzed his/her own data based on a commonly designed procedure. Data were analyzed in light of an international comparison. Based on previous findings (Bagiati et.al. 2011) and given the complexity of the nature of the present study, the following procedure was put in place for the data collection and analysis. In order to establish a common scheme for the collection and analysis, individual researchers brought their extensive knowledge of their educational system and their understanding of OER to the discussion. Definitions were agreed upon and a common analysis plan was designed. When all analyses were completed, crosschecking of the results occurred in the cases that knowledge of each other's native language allowed for it, and data and reports were examined across languages.

Data collection

Initial data collection took place in spring of 2014 and updated most recently in August 2014. Researchers conducted a systematic Internet search through the Google and Yahoo search engines, using the keywords, *PreK-12 engineering curriculum,* and proceeded using the combination of keywords, including *engineering curriculum, prekindergarten, kindergarten, elementary, middle school, high school, and PreK-12* in their own language. Following the initial exploration, modifications in the search terms were inevitable from language to language, given

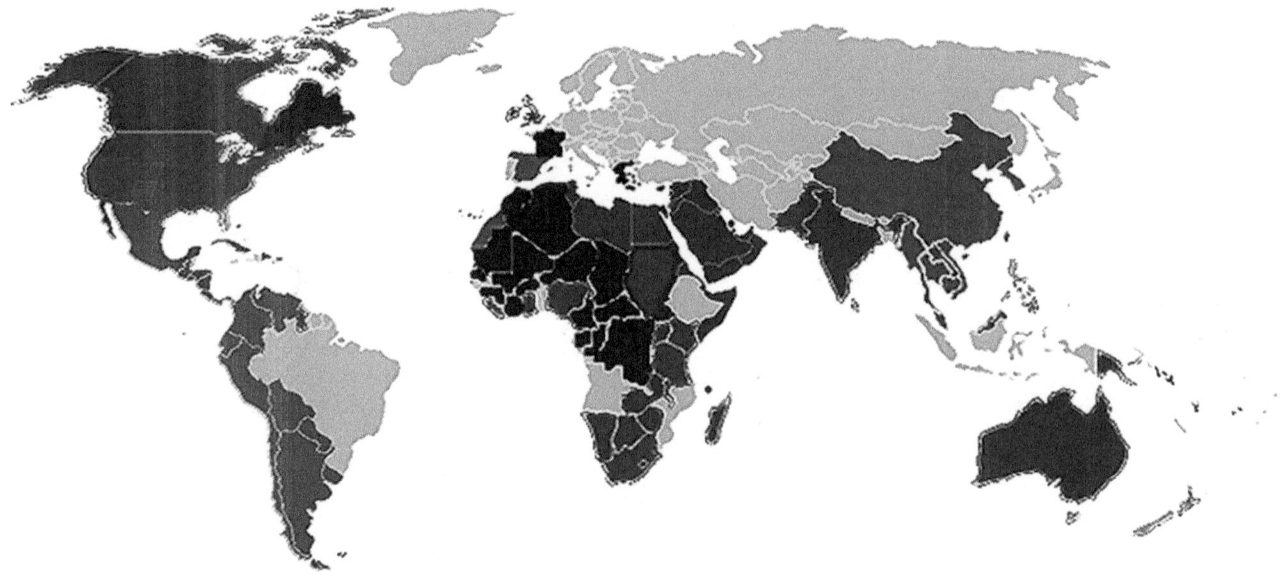

Figure 1 Countries around the globe where the seven languages are being used in the formal education system. Dark shades representing the countries that use Arabic, Chinese (Mandarin), English, French, Greek, Korean, and Spanish as one of the main languages.

the variation in STEM terminology used across the different languages/contexts.

In a second round of discussions of preliminary findings, key terms that resulted in relevant outcomes were shared, namely in educational resources that reflect engineering content. Subsequently, non-English speaking researchers used additional keywords, such as *science, technology, design, creativity,* and *innovation,* as the researchers expected that these words would lead them to the desired websites in some cultures. Table 2 presents all terms used from the research group in order to complete the search. The right column presents the terms that returned desired results in each language case.

The following variables on each website containing engineering content were collected.

- Title: The title of the website
- URL: The website URL
- Entity: Type of organization that provides engineering content

Table 1 Estimates of the top ten languages in the Internet (as of 2011)

	Top ten languages in the Internet	Internet users by language	Internet users (% of total)	World population	Internet accessibility (%)
	English	565,004,126	26.8%	1,302,275,670	*43.4*
	Chinese	509,965,013	24.2%	1,372,226,042	*37.2*
	Spanish	164,968,742	7.8%	423,085,806	*39.0*
	Japanese	99,182,000	4.7%	126,475,664	78.4
	Portuguese	82,586,600	3.9%	253,947,594	32.5
	German	75,422,674	3.6%	94,842,656	79.5
	Arabic	65,365,400	3.3%	347,002,991	*18.8*
	French	59,779,525	3.0%	347,932,305	*17.2*
	Russian	59,700,000	3.0%	139,390,205	42.8
	Korean	39,440,000	2.0%	71,393,343	*55.2*
Top ten languages		1,615,957,333	82.2%	4,442,056,069	36.4
Rest of the languages		350,557,483	17.8%	2,403,553,891	14.6
World total		2,099,926,965	100.0%	6,930,055,154	30.3
Total of six languages		1,404,522,806	67.10%	3,863,916,157	36.3

Languages in italics are the languages examined in this paper. Source: Internal World Stats: Usage and Population Statistics. Retrieved from http://www.internetworldstats.com/stats7.htm.

Table 2 Searched keywords related to PreK-12 engineering education web resources

Language	Terms that did not work	Terms that worked
Arabic	Engineering, activities, projects	Science technology:تكنولوجيا التعلم, educational technology (تكنولوجيا التعلم), learning site, interactive site (مواقع تفاعلية للأطفال)
Chinese	Engineering education, Engineers' education, middle/high school, kindergarten	Science education (科学教育), science and technology education (科学技术教育), youngsters (青少年), child (儿童/幼儿), science and technology museums (科技馆), science popularization (科普), work and technological education (劳动技术教育), practicality (实践能力)
English	Creativity, innovation, invention	K-12, engineering, science, technology, STEM, design, curriculum
French	Engineering education	Ingenieur (engineer), ressource pedagogiques pour l'ingenieur préscolaire (educational resources for the preschool engineer), science (science), ministere de l'education, technologie (technology), enseignement préscolaire (preschool education/teaching), ateliers scientifiques (scientific workshop), musee scientifiques (scientific museum), sciences a l'ecole (science at school), sites scolaires de sciences et technologie (academic sites for science and technology), resources academiques (academic resources), culture scientifique ou technologique (scientific or technologic culture), sites nationales de sciences et de technologie (National sites of science and technology), projets scientifiques (scientific projects), projets de sciences (science projects), exposciences (science exposition)
Greek	Engineering education, PreK-12 innovation, invention	Science (Θετικές Επιστήμες), engineering (Μηχανική), technology (Τεχνολογία), design (Σχέδιο/σχεδιασμός), mechanics (Μηχανική), electronics (Ηλεκτρονική), computer science (Πληροφορική), physics (Φυσική), chemistry (Χημεία), biology (Βιολογία), creativity (Δημιουργικότητα), curriculum (Πρόγραμμα σπουδών), kindergarten (Νηπιαγωγείο), elementary (Δημοτικό), middle school (Γυμνάσιο), high school (Λύκειο).
Korean	PreK-12 engineering education	Engineering (공학), science education (과학교육) , STEAM, STEM, science education (과학교육), technology education (기술교육), block building (쌓기), machines (기계), tools (도구), invention (발명), creativity (창조), pre-engineering education (예비공학교육), STEAM (science, technology, engineering, arts, and mathematics) integrated education (융합인재교육)
Spanish	Engineering education, curriculum	Science and technology museums (Museos de Ciencia y Tecnologia), science projects (Proyectos de Ciencia), school technology projects (Proyectos Escolares de Tecnologia), engineering school projects (Proyectos Escolares de Ingenieria), didactic materials for technology education (Materiales Didacticos en Educacion en Tecnologia), didactic materials for engineering education (Materiales Didacticos para Educacion en Ingenieria), engineering activities for elementary education (Actividades de Ingenieria para Educacion Primaria), engineering experiments (Experimentos de Ingenieria), engineering projects for children (Proyectos de Ingenieria para Ninos).

- Education level: Target students' age or grade level for the content
- Terms: Terms related to STEM used by the developers while introducing the content in the web resources
- PreK-3 and grades 4 to 12 resources: Type of content presented on the website, namely single activities, learning plans, or full curricula in grades PreK-3 and grades 4 to 12.

Previous studies have shown that although many websites claim to present PreK-12 content, they typically only target older students, while web resources for the early education students are very limited or absent (Bagiati et.al. 2010; Bagiati et.al. 2011). Content was carefully examined to ascertain which websites actually made available content targeting early ages and to identify such relevant content.

In many cases, the Internet searches led to websites that were portals redirecting users to other websites containing the desired educational content. Furthermore, although many websites claimed to contain curricula, they included individual lesson plans or scattered activities. Therefore, researchers recorded the content of each website's homepage and examined the actual type of content presented. As many web searches led to websites that served as portals to other sites containing the actual educational material, the researchers kept track of the existing portals but did not add them to the final data set for analysis. In addition, many websites that appeared through the searches only contained information regarding engineering outreach programs, while others were websites not openly presenting but selling the desired educational resources. Commercial websites and websites presenting outreach programs, without presenting any educational resources, were also not included in the study.

The engineering resources identified were classified as: (a) *activity*, small scale, stand-alone, designed for use in or out of class, and not presenting any particular learning objectives or assessment mechanism, (b) *lesson plan*, a structured process, typically outlining step-by-step instructions for teachers, including learning objectives accompanied by an assessment mechanism, or (c) *curriculum*, defined by Toombs and Tierney (1993) as 'an intentional design for learning negotiated by faculty in light of their specialized knowledge and in the context of social expectations and students' needs' (p. 183).

In order to enhance the validity of the search, our data sample was limited to web resources only offered by credible organizations, such as universities, museums, foundations, institutions, and similar entities formally recognized as relevant to engineering, as well as educational and curriculum topics. Furthermore, during our data collection, we paid careful attention in order to include websites that would present resources related to engineering concepts and the design process and to exclude STEM websites that were actually only addressing a traditional scientific discipline, e.g., only biology, chemistry, physics. Additional file 1 presents the complete data set of the websites that were analyzed.

At this point, it should be noted that data collection and analysis in this paper represents the OER available on the web in August 2014, we do understand though that due to the very nature of the Internet, many websites analyzed have probably updated their content by now.

Data analyses

Data analysis was performed using descriptive statistics, and data were summarized in graphs for frequency comparisons. Initially, we compared the number of web resources containing PreK-12 and PreK-3 engineering content. The following themes were identified: (a) types of organizations, (b) numbers of websites and type of content presented, and (c) accessibility. In Table 3, additional criteria on the quality of the resources according to understanding by design (Wiggins and McTighe 1997, 2005) are presented. Understanding by design is a way of thinking about curricular design and implementation that emphasizes three main components: (a) the content of the lesson including learning outcomes, credibility, or validity of the content, explanations of how to implement the content, and so on; (b) determining the acceptable evidence of learning including methods of assessing learning while providing formative feedback to learners or providing learners with an opportunity to reflect about their learning; and (c) the instructional approach or pedagogy considering aspects, such as teamwork, hands-on activities, inquiry learning, and design- or inquiry-based learning. We used understanding by design as a framework for this part of the study because it encompasses all elements that should be involved in any instructional intervention.

Table 3 Criteria used to establish validity of web resource for engineering education

Topic to examine	Relevant questions to ask
Regarding content:	
	• What are the credentials of the author/sponsor of the site?
	• How updated is the content?
	• Is there a feature that will allow you to get your questions answered such as a direct contact for the developer or a discussion forum?
	• Has the content presented ever been implemented in a class and if so what was the evaluation?
	• Has the content been assessed?
Regarding instruction:	Does it present
	• A curriculum (if not then lesson plans…)?
	• Clear learning objectives?
	• Clear instructions for implementation in class?
	• Ways to assess student learning during class or rubrics?
	• Tests/homework sample and grading method?
Regarding pedagogy appropriate for engineering:	Does it allow opportunities for
	• Design based learning or project based learning?
	• Hands on activities?
	• Individual as well as teamwork?
	• Discussion and reflection?
	• Student Feedback?
	• Presentation of the final product to external audience?

Results

Results are based on the factors that emerged throughout the data analyses to highlight differences or similarities across the seven languages. Considered factors include frequency of identified websites, types of entities that developed engineering educational resources, types of engineering contents by grade level, terms searched to identify engineering educational resources by language, and accessibility to the websites. Therefore, the results assisted us to better understand the global landscape of PreK-12 engineering education web resources and to start identifying global trends.

Web resources

The number of websites containing educational resources per language was identified first. Figure 2 shows a summary chart that compares the number of websites with OER that contain engineering content targeting PreK-12 and PreK-3 students. Figure 3 shows the percentage of PreK-3 websites with resources within the PreK-12 ones. Since each country using one of the languages has different infrastructure and accessibility regulations for the use of educational web resources, there are two underlying issues that need to be accounted for: first, even if there is no

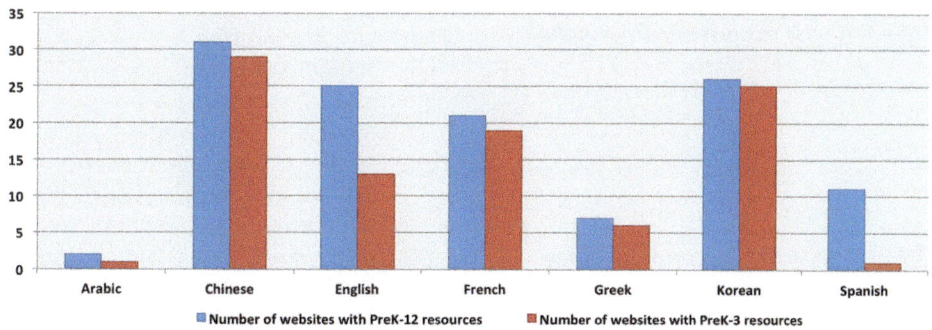

Figure 2 Number of websites presenting PreK-12 educational engineering resources identified per language.

language barrier, resources might still not be visible or accessible to the public or users out of a country. Second, different resources might have varied emphasis on each of the four components of PreK-12 STEM education, as well as on the ages they are targeting. Thus, there is a chance that the number of websites could be impacted by those conditions. Despite the disparity, results of this study provide insight into the contemporary landscape of engineering education for PreK-12 students in the countries using the corresponding languages.

Entities developing PreK-12 engineering resources

In Table 4, we present the entities, officially related to education, that appear to work towards development of PreK-12 engineering content. The identified entities were Ministries of Education, usually in collaboration with various government-related organizations, private organizations formally recognized to be related to educational content development, foundations, universities, teacher organizations, and museums. Furthermore, in Table 5, we present if these resources were open to all users or if there were restrictions that apply.

Types of educational engineering content

Taking a look at the type of PreK-12 contents developed by the aforementioned entities, curricula - learning resources that provide a lesson plan to help the teacher implement the activity in the classroom, and assessment instruments, so teachers can evaluate knowledge gain - were rare, if any, in all seven languages. As presented in Figure 4, individual, small-scale activities were the most common type of resource identified, followed by individual one- or two-session-long lesson plans. Among the seven languages, Arabic was the language in which websites with only activities were found. In the cases of Korean, Greek, and Spanish, in addition to individual activities, there were a few websites with lesson plans and one or two websites with curricula. Examining the other end of the spectrum, Chinese and English, followed by French, are the languages in which the largest numbers of websites with curricula have been developed. Similarly, as presented in Figure 5, the PreK-3 level resources are mainly comprised of individual activities, with rare lesson plans and even fewer curricula.

Terminology

Careful examination of the terms used in web searches and identification of PreK-12 engineering resources revealed that similar types of content were addressed in many different ways around the world. Table 2 presents the terms used by the researchers in order to identify the engineering educational resources. As expected, according to the nomenclature of the languages represented in this study, the web searches leading to the desired data had to include different terms.

As Table 2 indicates, in alignment with the plurality of the search terms, the terms used in the websites also vary among the different languages. The terms that appear in

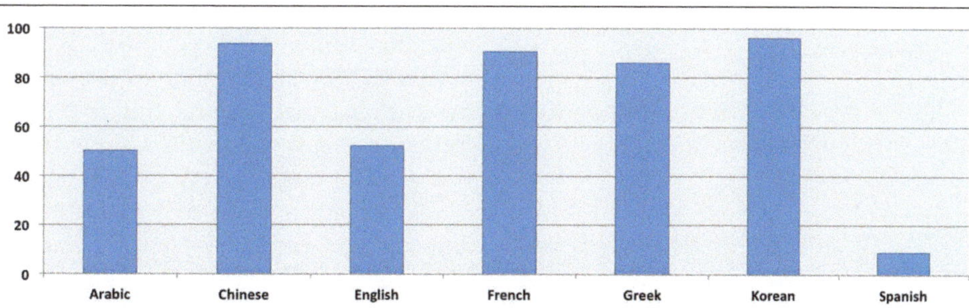

Figure 3 Percentage of websites with PreK-3 resources within the websites with PreK-12 resources.

Table 4 Types of organizations (entities) that develop and distribute engineering web resources per language

Language	G	P	F	U	T	M
Arabic		X			X	
Chinese	X				X	
English	X	X	X	X	X	X
French	X			X		X
Greek	X		X			
Korean	X	X	X			X
Spanish	X	X			X	

Note: X = exists; G = government organization/ministry of education; P = private organization formally related to education; F = foundation; U = university organization; T = organization by teachers; M = museum.

the websites are primary, *Science, Technology, Engineering,* and *Mathematics,* followed by *STEM, Invention, Creativity, Design,* and then *Physics, Biology, Chemistry, Electrical, Mechanical,* and *Computer Science.* As presented in Figure 6, the terms *Science* and *Technology* were commonly represented in all languages. The term *Engineering* appears mainly in English resources followed by Greek and Korean. We should note here that United States developers offered all English resources but one, which was British. The term *STEM* was, as expected, only used in the United States resources.

At the point of data collection for this study, *engineering for P-12 education* or *P-12 engineering education* rarely returned Korean web resources. Instead, *pre-engineering education* (예비공학교육) or science, technology, engineering, arts, and mathematics (*STEAM*) *integrated education* (융합인재교육) have started to appear to address integrated education across several disciplines that include engineering. In addition, many engineering activities have been conducted under the name of science education or programs for creativity and invention. The term *Invention* was predominantly used in Chinese and it also appears in French and Korean web resources, and *Creativity* appears a few times in Greek and Korean websites. For Spanish, the terms *Technology* or *Science and Technology* were the most successful ones. Greek is also the language that, when it comes to the content distributed to the schools by the Ministry of Education, no aggregate terminology, such as *STEM* or *Science,* is used, and web resources are only categorized under the individual disciplinary descriptive terms of *Design, Physics, Chemistry, Biology, Math, Electrical, Mechanical,* and *Computer Science.* There was also one case in Arabic in which the content was also described as general information.

Table 5 Accessibility and openness of the engineering education websites by language

Language	Openness
Arabic	All resources were open
Chinese	Most websites have resources readily available without login process, 6/31 sites request login
English	Most websites have resources readily available without login process, 3/25 sites request a free registration and login
French	Most websites have resources readily available without login process, 1/21 sites requests login
Greek	All resources were open
Korean	Even though the use of web resources are free, most websites require a free registration and a login process to access the resources
Spanish	Most websites have resources readily available without login process, 3/11 sites request login

Accessibility

As a final factor, examining the open availability of these resources to teachers or other potential users made some discrepancies apparent. Discrepancies can be explained by the facts that different countries have adopted different standpoints in terms of (a) offering open resources and (b) allowing particular platforms supporting share of content to be accessible within their country.

Discussion

Findings are summarized into four main points below.

- Across all languages, web resources on learning materials about engineering were easy to locate. However, developmental appropriateness and content validity were hard to establish. Searching for such content requires painstaking attention.
- Web resources presenting scattered activities and lesson plans are well developed. Engineering curricula (e.g., containing additional resources, such as indications of pedagogical strategies and assessment instruments) are significantly fewer.
- The number and type of resources developed to first introduce early education students to engineering content differ significantly across languages.
- All languages revealed the availability of engineering content but different terminology was employed.

The search for web-based *PreK-12 engineering curricula* revealed a wide variety of resources developed by different education-related entities, as well as individuals and corporations. However, resources presenting valid engineering curricula were limited, and in some cases, they were particularly hard to identify among the plethora of information. The large variety of uncategorized and difficult to validate information may result in teachers being discouraged and confused when they attempt to familiarize themselves with engineering. Furthermore, the uneven distribution in regards to the language used to describe the content made the resources widely available to some

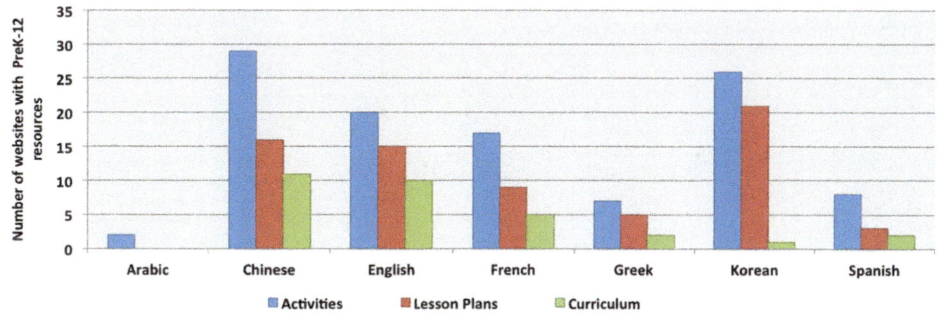

Figure 4 Number of websites presenting PreK-12 activities, lesson plans, and curricula per language.

target groups, while still a large number of teachers cannot take advantage of this shared information.

International findings regarding the type of content remained consistent with the group's prior research findings based on the English websites' analysis (Bagiati et.al. 2010). Most resources were comprised of individual activities, while well-organized lesson plans or long-term curricula were harder to find, if at all. For a PreK-12 teacher, identifying some engineering activities to bring in class is always a good first step. The lack of further instruction in regards to how to make visible and assess engineering-related learning, or how to proceed in a subsequent class in order to provide the students a more holistic experience, still leaves the teacher's preparation incomplete. However, the increasing level of global activities, the interactive nature of the Internet, and the global desire to share educational resources will surely be positive forces in improving the quality of available resources, thus facilitating teacher access and adaptation of engineering content in the PreK-12 engineering relevant education in schools.

Availability of early engineering web-based materials was uneven around the globe but well under way in multiple contexts, languages, and cultures. When considering early education of engineering, China appeared to be the country that has the most web resources regarding PreK-3 engineering resources, followed by Korean, French, and English-speaking countries. English web-resources appeared to have a strong presence in the PreK-12 level, but when comparing proportions within those websites for the PreK-3 alone, they appeared to be significantly less. In the case of Arabic-speaking countries, only two websites with OER were identified, and one of them also contained some PreK-3 STEM activities. In the case of Greece, it is particularly interesting that although there were not as many resources compared to other languages, all but one website included content targeting the PreK-3 group, probably indicating a particular value placed onto early education. Spanish was the language that showed a very weak presence of PreK-3 content among the seven languages.

Although the Internet allows for access to curricula developed and offered to a global audience, the terminology used in seven languages in which this content is presented appeared to be a barrier. Users start using the search engines by looking up for terms that represent their own educational nomenclature. A direct translation of these terms most probably would lead to a very small number of relevant entries. Different educational systems present similar educational content but employ different

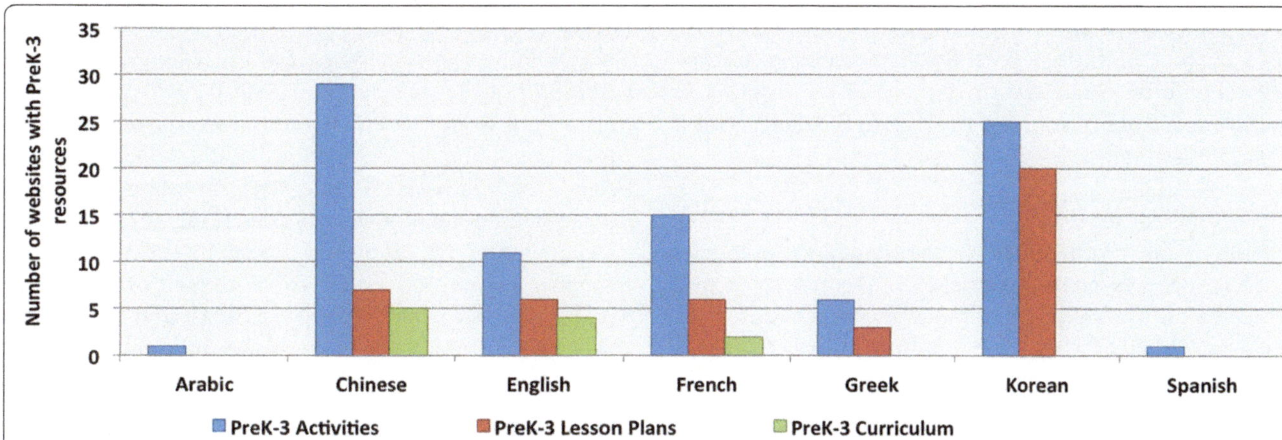

Figure 5 Number of websites presenting PreK-3 activities, lesson plans, and curricula per language.

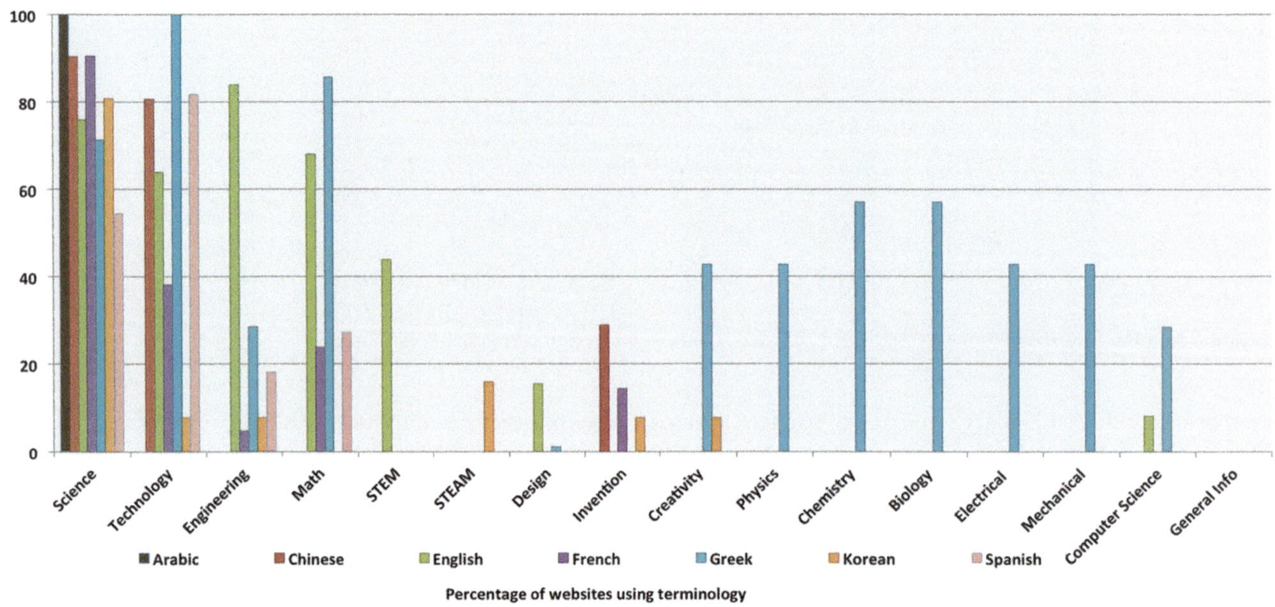

Figure 6 Percentages of websites using engineering-related terminology per language.

terminology, and although web translators are returning quite accurate results when it comes to direct translation, such differences in conceptual interpretations cannot be accurately represented yet. In the United States, the terms *Engineering, STEM,* and *Science* are the predominant ones. In Arab, European, and Latino cultures represented by Arabic, Greek, French, and Spanish, the labels of *Science* and *Technology* are used more often. Asian cultures using Chinese and Korean refer to similar content using terms such as *Creativity* and *Invention.*

Although it does not appear to be a serious issue, we also observed a small disparity in the availability of these types of resources across seven languages. Internet accessibility, and also different trends regarding content accessibility that appear to be the norm among different cultures and countries (open source content vs. content available for citizens only), may also influence the spread of the educational content. Therefore, for teachers to remain current or further promote their leaning, accessibility should be considered in the use of the Internet to openly distribute resources through individual professional initiatives.

Implications for teaching

Examining our resources within the framework presented in Table 3, researchers have selected the resources presented below as a sample that meets most criteria in every language. Quality PreK-3 resources have also been identified and are presented due to the group's particular interest in early education resources and due to the different developmentally appropriate pedagogies required for this age level. However, such content could not be identified in all languages. Taking into consideration the pace at which online content appears or changes daily, the audience is not suggested to consider the selected resources presented as the state-of-the-art contents at the time this paper is published or read but as a good example of a high-quality resource. We hope that teachers can easily use the criteria, presented in Table 3, for future references, as they will be attempting to evaluate content on their own.

Arabic

Regarding the Arabic websites, there were no comprehensive websites presenting curricula or even lesson plans. As presented in Figure 4 above, resources would present small-scale individual activities with no further information regarding assessment or evaluation of the content or the pedagogy used.

Chinese

To provide a starting point for the Chinese language, while noting that the term *engineering* was not used in this culture to describe the content, we suggest the website of the Shanghai Association for the Advancement of Science for Youths as an example to showcase our criteria in discerning a quality website presenting content related to engineering education. As noted in the website, the Shanghai Association for the Advancement of Science for Youths is a part of the Shanghai Science and Technology Association. The association's aim is to promote educational reform in Science education, by enhancing scientific attributes among youths, and their website includes a list of scientific and technological teaching materials, including curricula, lesson plans, and formal and informal activities. These materials are organized in different topics, such as, 'Learning Science by Doing,' 'Innovation and DIY in Science Education,' etc. They also provide a forum for posting excellent examples in science teaching and scholarly papers which are geared toward the need of teachers in science and technology. Well-organized curriculum/ lesson plans/activities are found within the list of examples in science teaching. Scholarly papers offer ideas and suggestions to teachers regarding different aspects in science teaching, such as teachers' roles in guiding students' innovative scientific and technological innovation, creative thinking among youths, etc. Their website is open to general public without any requirement for registration or login process.

English

A great starting point while searching in English would be the resources developed and presented by the Museum of Science in Boston. Through their National Center for Technological Literacy website (http://legacy.mos.org/nctl/k12_curricula.php), people can find information and resources regarding various K-12 programs and curricula related to engineering, such as Engineering is Elementary (EiE) or Engineering the Future (EtF), and more. The website presents various resources for teachers, students, and parents; instructional videos to facilitate and guide the teachers on how to implement the lessons and activities in class based on research studies conducted on the curricula. The full curricula though are not always available online are for free. Teach Engineering - Resources for K-12 (http://www.teachengineering.org) and Engineering - Go for it! (http://www.egfi-k12.org) are two more website teachers can use in order to find validated K-12 content. However, as both sites contain few curricula but a very big number of lesson plans or individual activities targeting almost all student ages from upper elementary all the way to high school, not all resources are presented in the same way, or provide the same level of information and support to the teacher. Regarding the early education level, website presenting a developmentally appropriate early engineering curriculum is Puppeteering to Engineering (P2E) (http://puppetengineering.com). P2E is a semester-long, age-appropriate design-based curriculum, designed by two of the researchers participating in the current study, aiming to achieve higher knowledge integration of STEM in the preschool classroom and is addressing the STEM integration, with primary emphasis on the engineering component. Twenty-four lessons comprising the curriculum are available online in PDF format, including instructions for classroom implementation and assessment. The curriculum has been implemented in a preschool classroom, and the evaluation is also presented online.

French

Sciences et Technologie - Lot http://pedagogie.ac-toulouse.fr/lotec/Sciences/SPIP/ website appears to be one of the most comprehensive web resources within the French websites researched. It targets early, middle and high school students, as well as teachers of all science professions (biology, archeology, physics, math, natural science, environmental science, and numerous others). It can also be a good resource for parents. This website promotes hands-on scientific investigation based on four main concepts: energy, planet Earth, living organism, and unity and diversity of the living organism. The site is quite interactive, consisting of videos, articles, interesting visuals for anyone accessing the website for information about the specified concepts - it should be noted that within each concept, under the broader concepts mentioned, there are more detailed resources under each component.

There are examples of lesson plans that are also supported with further complementary resources. Every example of lesson plan is presented in PDF format - for each age group or cycle; there are sample lesson plans that include a detailed step-by-step elaboration on a particular scientific concept to include the objectives, expected outcomes for the particular age group, and certain strategies that can be used to elaborate learning of certain concepts. All can enjoy the site for free. Also, given that this is a governmental website, each focus area ties in the topic to an ongoing initiative or project that is happening in a particular region - this is open for all to be aware of the ongoing events in the country, encouraging all the viewers to be more active members of their environment, making learning more fun.

La main à la pate, http://lamap.inrp.fr// is another example of a comprehensive website that aims to develop inquiry-based science education in primary and lower-secondary schools, with a hands-on approach being the pedagogical principle. Launched in 1996, initiated by the Nobel Laureate in Physics, Georges Charpark, La main à la pate became a foundation for scientific cooperation in 2012 founded by the Académie des sciences, the Ecole normale supérieure (Paris), and the Ecole normale supérieure of Lyon. The La main à la pâte foundation pursues and develops the activities carried out in France and the rest of the world. The website is translated into six languages, English, German, Spanish, Chinese, Serbian, and Arabic. Taken from the website, there are nearly 400 class activities available online with ten educational projects that have been freely distributed to 55,000 teachers worldwide. This website has provided support in terms of resources engaging 160 middle schools in integrated science education projects. Their priorities include producing and disseminating pedagogical and scientific resources and contributing to the training of teachers and trainers. With their international cooperation around science education, they have scientists and industrialists in the development of science education.

Greek

Regarding the Greek language, the Digital School (DS) (το Ψηφιακό Σχολέιο), dschool.edu.gr, developed by Greece's Ministry of Education, appears to be the main platform offering curricula and additional recourses. Greece is one of the countries that use national curricula. Teachers have to follow the curricula provided by the Ministry of Education, but can enhance their teaching with material of their choice as well. On the Digital School's website (http://digitalschool.minedu.gov.gr), teachers and students can find electronic books, curricula to be used at all classes and courses as well as additional resources that could be used to enhance a course, or links to other websites that may be helpful to teachers. When it comes to the early education level, no engineering curriculum is there to find. The Ministry of Education for this age level is offering some generic suggestions on how an early education teacher could introduce the use of a computer, other digital devises, and new technologies in the classroom.

Korea

When it comes to Korean, as Korea has a large proportion of the Internet users, various educational web resources were available. Particularly, each provincial office of education in Korea provides a website that contains all grade levels (K-12) of educational resources under the name of Education Supporting Center (ERC). As a quality example for a website, the KARI (Korea Aerospace Research Institute) school website (http://www.karischool.re.kr/) provides teachers with lesson plans appropriate for teaching elementary and middle school students. In detail, the website contains educational resources about four main topics related to aerospace engineering: aeronautics, rockets, space science, and space exploration. For each topic, a series of lesson plans consisting of three or four lesson plans, including various hands-on activities are prepared for elementary students and middle school students, respectively. All the lesson plans are presented in PDF files. Each lesson plan provides descriptions of the target grade level of students, lesson goals, and introduction and concepts for the topic, time estimates for each unit, materials for preparation, key vocabulary, instructions for activities, tips for teachers to deliver the lesson, worksheets for students that can be used for assessment, and reading materials. To use those resources, teachers need to create an account to login so that they can download the PDF documents.

Examining the early education space in Korean, in addition to the official websites by the government, private organizations run websites providing educational resources, specifically targeting young learners, in various subject areas that include engineering topics, too. While educational resources for PreK and kindergarten were presented in the form of activities for the use of both parents and teachers, educational resources for early elementary students (grades 1~3) were better structured to be lessons and aligned well with the formal standards and curriculum of each grade level. Usually, engineering topics were presented under the name of science, creativity, or invention activities. Recently, the Korean Ministry of Education has adopted the term STEAM to initiate integrated education that embraces concepts across five subject areas, and STEAM education is becoming an integral part of K-12 education across the nation (Kim et al. 2013).

Spanish

An example in the Spanish language that meets the criteria presented in Table 3 is the website Exploradores (http://www.exploradores.org.pe), hosted by the National Society of Mining, Petroleum and Energy (Sociedad Nacional de Mineria Petroleo y Energia) in Lima, Peru. This website is organized in four related topics including mining, hydrocarbons, electricity, and environment. For each of these topics, several resources are provided targeting students and teachers. Resources for students include an interactive multimedia scene where students can explore its components through an interactive map. Each component of the scene provides a link to a sub-topic that provides additional information in the form of text, images, frequently asked questions, and additional related links to other websites. Additional resources available for both teachers and students are educational slides and downloadable and printable glossary of terms in the form of pictures and text.

Resources for teachers include lesson plans organized by grade levels (elementary and secondary education) and topic (energy, mining, hydrocarbons). The organization of the lesson plan follows a logical progression by first introducing the topic and associated relevant concepts and processes, and then transitions into applications. In addition, the lesson plan provides teachers with activities for students to do (e.g., hand-outs). These activities are organized in a series of steps and are accompanied with guidelines of pedagogical strategies and materials students will use. These hand-outs are meant to be used to prompt students to reflect and, at the same time, assess what they have learned. The lesson plan also provides extensive materials for teachers to do reflection and formative evaluation of their lesson implementation. The lesson plan concludes with a glossary of terms, list of references, and complementary readings.

Limitations and future research

While we attempted to investigate PreK-12 engineering resources for teachers around the world, the searched languages were limited to seven languages; thus, we could not identify the current status of online PreK-12 engineering resources available in other languages. Considering the population presenting academic work relevant to PreK-12 engineering education curricula in scholarly settings, there is expectation that more relevant content could be identified in northern European languages and probably others as well. Furthermore, even though we discussed differences in searching strategies for every language, there might be a sampling error in identification of the online resources because of the massive websites containing the keywords.

Acknowledging the fact that one language does not only represent one country (e.g., French is spoken in more than 30 countries), we have tried to identify resources and information regarding STEM or engineering standards in many countries. However content available on the Internet was heavily available only from a small number of countries. A local nomenclature or a different educational standpoint towards STEM in PreK-12 may exist in other countries, but resources were not available on the web and therefore it is not represented in this paper.

In addition to the language and terminology limitations, the group made the deliberate choice to examine content developed by entities formally associated with education and curriculum development, to establish a first level of validation regarding the content examined. Searching on the web, there appeared to be dozens, and in some languages even hundreds, of additional web resources developed by individuals (teachers, students, and professional engineers). Lack of credentials in many cases placed content validity and pedagogical appropriateness of the content under question and requires further inquiry.

When examining the content, our group was aiming to identify engineering-related resources. Given that in many languages these recourses were to find under different terminology, e.g., science or creativity, we were excluding the cases where activities would only refer to a traditional scientific discipline or were just referring to an arts and crafts project. However, we understand that since no firm boundaries exist, especially when discussing STEAM topics, results are reflecting the researchers' perceptions on whether an activity should be categorized as *engineering*.

Last but not least, by going through the resources identified, it is the group's first impression that not all resources are of the same quality or would have the same impact when used. Although data related to implementation and assessment of the identified resources would be a valuable validation mechanism, relevant data was not available for most of the websites identified.

Conclusions

Based on the aforementioned themes identified, we conclude that although the advent of the Internet has made educational content globally available, the barriers related to language, terminology, content validity, and accessibility are tough to overcome, and currently may significantly limit single language users and teachers from taking full advantage of available content. Realizing how challenging it is for a teacher, student, or parent to navigate through such a chaotic cloud of educational resources, this calls to the community of engineering education for the question of who or what could be an authoritative body legitimated to produce and disseminate this kind of material. What would be the appropriate process for this dissemination? Then, should it be at a national or international level? Should one or more entities be responsible for validation of content and pedagogy? Furthermore, while attempting to disseminate the existing information, would it even be appropriate to attempt to impose a dominant terminology in hopes of structuring the future of engineering-related curriculum development more efficient for a global audience to identify, or should we, as a global community of scholars, focus on exposing and embracing all different terminologies currently used?

On a more immediate tone, the implications of this study could relate to the creation of collections for engineering education resources specifically, and STEM education in general. We suggest that these collections should not only include the name of the resource and the audience but that such resources should include metadata or descriptors, such as associated learning outcomes, target audience, scope, and overall measures of quality of the identified resources, to help teachers and students better navigate during their search.

Additional file

Additional file 1: Complete data set of the websites that were identified and analyzed. Websites for engineering education for the seven languages studied.

Abbreviations

OER: Open educational resources; PreK-12: Prekindergarten through 12th grade; STEAM: Science, technology, engineering, arts, and math; STEM: Science, technology, engineering, and math.

Competing interests

One of the curricula mentioned in the study as an example (the Puppeteering to Engineering Curriculum) has been developed by the first author, Dr. Aikaterini Bagiati, as her doctoral study under the supervision of Dr. Demetra Evangelou.

Authors' contributions

AB conceived the study, participated in its design and coordination, and helped to draft and revise the manuscript. She also worked on data collection, analysis, and interpretation of the English and Greek resources. SY helped to draft and revise the manuscript. She also worked on data collection, analysis, and interpretation of the Korean resources. DE conceived the study, participated in its design and coordination, and helped to draft and revise the manuscript. AM helped to draft and revise the manuscript. She also worked on data collection, analysis, and interpretation of the Spanish resources. GK helped to draft and revise the manuscript. She also worked on data collection, analysis, and interpretation of the French resources. JZ helped to draft and revise the manuscript. She also worked on data collection, analysis, and interpretation of the Chinese resources. All authors read and approved the final manuscript.

Author details

[1]MIT-SUTD Collaboration Office, Massachusetts Institute of Technology, Cambridge, MA, 02139, USA. [2]Texas A&M Engineering Experiment Station, Texas A&M University, College Station, TX 77843, USA. [3]Department of Education Sciences in Early Childhood, Democritus University, Alexandroupolis 69100, Greece. [4]Computer and Information Technology Department, Purdue University, West Lafayette, IN 47907, USA. [5]Department of Education, Lebanese American University, Beirut, Lebanon. [6]Graduate School of Education, Shanghai Jiao Tong University, Shanghai City, P. R. China.

References

American Association of Colleges for Teacher Education. (2013). *The changing teacher preparation profession: a report from AACTE's professional educational data system (PEDS)*. http://blogs.edweek.org/edweek/charterschoice/AACTE.pdf. Accessed March 22 2014.

Bagiati, A. (2011). *Early engineering: a developmentally appropriate curriculum for young children (Dissertation)*. West Lafayette: Purdue University.

Bagiati, A, & Evangelou, D. (2008). An examination of web-based P-12 engineering curricula: issues of pedagogical and engineering content fidelity. In *Proceedings of the Research in Engineering Education Symposium.*

Bagiati, A, Evangelou, D (in press (a)). Engineering curriculum in the preschool classroom: the teacher's experience. *European Early Childhood Education Research Journal, 23*(1).

Bagiati, A, Evangelou, D, (in press (b)) Practicing engineering while building with blocks: identifying engineering thinking. *European Early Childhood Education Research Journal, 24*(1).

Bagiati, A, Yoon, SY, Evangelou, D, Kaloustian, G, Cekic, O, Zhu, J Magana, AJ (2011). Engineering in early education: A multicultural comparison of web resources. Proceedings of the American Society for Engineering Education Annual Conference, Vancouver, BC, Canada.

Bagiati, A, Yoon, SY, Evangelou, D, & Ngambeki, I. (2010). Engineering curricula in early education: Describing the landscape of open resources. *Early Childhood Research & Practice, 12*(2), 1–15.

Bairaktarova, D, Evangelou, D, Bagiati, A, & Dobbs-Oates, J (2012). The role of classroom artifacts in developmental engineering. In *Proceedings of the American Society for Engineering Education Annual Conference, San Antonio, TX.*

Becker, SB. (2010). Why don't young people want to become engineers? Rational reasons for disappointing decisions. *European Journal of Engineering Education, 35*(4), 349–366.

Borko, H, Whitcomb, J, & Liston, D. (2009). Wicked problems and other thoughts on issues of technology and teacher learning. *Journal of Teacher Education, 60*(1), 3–7.

Brophy, S & Evangelou, D (2007). Precursors to engineering thinking (PET). In Proceedings of the American Society for Engineering Education Annual Conference. Honolulu, Hawaii. June 24–27.

Brophy, S, Klein, S, Portsmore, M, & Rogers, C. (2008). Advancing engineering education in P-12 classrooms. *Journal of Engineering Education, 97*(3), 369–387.

Bybee, RW. (2011). K-12 engineering education standards: opportunities and barriers. *Technology and Engineering Teacher, 70*(5), 21–29.

Campos, BP, Kallos, D, & Stephenson, J. (2000). *Green paper on teacher education in Europe*. Urnéa, Sweden: TNTEE.

Copple, C, & Bredekamp, S (Eds.). (2009). *Developmentally appropriate practice in early childhood programs serving children from birth through age 8* (3rd ed.). Washington, DC: National Association for Education of Young Children.

Dimopoulos, C, Katzis, K, & Hawwash, K. (2011). *Attracting students to engineering education studies: a survey of practices*. Lisbon, Portugal: European Society for Engineering Education (SEFI).

Giordan, A. (2010). Nouveaux contenus, nouvelles pratiques, peut-on mutualiser les problèmes et les acquis? In A. Hasni, & J. Lebeaume (Éds). Nouveaux enjeux de l'éducation scientifique et technologique: visées, contenus, compétences et pratiques (pp. 17-49). Ottawa : Presses Universitaires.

Gounari, P. (2009). Rethinking critical literacy in the new information age. *Critical Inquiry in Language Studies, 6*(3), 148–175.

Graziano, WG, Habashi, MM, Evangelou, D, & Ngambeki, I. (2012). Orientations and motivations: are you a "people person", a "thing person", or both? *Motivation and Emotion, 36*(4), 465–477.

Hedtke, R, Kahlert, J, & Schwier, V. (2001). Service industry for teachers? Using the Internet to plan lessons. *European journal of education, 36*(2), 189–193.

Hsu, M-C, Purzer, S, & Cardella, ME. (2011). Elementary teachers' views about teaching design, engineering, and technology. *Journal of Pre-College Engineering Education Research (J-PEER), 1*(2), 31–39.

Johnstone, S. (2005). *Open educational resources serve the world. Sharing educational resources over the Internet provides multiple benefits, from academic collaboration to economic development*. Boulder, Colorado: EDUCAUSE Quarterly.

Jung, I. (2005). ICT-pedagogy integration in teacher training: application cases worldwide. *Educational Technology & Society, 8*(2), 94–101.

Katehi, L, Pearson, G, & Feder, M. (2009). The status and nature of K-12 engineering education in the United States. *The Bridge, 3*(3), 5–10.

Kim, KS, Hong, JH, Huh, CS, Moon, DY, Kim, MY, Lee, CH, Kim, KY, Choi, EK, & Kim, YM. (2013). *A study on the reinforcement strategies of engineering education in elementary and secondary school [초중등 공학교육 강화방안 정책연구]*. Daejeon, South Korea: Korea Ministry of Education, Science, and Technology [한국교육과학기술부], Korea Foundation for the Advancement of Science & Creativity [한국과학창의재단].

Kuenzi, JJ. (2008). CRS report for congress: science, technology, engineering, and mathematics (STEM) education: background, federal policy, and legislative action. *Congressional Research Service, Library of Congress*, RL33434, Washington, DC. Retrieved on December 30th 2014 from https://www.hsdl.org/?view&did=715973

Lebeaume, J. (2011). Integration of Science, Technology, Engineering and Mathematics: Is This Curricular Revolution Really Possible in France? *Design and Technology Education, 16*(1), 47–52.

Lock, JV. (2006). A new image: online communities to facilitate teacher professional development. *Journal of Technology and Teacher Education, 14*(4), 663–678.

Moore, TJ. (2010). Implementing K-12 engineering standards through STEM integration. In *National Science Foundation (NSF) Faculty Early Career Development (CAREER) Program, Engineering Education Division, Award # 1055382.*

National Research Council. (2009). *Engineering in K-12 education: understanding the status and improving the prospects*. Washington, DC: The National Academies Press.

Perrault, AM (2007). An exploratory study of biology teachers' online information seeking practices. School Library Media Research (pp. 10).

Pimienta, D, Prado, D, & Blanco, A. (2009). *Twelve years of measuring linguistic diversity in the Internet: balance and perspectives*. Paris: United Nations Educational, Scientific and Cultural Organization.

Punie, Y. (2012). Preface. In *Joint Research Centre of the European Commission Innovating Learning: key elements for developing creative classroom in Europe (p. 1)*. Luxemburg: Publications Office of the European Union.

Recker, M. (2006). Perspectives on teachers as digital library users: consumers, contributors, and designers. *D-Lib Magazine, 12*(9), 2.

Recker, M, Dorward, J, & Nelson, LM. (2004). Discovery and use of online learning resources: case study findings. *Journal of Educational Technology and Society, 7*, 93–104.

Sanders, M. (2009). STEM, STEM education, STEMmania. *The Technology Teacher, 20*, 20–26.

Shulman, LS. (1986). Those who understand: knowledge growth in teaching. *Educational Researcher, 15*(2), 4–14.

Toombs, WE, & Tierney, WG. (1993). Curriculum definitions and reference points. *Journal of Curriculum and Supervision, 8*(3), 175–195. Retrieved from http://www.ascd.org/publications/jcs/spring1993/Curriculum-Definitions-and-Reference-Points.aspx.

Wang, H-H, Moore Tamara, J, Roehrig, GH, & Park, MS. (2011). STEM integration: teacher perceptions and practice. *Journal of Pre-College Engineering Education Research, 1*, 2.

Watt, HM, Richardson, PW, & Pietsch, J. (2007). Choosing to teach in the "STEM" disciplines: characteristics and motivations of science, ICT, and mathematics teachers. In mathematics: essential research, essential practice. In *Proceedings of the 30th Annual Conference of the Mathematics Education Research Group of Australasia* (2nd ed., pp. 795–804). Adelaide: MERGA.

Wiggins, G, & McTighe, J. (1997). *Understanding by design*. Alexandria, VA: Association for Supervision and Curriculum Development.

Wiggins, G, & McTighe, J. (2005). *Understanding by design* (2nd ed.). San Francisco, CA: Pearson Education.

Yaşar, Ş, Baker, D, Robinson-Kurpius, S, Krause, S, & Roberts, C. (2006). Development of a survey to assess K-12 teachers' perceptions of engineers and familiarity with teaching design, engineering, and technology. *Journal of Engineering Education, 95*(3), 205–216.

5

STEM education K-12: perspectives on integration

Lyn D. English

Abstract

This commentary was stimulated by Yeping Li's first editorial (2014) citing one of the journal's goals as adding multidisciplinary perspectives to current studies of single disciplines comprising the focus of other journals. In this commentary, I argue for a greater focus on STEM integration, with a more equitable representation of the four disciplines in studies purporting to advance STEM learning.

The STEM acronym is often used in reference to just one of the disciplines, commonly science. Although the integration of STEM disciplines is increasingly advocated in the literature, studies that address multiple disciplines appear scant with mixed findings and inadequate directions for STEM advancement. Perspectives on how discipline integration can be achieved are varied, with reference to multidisciplinary, interdisciplinary, and transdisciplinary approaches adding to the debates. Such approaches include core concepts and skills being taught separately in each discipline but housed within a common theme; the introduction of closely linked concepts and skills from two or more disciplines with the aim of deepening understanding and skills; and the adoption of a transdisciplinary approach, where knowledge and skills from two or more disciplines are applied to real-world problems and projects with the aim of shaping the total learning experience.

Research that targets STEM integration is an embryonic field with respect to advancing curriculum development and various student outcomes. For example, we still need more studies on how student learning outcomes arise not only from different forms of STEM integration but also from the particular disciplines that are being integrated. As noted in this commentary, it seems that mathematics learning benefits less than the other disciplines in programs claiming to focus on STEM integration. Factors contributing to this finding warrant more scrutiny. Likewise, learning outcomes for engineering within K-12 integrated STEM programs appear under-researched. This commentary advocates a greater focus on these two disciplines within integrated STEM education research. Drawing on recommendations from the literature, suggestions are offered for addressing the challenges of integrating multiple disciplines faced by the STEM community.

Keywords: STEM integration, STEM research, Multidisciplinary, interdisciplinary, and transdisciplinary integration, Mathematics education, Engineering education

Background

International concerns for advancing STEM education have escalated in recent years and show no signs of abating. Educators, policy developers, and business and industry organizations, to name a few, are highlighting the urgency for improving STEM skills to meet current and future social and economic challenges (e.g., Caprile et al., 2015; Honey et al., 2014; Marginson et al., 2013; Prinsley and Baranyai, 2015; The Royal Society Science Policy Centre, 2014). The almost universal preoccupation with STEM education in shaping innovation and development is evident in numerous reports. In the USA for example, the 2013 report from the Committee on STEM Education stressed that "The jobs of the future are STEM jobs," with STEM competencies increasingly required not only within but also outside of specific STEM occupations (National Science and Technology Council, 2013, p. vi). Developing competencies in the STEM disciplines is thus regarded as an urgent goal of many education systems, fuelled in part by perceived or actual shortages in the current and future STEM workforce (e.g., Caprile et al., 2015; Charette, 2013;

Correspondence: l.english@qut.edu.au
Faculty of Education, Queensland University of Technology, S Block, Victoria Park Road, Kelvin Grove, Brisbane, Queensland 4059, Australia

Hopkins et al., 2014; The Royal Society Science Policy Centre, 2014), as well as by outcomes from international comparative assessments (e.g., OECD, 2013).

Although global interest in STEM from educational and workforce perspectives has proliferated in recent years, the acronym was coined in the USA during the 1990s by the National Science Foundation (USA). The combining of the disciplines was seen as "a strategic decision made by scientists, technologists, engineers, and mathematicians to combine forces and create a stronger political voice" (STEM Task Force Report, 2014, p. 9). Since this time, the debates and dilemmas surrounding STEM employment shortages and STEM education in general have compounded.

Perspectives on the nature of STEM education and on the competencies requiring development are mixed, however. With the increased focus on STEM integration (e.g., Honey et al., 2014; Johnson et al., 2015), it appears timely to consider issues pertaining to STEM and its disciplinary integration and consider some research recommendations for advancing the field.

Perspectives on STEM and STEM integration

One of the problematic issues for researchers and curriculum developers lies in the different interpretations of STEM education and STEM integration. As indicated in numerous articles, STEM education has been defined variously ranging from disciplinary through to transdisciplinary approaches (e.g., Burke et al., 2014; Honey et al., 2014; Moore and Smith, 2014; Rennie et al., 2012; Vasquez, 2014/2015; Vasquez et al., 2013). In acknowledging the lack of an agreed-upon definition, the California Department of Education (2014) provides a broad perspective on STEM education, namely, "[STEM]... is used to identify individual subjects, a stand-alone course, a sequence of courses, activities involving any of the four areas, a STEM-related course, or an interconnected or integrated program of study" (http://www.cde.ca.gov/PD/ca/sc/stemintrod.asp).

In his editorial for the journal's first issue, Yeping Li introduced the publication as "a brand new, forward looking journal that will add the multidisciplinary perspectives needed to complement current disciplinary-focused journals in the field of STEM education" (Li, 2014, 1:1). In doing so, Li emphasized the need for researchers to "span disciplinary boundaries." Boundary crossing is a primary feature of integrated STEM perspectives, although the extent of disciplinary crossing in definitions of integration varies considerably. In their National Academies Press report, *STEM integration in K-12 education: Status, prospects, and an agenda for research,* Honey et al. (2014) provide a basic definition of integration as "working in the context of complex phenomena or situations on tasks that require students to use knowledge and skills from multiple disciplines" (p. 52). A more comprehensive perspective on STEM integration is featured in Vasquez et al.'s work (2013; Table 1), where different forms of boundary crossing are displayed along a continuum of increasing levels of integration, with progression along the continuum involving greater interconnection and interdependence among the disciplines.

An increased commitment to interdisciplinary and transdisciplinary STEM integration has appeared in recent years in several US documents. For example, the STEM Task Force Report (2014) adopts the view that STEM education is far more than a "convenient integration" of its four disciplines, rather it encompasses "real-world, problem-based learning" that links the disciplines "through cohesive and active teaching and learning approaches" (p. 9). The Report argues that the disciplines "cannot and should not be taught in isolation, just as they do not exist in isolation in the real world or the workforce" (p.9). Likewise, the California Department of Education adopts the axiom that "the whole is more than the sum of the parts" in its call for an increased focus on STEM integration (http://www.cde.ca.gov/PD/ca/sc/stemintrod.asp). More in-depth connections among the STEM disciplines are further advocated in the US *Common Core State Standards for Mathematics* (http://www.corestandards.org/Math/) as well as the *Next Generation Science Standards* (http://www.nextgenscience.org/).

Given the various interpretations of STEM education and STEM integration, it is little wonder that confusion can arise when researchers and policy developers refer to STEM education but differ considerably in their perspectives. Although the STEM acronym was initially coined to highlight the importance of the respective disciplines, the interdisciplinary nature of the world in

Table 1 Increasing levels of integration (adapted from Vasquez et al., 2013)

Form of integration	Features
1. Disciplinary	Concepts and skills are learned separately in each discipline.
2. Multidisciplinary	Concepts and skills are learned separately in each discipline but within a common theme.
3. Interdisciplinary	Closely linked concepts and skills are learned from two or more disciplines with the aim of deepening knowledge and skills.
4. Transdisciplinary	Knowledge and skills learned from two or more disciplines are applied to real-world problems and projects, thus helping to shape the learning experience.

which we live and work demands a broadening of STEM education and research (Hoachlander, 2014/2015). Interdisciplinary and transdisciplinary approaches to STEM research are emerging in the literature; however, the presence of integration as a distinct field of study is in its embryonic stages (Honey et al., 2014).

Inequitable STEM discipline representations

Although each of the integrative approaches in Table 1 has value in advancing learning, as Vasquez et al. (2013) pointed out, a major concern is that of inequitable discipline representations in STEM research and learning outcomes (English, 2015; English and Kirshner, 2016; Hoachlander, 2014/2015; Honey et al., 2014; Marginson et al., 2013; Moore et al., 2014; Shaughnessy, 2013). As one example of this uneven representation, of the 141 regular papers presented at the 2014 STEM conference in Vancouver, 45 % were devoted to science, 12 % to technology, 9 % to engineering, 16 % to mathematics, and interestingly, the remaining 18 % were classified as "general" with several papers in this category addressing two or more of the STEM disciplines (http://stem2014.ubc.ca/presentations/).

As several researchers have lamented (e.g., Barrett et al., 2014; Honey et al., 2014), the effectiveness of integrated STEM education in developing students' knowledge of core content is relatively under-researched. More studies are needed to identify ways in which learning across the disciplines might be more evenly distributed so that student achievement in one area does not overshadow or reduce gains in others. As Marginson et al. (2013) expressed metaphorically, "we need to lift the level of the peaks of the STEM mountain range, and broaden and elevate the whole of the range at the same time" (p. 72).

While acknowledging that reference to science could be interpreted as encompassing the other disciplines, especially mathematics, the STEM acronym itself is frequently defined as simply "science" (e.g., Office of the Chief Scientist, 2014). Many nations also refer to the role of STEM education as one that fosters "broad-based scientific literacy," with a key objective in their school programs being "science for all" in efforts to lift science education in the elementary, middle, and secondary school curricula (Marginson et al., 2013, p. 70). As Marginson et al. indicated, STEM discussions rarely adopt the form of "mathematics for all," even though mathematics underpins the other disciplines: "the stage of mathematics for all should be shifted further up the educational scale" (p.70). Likewise, Shaughnessy (2013) warned of programs that are merely a STEM veneer, that is, where approaches do not genuinely integrate the disciplines and thus may be devoid of important learning especially in mathematics. Even the rise in engineering education, beginning in the early school years (e.g., Lachapelle & Cunningham, 2014), would appear to be oriented towards the science strand with less emphasis on mathematics. Hoachlander (2014/2015) reiterates the above concerns:

> Despite more than a decade of strong advocacy by practitioners, employers, and policymakers, STEM education in US schools leaves a great deal to be desired. In too many schools, science and math are still taught mostly in isolation from each other, and engineering is absent (p. 74).

Although several policy and curriculum documents are now recognizing the important role of the respective disciplines in STEM integration, including engineering, a focus on connecting core content knowledge and processes across the disciplines still appears limited.

Advancing integrated STEM education research

Given the global importance accorded to STEM achievements as measured by national and international assessments, it is not surprising that many nations are questioning the quality of their curricula and the strategic actions needed to enhance the STEM disciplines. If we are to advance STEM integration and lift the profile of all of its disciplines, we need to focus on both core content knowledge and interdisciplinary processes. Nations that enjoy high international testing outcomes as well as strong STEM agendas have well-developed curricula that concentrate on twenty-first century skills including inquiry processes, problem-solving, critical thinking, creativity, and innovation as well as a strong focus on disciplinary knowledge (English and Gainsburg, 2016; Marginson et al., 2013; Partnership for 21st Century Skills, 2011). The need to nurture generic skills, in-depth conceptual understandings, and their interdisciplinary connections is paramount.

Making STEM connections more apparent

Developing students' understanding and appreciation of how integrated content, skills, and modes of thinking interact, including how they support and complement one another, is not an easy task (Honey et al., 2014; Moore et al., 2014). As Moore et al. (2014) noted, just because these connections might be emphasized in a curriculum, there is no guarantee that students will identify them or make the connections on their own. Consequently, the desired integrated STEM learning may well be lost. Likewise with respect to mathematics, Shaughnessy (2013) stressed that the "M" must be made "transparent and explicit." We cannot assume that all students will "see" the mathematics that is inherent in a particular problem (p. 324). More research is called for on ways to help students make STEM connections more transparent and meaningful across disciplines, including how this might be achieved at different grade levels. At the same time, further research is required on ways of assisting teachers to foster these connections, especially when appropriate curriculum frameworks and resources might be lacking.

Targeting student outcomes

Research on student outcomes in STEM integration appears limited and inconclusive, especially from a long-term perspective. A number of research issues arise including how integrated STEM programs might encourage more student engagement, motivation, and perseverance (Honey et al., 2014). Unfortunately, Honey et al.'s review of research reports indicated that such aspects, especially from a long-term view, are rarely measured in evaluations of these programs. Their review revealed that "few data convincingly correlate integrated STEM education with student outcomes" (Honey et al., 2014, p. 136). This finding is of particular concern, especially with respect to students' achievements in each of the STEM disciplines at different grade levels. Studies have yielded varied results. For example, Becker and Park's (2011) meta-analysis of studies investigating the possible differential effects of integration types on students' learning showed a large effect size (1.76) when all disciplines were integrated. In contrast, the effect size for integrating engineering and mathematics was small (0.03), as was the case when mathematics was integrated with science and technology (0.23).

Given that a number of studies analyzed by Becker and Park (2011) did not report on students' mathematics achievements, there remains the problem of inadequate research on the effects of integrative approaches on mathematics learning. Honey et al.'s (2014) review suggests that mathematics achievement is difficult to promote through STEM integration. If this is the case, then possible reasons for this need further investigation including whether a sequenced and structured approach to mathematics instruction hinders in-depth learning within STEM integration (Honey et al., 2014; Lehrer and Schauble, 2000).

Lifting the profile of mathematics in STEM integration

Recent concerns for the often diminished focus on mathematics include how its concepts and practices can contribute more effectively to an understanding of the remaining STEM disciplines (e.g., English, 2015; English and Kirshner, 2016; Fitzallen, 2015; Rennie et al., 2012; Shaughnessy, 2013). As Fitzallen (2015) highlighted, many reports claim that STEM provides contexts for fostering mathematical skills but these reports do not acknowledge the reciprocal relationship between mathematics and the other STEM disciplines. That is, the ways in which "mathematics can influence and contribute to the understanding of the ideas and concepts of other STEM disciplines" (p. 241) are not being addressed.

Coupled with the above is how we might best develop in-depth understanding of core mathematics content and processes within STEM experiences, while at the same time acknowledge that not all of mathematics can or should be learned within an integrated program (Honey et al., 2014). An inadequate focus on assisting students (and teachers) to recognize and make mathematics connections to the remaining disciplines further contributes to undermining mathematics learning within STEM. Making explicit the role of mathematics by repeatedly foregrounding the desired content and temporarily backgrounding other STEM content is one way in which the discipline might be advanced (Silk et al., 2010).

One example of how mathematics could provide core foundations and promote learning in the other disciplines is through a focus on mathematical literacy (English, 2015). Mathematical literacy was a core feature of PISA 2012 (OECD, 2013), where "meeting life needs... through using and engaging with mathematics, making informed judgements, and understanding the usefulness of mathematics in relation to the demands of life" were emphasized (Thompson et al., 2013). Mathematical literacy is foundational to STEM education, where skills in dealing with uncertainty and data are central to making evidence-based decisions involving ethical, economic, and environmental dimensions. Furthermore, with the exponential rise in digital information within STEM, the ability to handle contradictory and potentially unreliable online data is critical (Lumley and Mendelovits, 2012). Mathematics thus warrants increased recognition for its role in developing students' abilities to analyze and reason with data in making informed decisions and to engage in constructive debate about local and global issues (The Royal Society Science Policy Centre, 2014).

Lifting the profile of engineering in STEM integration

Although engineering across K-12 is emerging as a significant research area in its own right (e.g., Johri and Olds, 2014; Purzer et al., 2014; *Journal of Pre-College Engineering Education*), its presence within integrated STEM education deserves heightening. Engineering design and thinking, recognized as major components of K-12 engineering education, provide foundational linking processes across the STEM disciplines and are not just confined to engineering (Bryan et al., 2015; Lucas et al., 2014; *Next Generation Science Standards [NGSS]*, 2014; The National Academies, 2014). The NGSS specifically includes core practices and concepts from engineering alongside those for science, highlighting the interrelated nature of science and engineering education.

Broadening the role of engineering design and elevating it to the same level as scientific inquiry, the NGSS defines engineering design practices as those that all citizens should develop. Core features of engineering design are commonly described as comprising iterative processes including (a) defining problems by specifying criteria and constraints for acceptable solutions, (b) generating a number of possible solutions and evaluating these to determine which ones best meet the given problem criteria and constraints, and (c) optimizing the solution by systematically testing and refining, including overriding less significant features for the more important. Although there is increasing research demonstrating ways in which engineering can link the mathematics, science, and technology disciplines, mathematics still requires greater recognition in these experiences. In the next section, I provide one example of how both mathematics and engineering can be elevated within a modeling with data activity.

Engineering-based modeling with data

Modeling with data addresses the mathematical literacy domain addressed previously and comprises important learning features that facilitate different forms of integration including the interdisciplinary and transdisciplinary approaches of Table 1. As displayed in Table 2, modeling with data involves several features that support engineering within integrated STEM approaches including design processes, problem-solving and thinking, and testing, revising, and improving generated products.

In a collaborative research project (English and Mousoulides, 2015), 48 students from two sixth-grade classes (12-year-olds) in a K-6 urban public school in Cyprus worked a problem that addressed the 2007 structural failure of the 35W Minneapolis Bridge in Minnesota (adapted from Guzey et al., 2010). Developing models to rebuild the damaged bridge was a new experience for the students.

The problem commenced with an introductory session (35–45 min) where students studied a newspaper article about the bridge collapse as well as a video clip; they then answered questions to establish their understanding of the context and its data. In the second session (1 h 20 min–1 h 30 min), students were presented with two tables of data, together with the problem description. The first table of data comprised the key characteristics of the four main bridge types (truss, arch, suspension, cable-stayed), namely, the advantages and disadvantages of each bridge, the span range, the main materials used in construction, and the design effort (low, medium, high). The second table contained two samples of each of the major bridge types and some of their key features including the total length, the number of car lanes, the construction difficulty, and the building costs (in current values).

Table 2 Features of modeling with data (adapted from English, 2015)

- Exploring, posing, and refining investigative questions within STEM contexts
- Applying discipline-based concepts and engineering design in formulating and solving problems
- Testing, revising, and improving products generated
- Planning and undertaking investigations
- Analyzing and representing data in multiple ways
- Developing, applying, and assessing evidence-based models
- Understanding informal inference involving variation and uncertainty
- Critically evaluating data-based arguments and conclusions
- Sourcing, evaluating, and communicating information
- Thinking in creative, flexible, and innovative ways

The problem stated that the Minnesota Public Works Department urgently needed to construct a new bridge in the same location given specific parameters including a highway length of approximately 1000 ft and a deck of four lanes with additional side lanes. Students were to assist the Department by creating a way (model) for comparing the different bridge types so as to choose the appropriate one to build across each span.

Working in small groups of 3–4 (mixed-achievement in school mathematics), the students drew on the given data to generate, refine, and document their models. The groups were to develop a model that (a) included calculating the cost for each one of the four bridge types (using the given characteristics of the four main bridge types) and (b) would enable selection of the best possible bridge type for the reconstruction of the collapsed bridge. All possible factors related to bridge type, materials used, bridge design, safety, and cost were to be taken into consideration. In the final session (40–50 min), each student group explained to their peers the models they had generated and their key findings, which they documented in a poster.

Data from 13 audiotaped student groups were analyzed together with videotapes of all whole-class discussions. The data sources also included students' worksheets and the researchers' field notes. Interpretive techniques (Miles & Huberman, 1994) were used to analyze the data, with detailed analysis of all data sources enabling identification of the mathematization and statistical reasoning processes students applied during solution. Students' phases of model development, reflecting aspects of engineering design, were identified through iterative refinement cycles of analyses to generate more in-depth evidence of students' learning (Lesh and Lehrer, 2000).

Students' models varied in the number of problem factors considered (cost per surface unit of bridge deck, aesthetics of the various bridge types, bridge design effort, construction difficulty, length), as well as in how they reasoned with these data, and in the sophistication of their models. Excerpts from one student group's model development, where they reasoned with multidisciplinary components, are presented next.

This group began the problem by excluding a truss-type bridge explaining that, "The collapsed bridge was a truss one" (student A) and "Selecting the truss type bridge would make people feel insecure and bring back all those bad memories" (student B). The group then decided that a cost model for ranking the different bridge types was needed, but after developing an initial model that involved calculating the average cost (money per ft^2) for each bridge type, they decided that it was not the most appropriate solution. The group concluded that the substantial variation in their results for bridges of the same type could be addressed by integrating more factors within their initial model:

Student C: Our calculations are correct. There is nothing wrong. The cost is very different.

Student D: There are other things (factors) that are important and influence the cost ... for those (bridges) that are close to sea it is more difficult.

Student C: Yes, like in the Golden Gate Bridge. It is so expensive and not that long.

Student B: Cost is not proportionally related to the surface of the bridge (deck), but also the level of difficulty in constructability, just like in the Golden Gate, is an important factor.

On returning to the key characteristics of the four major bridge types (advantages, bridge span etc.), the group concluded that all types had their advantages as well as disadvantages. It was thus decided that a suitable bridge type could not be determined from this set of data alone. This realization prompted the next phase of model development as students examined further data. Students' reflections on their prior discussion regarding an initial cost model also contributed to their movement towards a more comprehensive model.

The group's next phase of model development involved a consideration of engineering, scientific, and societal factors. The group decided that these should be incorporated within their earlier model. These additional data included the necessary extra lanes for bridges, bikes, and pedestrians, as well as the difficulty level for each bridge construction. The last factor was determined by dividing the estimated final cost per square feet by 1.5 for the given examples of the four major bridge types. The group referred to this as the "difficult constructability" factor, which they specifically created to provide the same basis of comparison for all bridge types.

The refined model ranked the bridge types from cable-stayed as most favored, followed by the arch, truss, and suspension bridge types. In deciding on their final model, however, the students were aware of scientific and engineering issues and thus selected the arch type as the best possible solution. They were still concerned about the stability of a cable-stayed bridge for long-span bridges.

Students' reasoning in working the above problem illustrates how they drew upon multiple disciplinary features, reflecting Charette's (2014/2015) sentiments on STEM integration: "If we truly want students who can think critically, solve problems, and communicate their thoughts clearly, then some kind of systematic, cross-disciplinary instruction is required" (p. 82).

Discussion

In this commentary, I have argued for a greater focus on STEM integration, with a more balanced focus on each of the disciplines. Specifically, I have maintained that mathematics and engineering are underrepresented in studies claiming to address STEM education. Identifying ways in which we might achieve a more equitable representation of the disciplines is a complex endeavor, especially given the lack of a globally accepted definition of STEM education, as well as the different perspectives on and approaches to STEM integration within and across nations. Vasquez et al.'s (2013) continuum of disciplinary through transdisciplinary approaches to integration, with increasing interconnection and interdependence among the disciplines, provides one framework for addressing STEM integration. Developing and implementing integrated STEM programs, however, is challenging especially if one is to ensure that the respective core concepts and skills are given due attention. Different approaches to teaching each of the disciplines, such as a sequenced and structured approach to mathematics, could hinder some learning outcomes during integrated experiences.

Although STEM integration is receiving increasing emphasis in many curriculum documents and policy reports, there appears inadequate research that yields substantive evidence of desired learning outcomes. Existing studies of integrated STEM education rarely document in sufficient detail the curriculum or program being implemented including the nature of the integration and ways in which it was supported. The form of evidence collected to demonstrate whether the intervention goals were achieved is also frequently lacking (Honey et al., 2014).

Clearly, there remain many research questions regarding STEM integration, as documented by Honey et al. (2014) and others (e.g., Kimmel et al., 2014). In an effort to provide much-needed direction to future research, Honey et al. (2014) developed a descriptive framework of core features and subcomponents of integrated STEM education incorporating *goals* and *outcomes* for students and educators, together with the *nature and scope of integration* and features of *implementation* (p. 32). Emanating from this framework, their recommendations include as a necessary starting point a consistent use of terminology that establishes a common STEM language. The development and application of substantial theoretical frameworks, and a better delineation of the nature of STEM integration programs, including how evidence for learning is gathered and the types of learning supports provided, are also essential to advancing the field.

With respect to program implementation, I noted previously the need to investigate ways to make connections among the STEM disciplines more transparent for both students and teachers. One expectation of effective STEM education programs is that students are encouraged to make new and productive connections across two or more of the disciplines, which may be evidenced in improved student learning and transfer as well as interest and engagement. These learning outcomes require students to be competent with specific discipline content as well as discipline representations, together with "representational fluency" in translating among these representations (Honey et al., 2014, p. 144). These competencies may require teacher scaffolding especially for younger learners. The research of Dorie et al. (2014) demonstrated how appropriate adult scaffolding can promote the "natural" engineering talents of young learners. The question of how much scaffolding should be provided, however, warrants further investigation. English and King (2015) recommend that such support needs to be balanced in terms of establishing an understanding of core concepts and allowing students to apply this learning in ways they choose during problem solution.

Conclusion

Integrated STEM education continues to raise more questions than there are presently answers. It is hoped that this commentary has prompted further avenues for research and discussion on how we can advance the STEM field including keeping abreast of the exponential growth in technology. The multifaceted ways in which technological advances can enhance student outcomes are expanding rapidly (Johnson et al., 2013), opening up new directions and challenges in our STEM research endeavors.

Competing interests

The author declares that she has no competing interests.

Acknowledgements

This commentary drew upon findings that have emanated from several research studies supported by grants from the Australian Research Council (ARC), including projects LP120200023 and DP DP120100158. Any opinions, findings, and conclusions or recommendations expressed in this commentary are those of the author and do not necessarily reflect the views of the ARC.

References

Barrett, B. S., Moran, A. L., & Woods, J. E. (2014). Meteorology meets engineering: an interdisciplinary STEM module for middle and early secondary school students. *International Journal of STEM Education, 1*, 6. doi:10.1186/2196-7822-1-6.

Becker, K., & Park, K. (2011). Effects of integrative approaches among science, technology, engineering, and mathematics (STEM) subjects on students' learning: a preliminary meta-analysis. *Journal of STEM Education, 12*(5/6), 23–37.

Bryan, L. A., Moore, T. J., Johnson, C. C., & Roehrig, G. H. (2015). Integrated STEM education. In C. C. Johnson, E. E. Peters-Burton, & T. J. Moore (Eds.), *STEM roadmap: A framework for integration* (pp. 23–37). London: Taylor & Francis.

Burke, L., Francis, K., & Shanahan, M. (2014). A horizon of possibilities: a definition of STEM education. Paper presented at the *STEM 2014 Conference*, Vancouver, July 12–15.

California Department of Education. (2014). *Science, technology, engineering, & mathematics (STEM) information*. http://www.cde.ca.gov/PD/ca/sc/stemintrod.asp. accessed December, 2014.

Caprile, M., Palmen, R., Sanz, & Dente, G. (2015). *Encouraging STEM studies for the labour market* (Directorate-General for Internal Policies: European Parliament).

Charette, R. N. (2013). *The STEM crisis is a myth*. Retrieved 23 December, 2014 from http://spectrum.ieee.org/at-work/education/the-stem-crisis-is-a-myth.

Charette, R. N. (2014/2015). Commentary: STEM sense and nonsense. *Educational Leadership*, December 2014/January 2015, 79–83.

Dorie, B. L., Cardella, M. E., & Svarovsky, N. (2014). Capturing the design thinking of young children interacting with a parent. Paper presented at the *121st SEE Annual Conference & Exposition*, Indianapolis, IN, June 15–18.

English, L. D. (2015). STEM: challenges and opportunities for mathematics education. In K. Beswick, T. Muir, & J. Wells (Eds.), *Proceedings of the 39th Conference of the International Group for the Psychology of Mathematics Education* (Vol. 1, pp. 3–18). Hobart, Australia: PME.

English, L. D., & Gainsburg, J. (2016). Problem solving in a 21st-century mathematics curriculum. In L. D. English & D. Kirshner (Eds.), *Handbook of international research in mathematics education* (3rd ed., pp. 313–335). New York: Taylor & Francis.

English, L. D., & King, D. T. (2015). STEM learning through engineering design: fourth-grade students' investigations in aerospace. *International Journal of STEM Education*, 2 (14). DOI: 10.1186/s40594-015-0027-7.

English, L. D., & Kirshner, D. (2016). Changing agendas in international research in mathematics education. In L. D. English & D. Kirshner (Eds.), *Handbook of international research in mathematics education* (3rd ed., pp. 3–18). New York: Taylor & Francis.

English, L. D., & Mousoulides, N. (2015). Bridging STEM in a real-world problem. *Mathematics Teaching in the Middle School, 20*(9), 532–539.

Fitzallen, N. (2015). STEM education: what does mathematics have to offer? In M. Marshman (Eds.), *Mathematics Education in the Margins*. Proceedings of the 38th annual conference of the Mathematics Education Research Group of Australasia, Sunshine Coast, June 28-July 2 (pp. 237–244). Sydney: MERGA.

Guzey, S. S., Moore, T. J., & Roehrig, G. H. (2010). Curriculum development for STEM integration: bridge design on the white earth reservation. In L. M. Kattington (Ed.), *Handbook of Curriculum Development* (pp. 347–366). Hauppauge, NY: Nova.

Hoachlander, G. (2014/2015). Integrating SET&M. *Educational Leadership*, (December 2014/January 2015), 74–78.

Honey, M., Pearson, G., & Schweingruber, A. (2014). *STEM integration in K-12 education: status, prospects, and an agenda for research*. Washington: National Academies Press.

Hopkins, S., Forgasz, H., Corrigan, D., & Panizzon, D. (2014). *The STEM issue in Australia: what it is and where is the evidence?* Paper presented at the STEM Conference. Vancouver, Canada (http://stem2014.ubc.ca).

Johnson, L., Adams Becker, S., Estrada, V., & Martín, S. (2013). *Technology outlook for STEM+ education 2013–2018: an NMC horizon project sector analysis*. Austin, Texas: The New Media Consortium.

Johnson, C. C., Peters-Burton, E. E., & Moore, T. J. (2015). *STEM roadmap: a framework for integration*. London: Taylor & Francis.

Johri, A., & Olds, B. M. (Eds.). (2014). *Cambridge handbook of engineering education research*. New York: Cambridge University Press.

Kimmel, H. S., Burr-Alexander, L. E., Hirsch, L., Rockland, R. H., Carpinelli, J. D., & Aloia, M. (2014). Pathways to effective K-12 STEM programs. In *Proceedings of the 2014 IEEE Frontiers in Education Conference*. Madrid, Spain.

Lachapelle, C. P., & Cunningham, C. M. (2014). Engineering in elementary schools. In S. Purzer, J. Stroble, & M. Cardella (Eds.), *Engineering in pre-college settings: Research in synthesizing research, policy, and practices* (pp. 61–88). Lafayette, IN: Purdue University Press.

Lehrer, R., & Schauble, L. (2000). Modeling in mathematics and science. In R. Glaser (Ed.), *Advances in instructional psychology* (Vol. 5, pp. 101–159). Mahwah, NJ: Lawrence Erlbaum Associates.

Lesh, R., & Lehrer, R. (2000). Iterative refinement cycles for videotape analyses of conceptual change. In R. Lesh & A. Kelly (Eds.), *Research design in mathematics and science education* (pp. 665–708). Hillsdale, NJ: Erlbaum.

Li, Y. (2014). Editorial: International Journal of STEM Education—a platform to promote STEM education and research worldwide. *International Journal of STEM Education*, 1:1.

Lucas, B., Claxton, G., & Hanson, J. (2014). *Thinking like an engineer: implications for the education system*. Royal Academy of Engineers. www.raeng.org.uk/thinkinglikeanengineer.
Lumley, T., & Mendelovits, J. (2012). *How well do young people deal with contradictory and unreliable information on line? What the PISA digital reading assessment tells us*. Vancouver: Presented at the Annual Conference of the American Educational Research Association.
Marginson, S., Tytler, R., Freeman, B., & Roberts, K. (2013). *STEM: country comparisons*. Melbourne: Australian Council of Learned Academies.
Miles, M., & Huberman, A. (1994). *Qualitative data analysis* (2nd ed.). London: Sage Publications.
Moore, T. J., & Smith, K. A. (2014). Advancing the state of the art of STEM integration. *Journal of STEM Education, 15*(1), 5–10.
Moore, T. J., Stohlmann, M. S., Wang, H., Tank, K. M., Glancy, A. W., & Roehrig, G. H. (2014). Implementation and integration of engineering in K-12 STEM education. In S. Purzer, J. Strobel, & M. Cardella (Eds.), *Engineering in pre-college settings: Research into practice* (pp. 35–60). West Lafayette, IN: Purdue University Press.
National Science and Technology Council. (2013). *A report from the committee on STEM education*. Washington, D.C: National Science and Technology Council.
Next Generation Science Standards (USA, 2014). http://www.nextgenscience.org/
OECD (2013). *PISA 2012 assessment and analytical framework: mathematics, reading, science, problem solving and financial literacy*. OECD Publishing (http://www.oecdilibrary.org/content/book/9789264190511-en).
Office of the Chief Scientist. (2014). *Benchmarking Australian science, technology, engineering and mathematics*. Canberra: Australian Government.
Partnership for 21st Century Skills. (2011). *Framework for 21st century learning 2-page*. Retrieved from http://www.p21.org/our-work/p21-framework.
Prinsley, R., & Baranyai, K. (2015). *STEM skills in the workforce: what do employers want?* Occasional Papers Series, issue 9, March. Office of the Chief Scientist.
Purzer, S., Stroble, J., & Cardella, M. E. (Eds.). (2014). *Engineering in pre-college settings: synthesizing research, policy, and practices*. Purdue: Purdue University.
Rennie, L., Venville, G., & Wallace, J. (2012). Reflecting on curriculum integration: seeking balance and connection through a worldly perspective. In L. Rennie, G. Venville, & J. Wallace (Eds.), *Integrating science, technology, engineering, and mathematics: Issues, reflections, and ways forward* (pp. 123–142). New York: Routledge.
Rennie, L., Wallace, J., & Venville, G. (2012). Exploring curriculum integration: why integrate? In L. Rennie, G. Venville, & J. Wallace (Eds.), *Integrating science, technology, engineering, and mathematics* (pp. 1–11). New York: Routledge.
Shaughnessy, M. (2013). By way of introduction: mathematics in a STEM context. *Mathematics Teaching in the Middle school, 18*(6), 324.
Silk, E. M., Higashi, R., Shoop, R., & Schunn, C. D. (2010). Designing technology activities that teach mathematics. *The Technology Teacher, 69*(4), 21–27.
STEM Task Force Report. (2014). *Innovate: a blueprint for science, technology, engineering, and mathematics in California public education*. Dublin, California: Californians Dedicated to Education Foundation.
The National Academies. (2014). *Next generation science standards: for states, by states*. Washington: National Academy of Sciences.
The Royal Society Science Policy Centre. (2014). *Vision for science and mathematics education*. London: The Royal Society.
Thompson, S., Hillman, K., & De Bortoli, L. (2013). *A teacher's guide to PISA mathematical literacy*. Melbourne: Australian Council for Educational Research.
Vasquez, J. (2014/2015). STEM: beyond the acronym. *Educational Leadership*, Dec./Jan.,10-16.
Vasquez, J., Sneider, C., & Comer, M. (2013). *STEM lesson essentials, grades 3–8: integrating science, technology, engineering, and mathematics*. Portsmouth, NH: Heinemann.

6

Incorporating effective e-learning principles to improve student engagement in middle-school mathematics

Kevin Mulqueeny[1*], Victor Kostyuk[1], Ryan S. Baker[2] and Jaclyn Ocumpaugh[2]

Abstract

Background: The expanded use of online and blended learning programs in K-12 STEM education has led researchers to propose design principles for effective e-learning systems. Much of this research has focused on the impact on learning, but not how instructional design impacts student engagement, which has a critical impact both on short-term learning and long-term outcomes. Reasoning Mind has incorporated the e-learning principles of personalization, modality, and redundancy into the design of their next-generation blended learning platform for middle-school mathematics, named Genie 3. In three studies, we compare student engagement with the Genie 3 platform to its predecessor, Genie 2, and to traditional classroom instruction.

Results: Study 1 found very high levels of student engagement with the Genie 2 platform, with 89 % time on-task and 71 % engaged concentration. Study 2 found that students using Genie 3 spent significantly more time in independent on-task behavior and less time off-task or engaged in on task conversation with peers than students using Genie 2. Students using Genie 3 also showed more engaged concentration and less confusion. Study 3 found that students using Genie 3 spent 93 % of their time on-task, compared to 69 % in traditional classrooms. They also showed more engaged concentration and less boredom and confusion. Genie 3 students sustained their engagement for the entire class period, while engagement in the traditional classroom dropped off later in the class session. In both study 2 and 3, Genie 3 students showed more growth from pre- to post-test on an assessment of key concepts in sixth-grade mathematics.

Conclusions: The incorporation of evidence-based e-learning principles into the design of the Genie 3 platform resulted in higher levels of student engagement when compared to an earlier, well-established platform that lacked those principles, as well as when compared to traditional classroom instruction. Increased personalization, the use of multiple modalities, and minimization of redundancy resulted in significant increases in time on-task and engaged concentration, but also a decrease in peer interaction. On the whole, this evidence suggests that capturing students' attention, fostering deep learning, and minimizing cognitive load leads to improved engagement, and ultimately better educational outcomes.

Keywords: Blended learning; E-learning; Middle-school mathematics; Time on-task; Engaged concentration; BROMP

* Correspondence: Kevin.Mulqueeny@reasoningmind.org
[1]Reasoning Mind, 2000 Bering Drive, Suite 300, TX,77057, Houston
Full list of author information is available at the end of the article

Background

As online and blended learning continues to see rapid expansion in K-12 (e.g., Horn and Staker 2011), particularly in Science, Technology, Engineering, and Mathematics (STEM) fields (e.g., Heffernan and Heffernan 2014; Koedinger and Corbett 2006), a growing body of research has begun to explore and develop design principles to ensure its efficacy (e.g., Betrancourt 2005; Clark and Mayer 2011; Garrison and Anderson 2003; Govindasamy 2002). Most of this research is based on empirical investigations of individual principles. This research strategy provides strong evidence about design features in isolation, but it is less informative when it comes to understanding how they function in concert.

In addition, little research has examined how these design principles influence not just immediate domain learning, but engagement as well, which may mediate long-term student outcomes. Indeed, many studies of the cognitive benefits of design principles do not consider how the removal of potentially appealing factors may (negatively) impact student engagement (see, for instance, Harp and Mayer 1998). Particularly in real-world settings where educational software must compete with many other activities, determining whether or not design features are engaging students is a necessary component of evaluating their effectiveness, leading many to investigate behavioral and affective indicators of student engagement in STEM learning systems. While findings suggest that some time off-task can refocus bored or frustrated students (Baker et al. 2011; Sabourin et al. 2011), students who completely disengage with educational software, spending large amounts of time off task, show lower learning (Goodman 1990), both in the short-term and in the long-term, the latter a result of aggregate effects from a loss of practice opportunities (Cocea et al. 2009). Other disengaged behaviors such as carelessness and gaming the system are also associated with poor learning outcomes (Cocea et al. 2009; Pardos et al. 2014). Furthermore, findings suggest engaged concentration (or Csikszentmihalyi's "flow") is positively associated with learning, while boredom leads to poor learning outcomes (Craig et al. 2004; D'Mello and Graesser 2012; Pardos et al. 2014). Confusion and frustration have more complex relationships to learning; while necessary for learning (D'Mello et al. 2014), spending a considerable amount of time confused or frustrated is associated with worse outcomes (e.g., Liu et al. 2013). In addition, both behavioral engagement and affect are associated with long-term student participation in STEM; for example, boredom, confusion, engaged concentration, gaming the system, and carelessness in middle school mathematics are predictive of eventual college attendance (San Pedro et al. 2013), and gaming the system and carelessness are predictive of whether or not a student enrolls in a STEM degree program (San Pedro et al. 2014). Researchers are beginning to explore the relationship between design features and engagement (e.g., Baker et al. 2009; Doddannara et al. 2013; D'Mello et al. 2014), but to date few studies have explored the causal impact of well-known and widely used design principles on engagement.

One of the more comprehensive discussions of designing for multimedia learning systems has been put forward by Clark and Mayer (2011), who present eight principles based on previous research. These include the following: (1) *Personalization*: Use a conversational style, polite speech, and virtual coaches (Moreno et al. 2001). (2) *Multimedia*: Use words and graphics, not words alone (Halpern et al. 2007). (3) *Contiguity*: Align words to corresponding graphics (Moreno and Mayer 1999). (4) *Coherence*: Limit extraneous information (Mayer et al. 2001). (5) *Modality*: Present words as audio, rather than text (Low and Sweller 2005). (6) *Redundancy*: Explain visuals with spoken word or text, not both (Mayer and Moreno 2003). (7) *Segmenting*: Present lessons in small, well-spaced units (Mayer and Chandler 2001). (8) *Pretraining*: Ensure that learners know the names and characteristics of key concepts (Kester et al. 2006). Each of these principles is designed to enhance learning by focusing students' attention and limiting cognitive load. Using design to focus the students' attention on the critical task of learning mathematics should minimize the attentional resources needed to inhibit distractions (Mayer and Moreno 2003), allowing for greater and more prolonged attention to be paid to learning.

In this paper, we investigate whether design changes that reflect three of Clark and Mayer's (2011) principles—*Personalization, Modality,* and *Redundancy*—improve student engagement with an online STEM learning system, Reasoning Mind. Developed by the nonprofit company of the same name, Reasoning Mind currently provides blended learning instruction in mathematics to over 100,000 students in the United States. Reasoning Mind works with expert teachers to design online learning experiences that recreate best-practices for instruction (Khachatryan et al. 2014), providing elementary and middle school curricula that focuses on fostering deep understanding of core mathematical topics necessary for students' later success in algebra. Having instruction delivered by the computer frees teachers to conduct the sort of targeted interventions with struggling students that research suggests is most effective at improving student learning (Bush and Kim 2014; Waxman and Houston 2012). In this paper, we study whether design changes to this platform, which reflect Clark and Mayer's principles, have a positive impact on student engagement.

Methods

The Reasoning Mind blended learning systems

In this article, we will study two generations of Reasoning Mind's online learning systems: Genie 2 and Genie 3, used by elementary and middle school students. Reasoning Mind developed the Genie 2 platform in 2005, designing instruction in line with the practices of expert teachers (Khachatryan et al. 2014) within a system where students receive immediate, individualized feedback while learning, primarily from a pedagogical agent known as the Genie. However, the design of this platform did not purposefully incorporate research-based principles of e-learning such as those in Clark and Mayer (2011). As of 2013, Reasoning Mind has been piloting the next-generation Genie 3 platform, which explicitly incorporates three instructional design principles previously found to increase learning gains in online instruction (Clark and Mayer 2011). The improvements made in Genie 3 to incorporate the *personalization*, *modality*, and *redundancy* principles are outlined in Table 1.

Genie 2

The Genie 2 platform presents students an online environment named RM City (see Fig. 1), where different buildings represent different types of learning activities. *Guided Study* is the main learning mode, where students study curriculum objectives. In *Homework*, students enter answers to mathematics problems chosen by the system based on the student's progress and prior performance. These problems are printed out and given as homework by the teacher. The student completes the problems at home and then types in the answers at the beginning of class. The *Office* allows teachers to assign individual objectives from Guided Study or practice problems for material that the student needs to focus on. The *Wall of Mastery* provides students opportunities to challenge themselves with more difficult problems. Throughout the system, the Genie acts as an empathic virtual guide, providing solutions and encouragement.

In *Guided Study*, where students spend the majority of their time in the Reasoning Mind system, the curriculum is divided into a series of objectives, or mathematical topics, for students to complete. Examples of objectives include "Numerical Expressions with Parentheses", "Comparing Fractions with Different Denominators", and "Rounding Decimals." Each objective consists of a sequence of pedagogical stages: warm up, theory instruction, a notes test, a series of increasingly difficult practice problems, and a review. As students progress through each stage of an objective, their progress is charted on a virtual map (Fig. 2). Objectives contain animated stories with a recurring cast of characters, as well as illustrations and animations that closely correspond to the problems students are solving. All instruction is delivered through text, with optional narration that reads out the text on the screen. Illustrations and accompanying explanatory text are positioned closely to facilitate comprehension (Moreno and Mayer 1999).

Objectives are strictly sequenced based on prerequisite skills, but a student's progress through an objective is self-paced, allowing the student to navigate forward and backward to review the material. Upon successful completion of an objective—defined by an accuracy cutoff—the student proceeds to the next objective in the sequence. When a student fails an objective, the system uses automatic diagnostics and remediation to fill in gaps in understanding that are hindering progress. Strong students move quickly and are challenged with more difficult problems.

Genie 3

The Genie 3 platform has a less cartoon-like home screen than Genie 2 (see Fig. 3). It includes some of the same learning activities from the earlier platforms (*Guided Study*, *Homework*, and *Wall of Mastery*) but it also adds the *Test Center*, where students complete tests and quizzes, and the *Math Journal*, a repository of the key rules and definitions provided by the system from the lessons the student has completed.

In the Genie 3 platform, *Guided Study* is redesigned to simulate ideal classroom experiences provided by expert teachers. As such, students control a customizable avatar (see Fig. 4), completing daily lessons in a virtual small-group session with a simulated tutor and two simulated peers. While Genie 2's characters, including the Genie, are used mainly for motivation, positive feedback, and emphasis of key points, Genie 3's rotating cast of three tutors and seven peers act as full pedagogical agents (cf.

Table 1 Improved implementation of e-learning principles in the Genie 3 platform

E-Learning principle	Genie 2	Genie 3
Personalization	"The Genie" is a limited pedagogical agent who only provides motivation, in text only, but does use a conversational style.	Virtual tutors and peers are full pedagogical agents and virtual coaches. They use conversational but polite speech, and are voiced by human narrators. Students have customizable avatars.
Modality	Entirely text-based with optional text-to-speech.	Prioritizes narrative, auditory instruction over text.
Redundancy	Audio is matched to on-screen text word for word.	Spoken narration and written text complement each other, and mostly do not match.

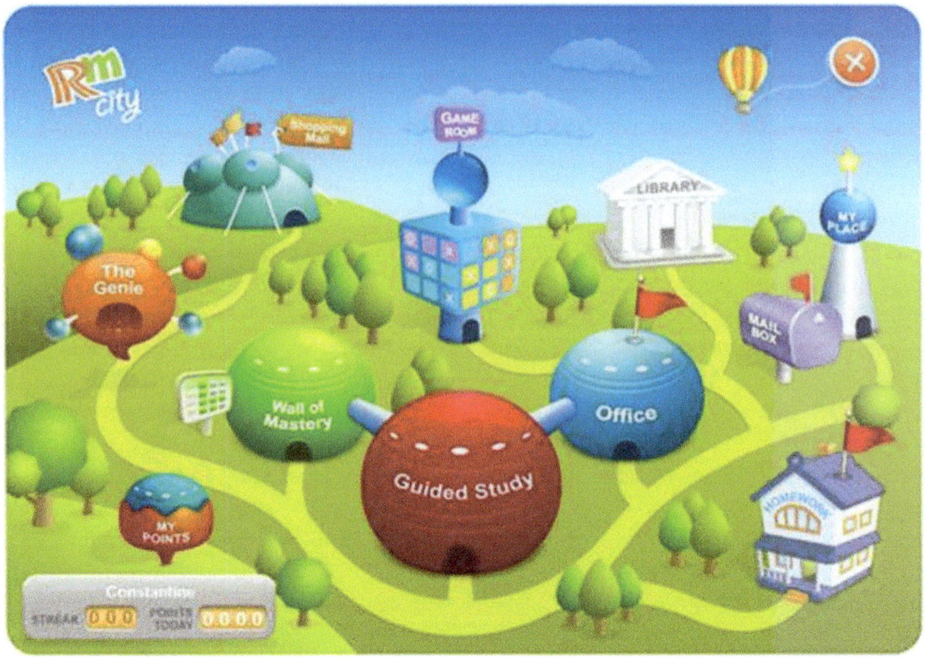

Fig. 1 Genie 2 home screen

Forsyth et al. 2014). The tutors lead the instruction of the lessons, ask the student or virtual peers to solve problems, and prompt the real student to evaluate the virtual peer's solution or work collaboratively, solving individual parts of a multi-step problem. Virtual peers model positive attitudes toward mathematics, demonstrate common misconceptions, and play a motivational role, encouraging the real student, sympathizing with difficulties, and emphasizing the value of persistence and hard work. All of the agents use an informal conversational style, in line with the principle of *personalization* (Moreno et al. 2001), and are narrated

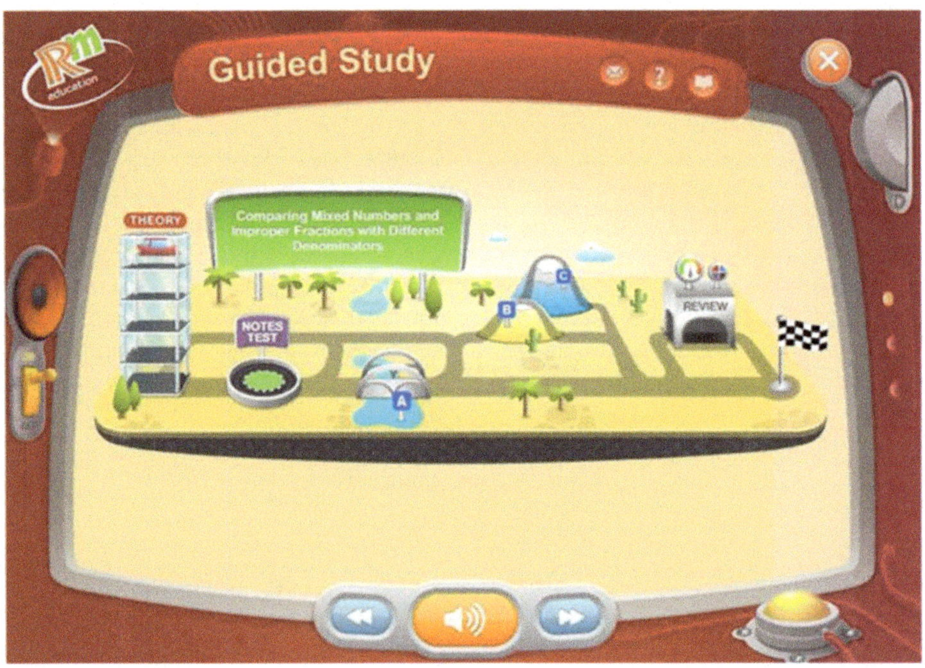

Fig. 2 Genie 2 Guided Study

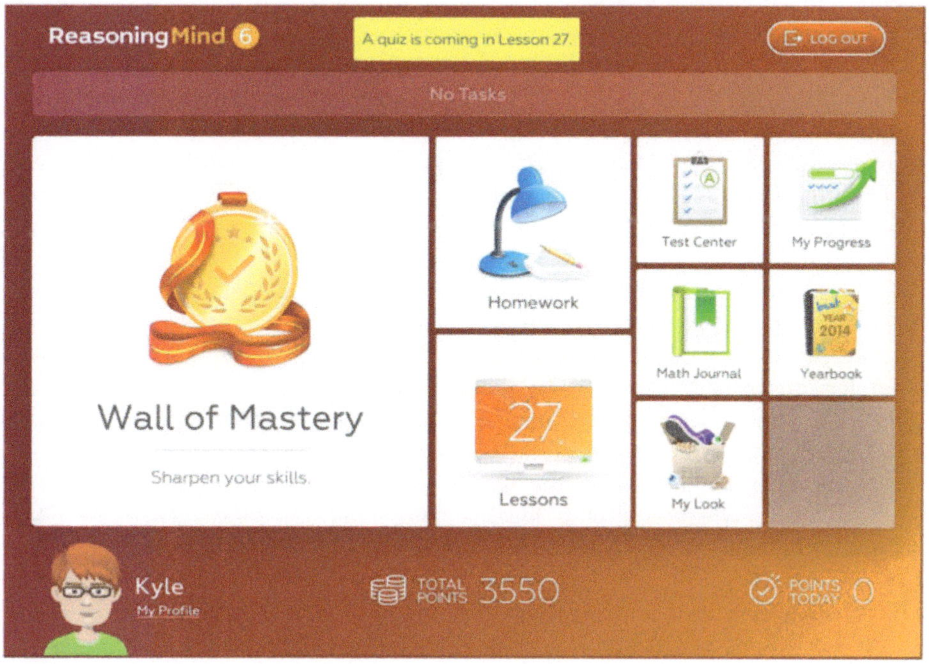

Fig. 3 Genie 3 home screen

by voice actors, supporting multiple *modalities* (Low and Sweller 2005).

The small-group lesson environment uses a shared virtual white board, where diagrams, problems, key definitions, rules, and statements are written, and where students work to solve problems. No other text is presented; spoken narration is used to carry the majority of instruction, a design choice in keeping with the principles of *modality* (Low and Sweller 2005) and *redundancy* (Mayer and Moreno 2003). Diagrams and illustrations are paired closely with explanatory labels and text, in line with the *continuity* principle (Moreno and Mayer 1999). Lessons are broken up into pedagogical segments corresponding to classroom lessons. Typically, lessons include

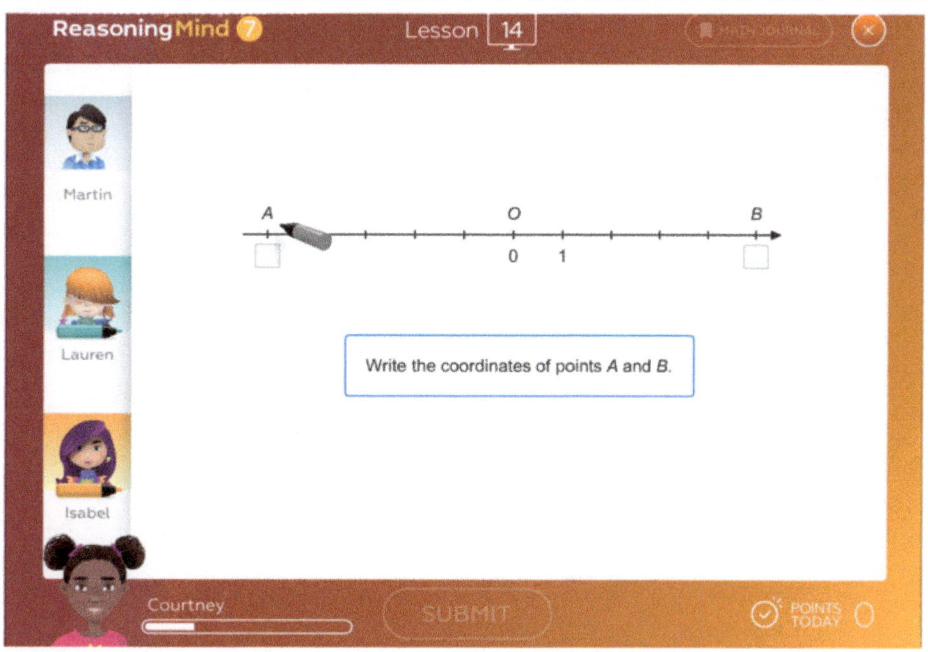

Fig. 4 Genie 3 Guided Study

a warm-up, introduction of new material, a series of practice problems, and review. Completion of the lesson is tracked on a progress bar at the bottom of the screen.

Measuring student engagement

Engagement is a concept that has been defined in many ways (see review in Fredricks et al. 2004). Finn and Zimmer (2012) outline four components of engagement thought to impact student learning and achievement: academic, social, cognitive, and affective. Both academic and social engagements are comprised of behavioral indicators (treated as a single construct in Fredricks et al. 2004). The former refers to behaviors related to the learning process, while the latter reflects whether or not the student follows written and unwritten rules for classroom behavior. Cognitive engagement involves the use of mental resources to comprehend complex ideas. Affective engagement is the emotional response and feelings of involvement in school.

Previous research has often examined these constructs using survey methods. For example, Finn et al. (1991) administered a questionnaire to teachers, finding that academic behaviors that reflect effort and initiative are positively correlated with end of year achievement test scores ($r = 0.40$ to 0.59), while inattentive behavior is negatively correlated with achievement ($r = -0.52$ to -0.34). More recently, research has found a significant relationship between academic and social engagement in fourth and eighth grades and high-school graduation (Finn and Zimmer 2012).

In this paper, student engagement measures (discussed more thoroughly in the next section) are investigated in series of three field observation studies that investigate the effect of the Reasoning Mind mathematics curricula on the prevalence of these indicators. Study 1 reports on observations of student engagement that were conducted when students were using the Genie 2 platform. Study 2 uses the same observation method to compare the engagement of students using Genie 2 to those using Genie 3. Finally, study 3 compares students using Genie 3 to students in a traditional mathematics classroom (with no technological support).

BROMP field observations

Quantitative field observations of student engagement were collected using the Baker Rodrigo Ocumpaugh Monitoring Protocol (or BROMP), an established observation method with over 150 certified coders in four countries (Ocumpaugh et al. 2015). BROMP has been used to investigate behavioral and affective indicators of student engagement in a number of different online learning environments (e.g., Baker et al. 2010; Paquette et al. 2014; Pardos et al. 2014; Rodrigo et al. 2008), including research on college attendance and engagement within ASSISTments (San Pedro et al. 2013, 2014).

Within this method, trained observers repeatedly record observations of educationally relevant behavior and affect of students individually, in a pre-determined order, ensuring roughly equal samples of each student's behavior. Observers record the first behavior and affect they see, but have up to 20 s to make that decision. In this study, behavior codes included *On Task—Independent* (i.e., working alone on an assigned task), *On Task—Conversation* (i.e., discussing work with a peer or teacher), *Off Task* (i.e., not working on their assigned task), and *Gaming the System* (i.e., systematic guessing or use of hints to obtain answers rather than learning)—all of which are typically coded for during BROMP observations. However in studies 2 and 3, the category of *On-Task Conversation* was split into two categories: *On-Task—Proactive Remediation,* which was coded when students received individual or small group interventions from the teacher (Miller et al., 2015), and all other *On-Task—Conversation* behaviors. Affective states included *Engaged Concentration, Boredom, Confusion, Frustration, and Delight* (D'Mello et al. 2010). Cases where the student had stepped out of class or their behavior or affect were otherwise impossible to classify or outside the coding scheme were coded as *Other* and are not included in the analysis. All observers in this study were BROMP-certified (Ocumpaugh et al. 2015), meaning that they had obtained an acceptable inter-rater reliability (Cohen's Kappa >0.6 on each coding scheme) with a previously certified BROMP coder during training sessions identical to the observations performed in all three studies.

Research questions

Research Question 1: Is the Reasoning Mind program more engaging than traditional classroom instruction? We hypothesize that students using these blended learning systems (both Genie 2 and Genie 3) will show greater levels of student engagement than students participating in traditional, face-to-face instruction.

Research Question 2: Is the Genie 3 platform more engaging than Genie 2? We hypothesize that the improvements to Genie 3 in the domains of *personalization, modality,* and *redundancy* (Clark and Mayer 2011) will lead to improved student engagement.

Method

Study 1 Method

In study 1, students who are using the Reasoning Mind Genie 2 platform were observed. In this first, pilot study, only one condition was observed; it is included here as it gave a baseline for engagement in the most established version of the Reasoning Mind blended learning system and inspired the remaining two studies.

Fifth-grade students from three different schools in the Texas Gulf Coast region were observed while using Genie 2 as their regular mathematics curriculum. Two schools were in urban areas with large class sizes (approximately 25 students each) and served predominantly minority populations (one mostly Latino and the other African American). The third was a suburban charter school with smaller classes (approximately 15 students each) and a predominantly White population. For each of the three schools, two classes were observed for one class period. Due to a data collection error, student IDs were not linked to the observations, in any form; as such, it is infeasible to conduct statistical significance tests of engagement without violating independence assumptions. However, each student was sampled an equal number of times, making averaging across students feasible.

Results and discussion

Results are given in Table 2. The overall incidence of behavior and affect indicates high engagement. Students were *on-task* 89 % of the time, which is higher than values observed in Cognitive Tutor classrooms in U.S. suburban middle schools (Baker et al. 2004) or traditional classrooms (Lloyd and Loper 1986; Lee et al. 1999). *Gaming the system*, where students misuse the software in order to succeed without learning, is almost non-existent, suggesting that students are taking the program seriously. Patterns of affect also indicated high levels of engagement, with students exhibiting high levels of *engaged concentration* (71 %) and relatively low levels of *boredom* (10 %). Low-to-moderate levels of *confusion* (9 %) and *frustration* (7 %) are on par with previous studies (Pardos et al. 2014) and suggest that students are being challenged to learn new material. These results demonstrate that Genie 2, which has been used annually by tens of thousands of elementary students over the last 10 years, is already quite engaging.

Table 2 Count and percentage of observations of each behavior and affective state

BROMP category		Number	%
Behavior	On Task	243	82
	On Task Conversation	20	7
	Off Task	31	10
	Gaming	2	1
Affect	Engaged Concentration	194	71
	Boredom	27	10
	Confusion	24	9
	Frustration	19	7
	Delight	9	3

Study 2 Method

Study 2 compares student engagement with the Genie 2 platform to the newly developed Genie 3. As explained above, this platform's design, which targets middle-school students, offers continuity with the Genie 2 platform, but incorporates improvements in several research-based e-learning principles, particularly including personalization, multimedia, and modality.

Study 2 employs a quasi-experimental design. Teachers within the same school were assigned to teach with the traditional or Genie 3 curriculum by the school principal, and students were non-randomly assigned to each group for the school year. Both groups were observed once in the fall semester and again in the spring. The observation procedure was similar to study 1. Two BROMP-certified coders conducted the observations. In this study, observers did not code for *Gaming the System*, which was all but non-existent in study 1, but they did include an additional behavioral category. Because one of the anticipated benefits of blended learning is that it frees teachers to engage more frequently in targeted interventions, BROMP observers also coded for *On Task—Proactive Remediation*, as discussed above. These cases were previously coded as *On Task—Conversation*, so we would expect a comparable reduction in that behavior compared to study 1.

The subjects we observed in this study were sixth-grade students in a small, central Texas City, with a student population that is one-third Latino and one-third White. We observed six classes (126 students in the fall and 125 in the spring) using the new Genie 3 platform and six classes (122 students in the fall and 123 in the spring) using the Genie 2 platform. The two groups performed equivalently on a pre-test measure of key topics in sixth-grade mathematics. The Genie 3 group scored an average of 32.63 % (SD = 17.06), while the Genie 2 group averaged 32.72 % correct (SD = 14.49), an effect size (Cohen's d) of 0.006.

Results and discussion

Observations (2966) were collected from the Genie 3 classrooms (1570 in the fall and 1396 in the spring) and 2764 observations were collected from Genie 2 classrooms (1510 in the fall and 1254 in the spring). Average distributions for these codes are given in Fig. 5.

Proportional data are constrained and tend not to be normally distributed; this was particularly the case here, with very many students having either very high or very low proportions of engagement in any one behavior or affective category. Table 3 shows the measurements of skewness and kurtosis for each of the behaviors and affects observed. Applying the rule of thumb that the ratio of skewness and kurtosis to the corresponding standard error should be within ±2.58, only the *On Task—Independent* behavior in Genie 2 classes had suitably low

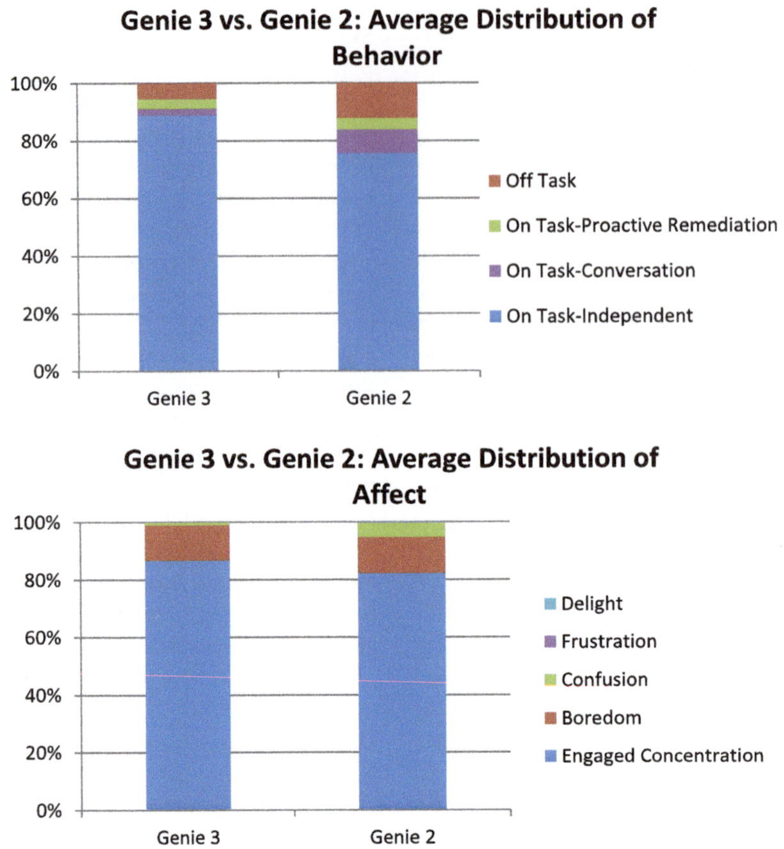

Fig. 5 Average distribution of behavior and affect, Genie 2 vs. Genie 3

kurtosis, but all distributions were skewed beyond normality. Because the proportional data was not normally distributed, we applied an arcsine transformation (calculating the arcsine of the square root) to the proportion of observations classified in a given behavioral or affective category. This transformation is used to normalize the distribution of proportional data, which are limited to values between 0 and 1. By extending this range, we expand the difference between extreme values (near 0 and 1) and compress the difference between central values (near 0.5; McDonald 2014). With more normally distributed data, we were able to perform an analysis of variance (ANOVA) for each behavior and affective state to compare the frequency in each group of students.

Table 3 Skewness and kurtosis of behavior and affect distributions for study 2

		Genie 3		Genie 2	
		Skewness (SE = 0.16)	Kurtosis (SE = 0.31)	Skewness (SE = 0.16)	Kurtosis (SE = 0.31)
Behavior	On Task—Independent	−1.98	7.10	−1.11	*0.60*
	On Task—Conversation	3.02	9.99	2.34	7.40
	On Task—Proactive Remediation	2.50	6.64	4.05	16.18
	Off Task	3.82	21.63	1.89	4.36
Affect	Engaged Concentration	−2.05	5.18	−1.09	0.97
	Boredom	2.19	5.69	1.53	2.90
	Confusion	3.96	17.50	2.34	5.98
	Frustration	15.75	248.00	12.64	167.15
	Delight	–	–	15.75	248.00

Acceptable ratios of skewness and kurtosis to SE are within ±2.58. Measures in italics are within the acceptable range

The ANOVA found that, for both semesters, students using Genie 3 spent more time in *On Task—Independent* (88.9 vs. 75.7 %, $F(1494) = 61.22$, $p < 0.001$) and less in *On-Task Conversations* (2.4 % vs. 8.3 %, $F(1494) = 62.44$, $p < 0.001$) and *Off Task* (5.4 % vs. 12.0 %, $F(1494) = 33.37$, $p < 0.001$). There was not a significant difference in the time spent in *On Task—Proactive Remediation* (Fall: 3.3 vs. 4.0 %, $F(1494) = 1.11$, $p = 0.293$, *ns*).

Similarly, we used an arcsine transformation of the proportion of each student's observations classified as each affective state. ANOVA found significantly higher levels of *engaged concentration* for Genie 3 students (86.8 vs. 82.3 %, $F(1494) = 9.90$, $p < 0.005$) and less *confusion* (1.0 vs. 5.0 %, $F(1494) = 46.19$, $p < 0.001$). There were not significant differences in *boredom* (12.2 vs. 12.5 %, $F(1494) = 0.27$, $p = 0.603$, *ns*), *frustration* (0.0 vs. 0.2 %, $F(1494) = 1.15$, $p = 0.283$, *ns*), *or delight* (0.0 vs. 0.0 %, $F(1249) = 1.00$, $p = 0.318$, *ns*).

In addition to determining whether engagement indicators differed across these two conditions, we were also interested in determining whether temporal dynamics might be influencing these results. Specifically, we evaluated whether engagement indicators shifted over the course of a lesson-period by comparing average distributions in the first 30 min of class and the second 30 min. Again, we performed an arcsine transformation of the proportional data, and used ANOVA to compare each behavior and affect category in the chosen timeframe.

There was a significant increase in the time *Off Task* in the Genie 3 classes during the second half of the class (3.8 vs. 7.3 %, $F(1469) = 5.18$, $p < 0.05$). This corresponded to a moderate decrease in *On Task—Independent:* (90.5 vs. 85.6 %, $F(1469) = 3.51$, $p = 0.062$, *ns*), but there were no changes in other behavior rates (*On Task—Conversation:* 2.0 vs. 3.2 %, $F(1469) = 1.92$, $p = 0.166$, *ns*; *On Task—Proactive Remediation:* 3.8 vs. 3.9 %, $F(1469) = 0.19$, $p = 0.665$, *ns*), nor among the affective states (*Engaged Concentration*: 88.7 vs. 85.0 %, $F(1469) = 2.38$, $p = 0.124$, *ns*; *Boredom:* 10.3 vs. 13.5 %, $F(1469) = 2.07$, $p = 0.151$, *ns*; *Confusion:* 0.9 vs. 1.5 %, $F(1469) = 0.47$, $p = 0.494$, *ns*; *Frustration:* 0.00 vs. 0.02 %, $F(1469) = 1.10$, $p = 0.294$, *ns*; *Delight:* No Variance).

These results contrast to the Genie 2 classes, where neither the behavioral nor the affective indicators of engagement changed from one-half hour to the next, for any construct (*On Task—Independent:* 76.7 vs. 79.6 %, $F(1465) = 2.09$, $p = 0.149$, *ns*; *On Task—Conversation:* 8.0 vs. 7.2 %, $F(1465) = 0.61$, $p = 0.437$, *ns*; *On Task—Proactive Remediation:* 3.37 vs. 3.36 %, $F(1465) = 0.02$, $p = 0.890$, *ns*; *Off Task*: 12.0 vs. 9.8 %, $F(1465) = 2.14$, $p = 0.144$, *ns*; *Engaged Concentration:* 84.0 vs. 83.0 %, $F(1465) = 0.02$, $p = 0.881$, *ns*; *Boredom:* 11.1 vs. 12.3 %, $F(1465) = 0.01$, $p = 0.934$, *ns; Confusion:* 4.69 vs. 4.66 %, $F(1465) = 0.75$, $p = 0.388$, *ns*; *Frustration:* 0.10 vs. 0.08 %, $F(1465) = 0.01$, $p = 0.942$, *ns*; *Delight:* 0.1 vs. 0.0 %, $F(1465) = 1.72$, $p = 0.191$, *ns*).

At the end of the school year, students in both groups completed the same assessment of key topics in sixth-grade mathematics that was given as a pre-test in the fall. Genie 3 students improved significantly more than Genie 2 over the course of the year, improving 25.41 percentage points on average compared to 16.47 ($t(209) = 4.60$, $p < 0.001$), an effect size of 0.63 standard deviations.

The improvements in the Genie 3 platform over Genie 2 improved students' *independent time on-task* and *engaged concentration* while reducing *time off-task*. The lack of a difference in time spent in *proactive remediation* suggests that design differences, which were aimed at changing the students' engagement, did not impact the frequency in which teachers offered help to individual students. This is not surprising, since teachers typically seek to maximize the time they can spend delivering this kind of instruction, regardless of the educational software students are using. The more frequent occurrence of *On-Task Conversation* in Genie 2 classes is likely due to the use of audio instruction in Genie 3 that requires students wear headphones, making it more difficult for students to talk to each other. It is possible that this is also the cause for the change in time *on-task* as well.

Study 3 Method

The design and procedure was identical to that of study 2, except for the use of a traditional instruction control, rather than the Genie 2 platform, and the number of subjects. Students were arbitrarily assigned to classes (i.e., not randomly), and the principal assigned two teachers to the traditional instruction condition and two to the Genie 3 condition, again not randomly. The traditional, face-to-face instruction classes included teacher lectures, individual worksheet exercises, whole-class work on an overhead projector, and work in pairs and small groups. Teachers did not use a complete, published curriculum, but pulled material from a variety of sources. The use of multimedia materials, such as videos or smart boards, was not observed, and the classrooms did not have computers present.

We observed 12 sixth-grade classrooms at one middle school in a majority Latino, urban Texas school district. In the fall, six classes (118 students) used the Genie 3 curriculum and four classes (95 students) received traditional classroom instruction. In the spring the same six classes using Reasoning Mind (109 students) and six classes using the traditional curriculum (132 students) were observed.[1] The two groups did not significantly differ on a Reasoning Mind-developed pre-test measure of key topics in sixth-grade mathematics, the Genie 3 group answered an average of 32.00 % of questions correct (SD = 13.11), while the traditional instruction group averaged 28.37 % questions correct (SD = 17.03), an effect size (Cohen's *d*) of 0.23.

Results and discussion

Observers collected 3085 observations from Genie 3 classes (1649 in the fall and 1436 in the spring) and 2879 observations from traditional classrooms (1131 in the fall and 1748 in the spring). Average distributions for these observations are given in Fig. 6. They show, broadly, that Genie 3 students spent more time on task and in engaged concentration.

Table 4 shows the measurements of skewness and kurtosis for each of the behaviors and affects observed in study 3. Applying the rule of thumb that the ratio of skewness and kurtosis to the corresponding standard error should be within ±2.58, only four of the ten distributions had suitably low kurtosis, but all distributions were skewed beyond normality. As in study 2, we used an arcsine transformation of the proportion of each student's observations classified as each behavioral category. ANOVA results show that the average proportions of all behavioral categories were significantly different when comparing the Genie 3 students to those in traditional classrooms. Genie 3 students spent more time in *On Task—Independent* (84.5 vs. 60.9 %, $F(1452) = 198.92$, $p < 0.001$), more time in *On Task—Proactive Remediation* (7.3 vs. 0.0 %, $F(1452) = 61.00$, $p < 0.001$), less time in *On-Task—Conversation* (1.5 vs. 7.8 %, $F(1452) = 106.17$, $p < 0.001$), and less time *Off Task* (6.7 vs. 31.3 %, $F(1452) = 380.99$, $p < 0.001$) than students in the traditional classroom.

As with the behavioral data, ANOVA results show that the two groups are significantly different in terms of their affective engagement measures. Genie 3 students showed higher levels of *engaged concentration* (74.8 vs. 66.2 %, $F(1452) = 23.72$, $p < 0.001$), less *boredom* (23.3 vs. 30.5 %, $F(1452) = 19.34$, $p < 0.001$), less *confusion* (1.8 vs. 3.1 %, $F(1452) = 16.02$, $p < 0.001$), and less *delight* (0.0 vs. 0.3 %, $F(1452) = 7.02$, $p < 0.01$) than students in the traditional classroom. Only *frustration* did not show a significant difference between conditions (0.1 vs. 0.0 %, $F(1452) = 3.73$, $p = 0.054$, *ns*).

As in study 2, we compared the behavior and affect observed in the first half hour of class against the second half hour (See Fig. 7). In this case, results show that

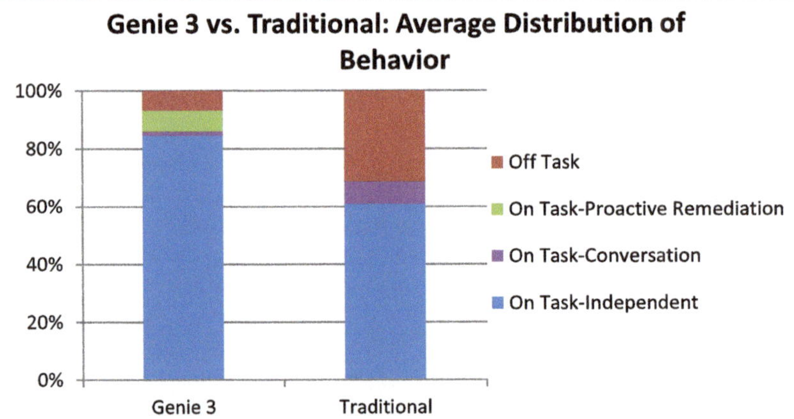

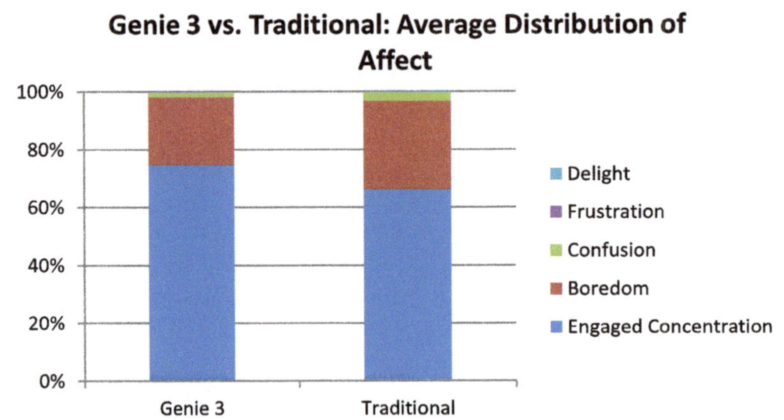

Fig. 6 Average distribution of behavior and affect, Genie 3 vs. traditional instruction

Table 4 Skewness and kurtosis of behavior and affect distributions for study 3

		Genie 3		Traditional classroom	
		Skewness (SE = 0.16)	Kurtosis (SE = 0.32)	Skewness (SE = 0.16)	Kurtosis (SE = 0.32)
Behavior	On Task—Independent	−1.67	2.71	−0.45	*0.10*
	On Task—Conversation	2.30	4.34	1.89	3.79
	On Task—Proactive Remediation	2.90	9.87	15.07	227.00
	Off Task	3.15	11.81	0.70	0.62
Affect	Engaged Concentration	−0.97	*0.22*	−0.72	*−0.21*
	Boredom	1.15	0.82	0.78	*0.03*
	Confusion	5.32	32.85	1.97	3.62
	Frustration	9.56	97.66	–	–
	Delight	–	–	6.29	41.13

Acceptable ratios of skewness and kurtosis to SE are within ±2.58. Measures in italics are within the acceptable range

Genie 3 students sustain high engagement throughout their lessons. In this condition, there were no significant changes in any behavioral or affective category from the first to second 30-min period (*On Task—Independent*: 87.2 vs. 82.9 %, $F(1411) = 1.96$, $p = 0.162$, *ns*; *On Task—Conversation*: 1.1 vs. 1.3 %, $F(1411) = 0.13$, $p = 0.724$, *ns*; *On Task—Proactive Remediation*: 6.2 vs. 9.1 %, $F(1411) = 1.41$, $p = 0.236$, *ns*; *Off Task:* 5.5 vs. 6.6 %, $F(1411) = 0.23$, $p = 0.633$, *ns*; *Engaged Concentration*: 76.2 vs. 76.6 %, $F(1411) = 0.50$, $p = 0.482$, *ns*; *Boredom:* 21.4 vs. 21.9 %,

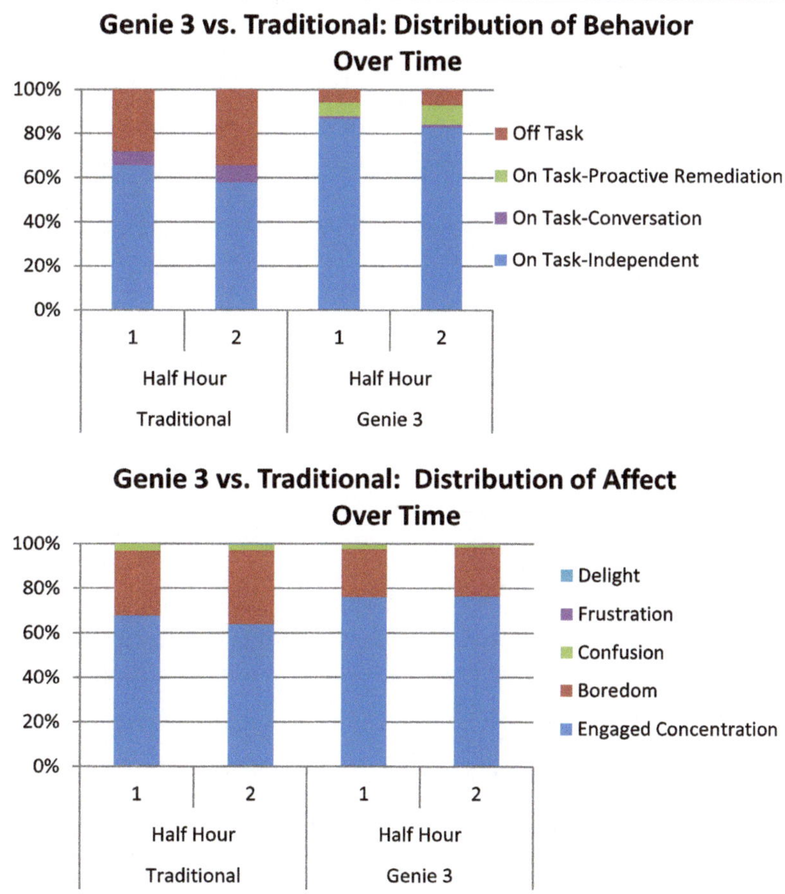

Fig. 7 Average distribution of behavior and affect by half-hour, Genie 3 vs. traditional instruction

$F(1411) = 0.09$, $p = 0.763$, *ns*; *Confusion:* 2.2 vs. 1.5 %, $F(1411) = 0.73$, $p = 0.395$, *ns*; *Frustration:* 2.9 vs. 2.2 %, $F(1411) = 0.67$, $p = 0.413$, *ns*; *Delight:* No variance).

Students in traditional classrooms, however, showed decreased engagement over the course of a lesson-period. Here, *independent on task behavior* dropped significantly in the second half hour, from 65.5 to 58 % ($F(1452) = 9.91$, $p < 0.005$), while *Off-Task behavior* increased from 28.2 to 34.2 % ($F(1452) = 9.02$, $p < 0.005$). There was a moderate increase in *On-Task Conversation*, from 6.2 to 7.8 % ($F(1452) = 3.88$, $p = 0.05$, *ns*) and no change in *proactive remediation* (0.00 vs. 0.04 %, $F(1452) = 1.00$, $p = 0.318$, *ns*). Among affective states, the traditional classroom students saw a significant increase in *delight* (0.0 vs. 0.3 %, $F(1452) = 5.98$, $p < 0.05$); however, this should not be seen as a positive development, as further investigation discovered that all cases of *delight* corresponded with *Off-Task behavior*. There was a moderate increase in *boredom*, from 29.0 to 33.1 % ($F(1452) = 3.05$, $p = 0.081$, *ns*), while *engaged concentration* (67.8 vs. 63.9 %, $F(1452) = 2.15$, $p = 0.144$, *ns*), *confusion* (3.2 vs. 2.7 %, $F(1452) = 0.00$, $p = 0.950$, *ns*), and *frustration* (0.0 vs. 0.0 %, no variance) did not change.

At the end of the school year, students in both groups completed the same assessment of key topics in sixth-grade mathematics that was given as a pre-test in the fall. Genie 3 students improved significantly more than traditional instruction over the course of the year, improving 21.70 percentage points on average compared to 9.81 ($t(221) = 6.03$, $p < 0.001$), an effect size of 0.81 standard deviations.

The Genie 3 students demonstrated consistently higher levels of engagement than students in the traditional classroom, and while engagement, particularly time on task, decreased over the course of the lesson in the traditional classrooms, Genie 3 students sustained engagement throughout the entire class.

Conclusions

In terms of Research Question #1, all three of these studies found very high levels of student engagement when using the Reasoning Mind blended learning program, in support of our initial hypothesis. In both the Genie 2 elementary school platform and the Genie 3 middle school platform, Reasoning Mind students demonstrated over 65 % of engaged concentration and over 85 % time on-task. These high levels of engagement are sustained for an entire hour-long mathematics lesson. Continued engagement creates a greater opportunity for student learning, and as discussed above, increases achievement (Finn et al. 1991) and odds of high-school graduation (Finn and Zimmer 2012). Several of the e-learning principles discussed in the introduction (Clark and Mayer 2011) serve to capture a student's focus, hold it, and minimize cognitive load (Chandler and Sweller 1991; van Merriënboer and Sweller 2005). A few principles are used similarly in both Genie 2 and 3. By the very nature of blended learning, both employ multimedia, with a mixture of words and graphics (Halpern et al. 2007), although Genie 3 uses significantly more audio than Genie 2. Lessons in both platforms use segmenting (Mayer and Chandler 2001) to allow for frequent mental breaks as the lesson is split up into chunks that are more easily digested and allow students to see the progress they are making. Contiguity (Moreno and Mayer 1999) and coherence (Mayer et al. 2001) limit the cognitive load of instruction by using visual information to support comprehension and restricting unnecessary information that would require the use of additional cognitive resources to inhibit (Pasolunghi et al. 1999).

Pre-post measures of mathematics achievement also found that increased engagement corresponded with greater mathematics learning gains. In both studies 2 and 3, Genie 3 students improved their performance approximately 10 percentage points more than the comparison groups. These findings lend further support to previous findings that increases in student engagement correspond with better learning outcomes (Craig et al. 2004; D'Mello and Graesser 2012; Pardos et al. 2014).

Research Question #2 considered the differences in the design of the two Reasoning Mind platforms. Several principles are emphasized in Genie 3 over Genie 2 that may account for the differences observed in study 2, where students were significantly more engaged in Genie 3, again, supporting our hypothesis. Applying the modality and redundancy principles, Genie 3 presents the instruction predominantly as audio and supplements it with text. This serves two purposes: to enhance learning through dual processing (Mayer and Moreno 1998) and to limit distractions to learning as students use headphones to listen to their own instruction. The personalization of Genie 3, in which students create their own avatar and engage in an informal virtual tutoring session with full pedagogical agents, encourages greater engagement than the cartoonish Genie 2 platform (Moreno et al. 2001). Further research is necessary to determine which of these improvements had the greatest impact on student engagement.

The Genie 2 platform did offer some advantages over Genie 3. For instance, although boredom was not significantly different between Genie 2 and Genie 3 in study 2, there appeared to be less boredom in Genie 2 in study 1. Future research should monitor boredom in particular to see if boredom is lower for Genie 2 within specific populations. Also concerning is the significantly lower levels of on-task conversation seen in Genie 3 compared to Genie 2, which suggests that there is little collaborative learning going on in the classroom. This is likely caused by the use of headphones to present spoken instruction. While this design choice had the benefit of reducing distractions, this benefit may come at the cost of discouraging conversation with peers. As such, it may be desirable for future versions of Genie 3 to add features which connect students with their actual peers, not just virtual ones.

It is also unclear why the consistency of behavior observed in Genie 3 students in study 3 was not seen in study 2. However, it is notable that the change in study 2 amounted to an increase in *Off-Task* behavior of 3.5 %, which, since it was almost double the rate of the first half hour, represents a statistical, but not necessarily a practical change in behavior. However, further study and replication should determine whether the consistency throughout the lessons is replicated in both Genie 2 and Genie 3.

Some limitations of the studies in this paper are that students were not randomly assigned to groups and there were no baseline measures of engagement. While this is typical of *in situ* studies, where researchers must be willing to work around the primary needs of the school, it does limit our ability to make full conclusions as to causality. On the other hand, since schools rarely make classroom assignments on a random basis, these results may be more typical of field conditions than a fully random trial would have been. Further large-scale studies will attempt to determine if the high levels of student engagement seen among Reasoning Mind students generalizes more broadly, but these results offer promising support for the engagingness of blended learning systems, particularly when they incorporate appropriate design principles.

Endnotes

[1]Note the discrepancy in the number of classes in the traditional classroom condition was due to an emergency at the school.

Abbreviations

ANOVA: analysis of variance; BROMP: Baker Rodrigo Ocumpaugh Monitoring Protocol; STEM: Science, Technology, Engineering, and Math.

Competing interests

Authors KM and VK are employed by Reasoning Mind, the nonprofit company that developed the Genie 2 and Genie 3 blended learning platforms that are the subject of this study.

Authors' contributions

KM was the primary author of the manuscript, led the data analysis, and collected data for studies 2 and 3. VK provided information about the design and implementation of the Reasoning Mind system. RB provided guidance on data analysis and substantial contributions to revising the manuscript critically. JO provided critical contributions to revision of the manuscript and interpretation of the findings. All authors read and approved the final manuscript.

Acknowledgements

We would like to thank the schools, teachers, students, and families for their cooperation with our study.

Thanks to Steven Gaudino, Matthew Labrum, and Travis Dezendorf for their help in collecting data for study 1, and Amy Altschuler for her help in collecting data for studies 2 and 3. Thanks to George Khachatryan for organizing the Genie 3 program pilot.

Author details

[1]Reasoning Mind, 2000 Bering Drive, Suite 300, TX,77057, Houston. [2]Teachers College, Columbia University, 525 West 120th Street, NY,10027, New York.

References

Baker, RS, Corbett, AT, Koedinger, KR (2004). Off-task behavior in the cognitive tutor classroom: When students game the system. *Proceedings of the SIGCHI Conference on Human Factors in Computing Systems*, 383-390. New York, NY: ACM.

Baker, RSJd, de Carvalho, AMJA, Raspat, J, Aleven, V, Corbett, AT, Koedinger, KR (2009). Educational software features that encourage and discourage "gaming the system". *Proceedings of the 14th International Conference on Artificial Intelligence in Education*. 475-482. Amsterdam, The Netherlands: IOS Press.

Baker, RS, D'Mello, SK, Rodrigo, MMT, & Graesser, AC. (2010). Better to be frustrated than bored: The incidence, persistence, and impact of learners' cognitive-affective states during interactions with three different computer-based learning environments. *International Journal of Human-Computer Studies, 68*(4), 223–241.

Baker, RSJd, Moore, G, Wagner, A, Kalka, J, Karabinos, M, Ashe, C, Yaron, D (2011). The dynamics between student affect and behavior occurring outside of educational software. *Proceedings of the 4th Bi-Annual International Conference on Affective Computing and Intelligent Interaction*, 14-24. Berlin, Germany: Springer Berlin Heidelberg.

Betrancourt, M. (2005). The animation and interactivity principles in multimedia learning. In RE Mayer (Ed.), *The Cambridge handbook of multimedia learning* (pp. 287–296). New York, NY: Cambridge University Press.

Bush, J & Kim, M (2014). Evaluation of Reasoning Mind Final Report 2013-14. Program Evaluation. *Dallas Independent School District*. http://www.dallasisd.org/cms/lib/TX01001475/Centricity/domain/98/evaluation/13-14/finalrpts/EA14-512-2-Reasoning-Mind-Program-Final.pdf. Accessed 1 March 2015.

Chandler, P, & Sweller, J. (1991). Cognitive load theory and the format of instruction. *Cognition and Instruction, 8*, 293–332.

Clark, RC, & Mayer, RE. (2011). *E-learning and the science of instruction: proven guidelines for consumers and designers of multimedia learning (3rd ed)*. San Francisco, CA: Pfeiffer.

Cocea, M, Hershkovitz, A, Baker, RSJd (2009). The impact of off-task and gaming behaviors on learning: Immediate or aggregate? *Proceedings of the 14th International Conference on Artificial Intelligence in Education*, 507-514. Amsterdam, The Netherlands: IOS Press.

Craig, S, Graesser, A, Sullins, J, & Gholson, B. (2004). Affect and learning: an exploratory look into the role of affect in learning with AutoTutor. *Journal of Educational Media, 29*(3), 241–250.

D'Mello, S, & Graesser, AC. (2012). Dynamics of affective states during complex learning. *Learning and Instruction, 22*(2), 145–157.

D'Mello, S, Lehman, BA, & Person, N. (2010). Mining collaborative patterns in tutorial dialogues. *Journal of Educational Data Mining, 2*(1), 1–37.

D'Mello, SK, Lehman, B, Pekrun, R, & Graesser, AC. (2014). Confusion can be beneficial for learning. *Learning & Instruction, 29*(1), 153–170.

Doddannara, LS, Gowda, SM, Baker, RSJ, Gowda, SM, & de Carvalho, AMJB. (2013). Exploring the relationships between design, students' affective states, and disengaged behaviors within an ITS. In HC Lane, K Yacef, J Mostow, & P Pavlik (Eds.), *Artificial intelligence in education (pp. 31-40)*. Germany: Springer Berlin Heidelberg.

Finn, JD, & Zimmer, KS. (2012). Student engagement: What is it? Why does it matter? In SL Christenson, AL Reschly, & C Wylie (Eds.), *Handbook of research on student engagement* (pp. 97–131). New York, NY: Springer Science + Business Media.

Finn, JD, Folger, J, & Cox, D. (1991). Measuring participation among elementary grade students. *Educational and Psychological Measurement, 51*, 393–402.

Forsyth, C, Li, H, & Graesser, AC. (2014). Learning by communicating in natural language with conversational agents. *Current Directions in Psychological Science, 23*(5), 374–380.

Fredricks, JA, Blumenfeld, PC, & Paris, AH. (2004). School engagement: potential of the concept, state of the evidence. *Review of Educational Research, 74*(1), 59–109.

Garrison, DR, & Anderson, T. (2003). *E-learning in the 21st century a framework for research and practice.* New York, NY: RoutledgeFalmer.

Goodman, L. (1990). *Time and learning in the special education classroom.* Albany, NY: SUNY Press.

Govindasamy, T. (2002). Successful implementation of e-learning pedagogical considerations. *Internet and Higher Education, 4*, 287–299.

Halpern, DF, Graesser, A, & Hakel, M. (2007). *25 learning principles to guide pedagogy and the design of learning environments.* Washington, DC: Association for Psychological Science Task Force on Life Long Learning at Work and at Home.

Harp, SF, & Mayer, RE. (1998). How seductive details do their damage: a theory of cognitive interest in science learning. *Journal of Educational Psychology, 90*, 414–434.

Heffernan, NT, & Heffernan, CL. (2014). The ASSISTments ecosystem: Building a platform that brings scientists and teachers together for minimally invasive research on human learning and teaching. *International Journal of Artificial Intelligence in Education, 24*(4), 470–497.

Horn, MB & Staker, H (2011). The rise of K-12 blended learning. Resource document. Innosight Institute. http://www.christenseninstitute.org/wp-content/uploads/2013/04/The-rise-of-K-12-blended-learning.pdf. Accessed 10 March 2015.

Kester, L, Kirschner, PA, & van Merriënboer, JJG. (2006). Just-in-time information presentation: improving learning a troubleshooting skill. *Contemporary Educational Psychology, 31*, 167–185.

Khachatryan, GA, Romashov, AV, Khachatryan, AR, Gaudino, SJ, Khachatryan, JM, Guarian, KR, & Yufa, NV. (2014). Reasoning Mind Genie 2: an intelligent tutoring system as a vehicle for international transfer of instructional methods in mathematics. *International Journal of Artificial Intelligence in Education, 24*(3), 333–382.

Koedinger, KR, & Corbett, AT. (2006). Cognitive tutors: technology bringing learning science to the classroom. In RK Sawyer (Ed.), *The Cambridge handbook of the learning sciences* (pp. 61–77). New York: Cambridge University Press.

Lee, SW, Kelly, KE, & Nyre, JE. (1999). Preliminary report on the relation of students' on-task behavior with completion of school work. *Psychological Reports, 84*, 267–272.

Liu, Z, Pataranutaporn, V, Ocumpaugh, J, Baker, RSJd (2013). Sequences of frustration and confusion, and learning. *Proceedings of the 6th International Conference on Educational Data Mining,* 114-120. Memphis, TN: International Educational Data Mining Society.

Lloyd, JW, & Loper, AB. (1986). Measurement and evaluation of task-related learning behavior: attention to task and metacognition. *School Psychology Review, 15*(3), 336–345.

Low, R, & Sweller, J. (2005). The modality effect in multimedia learning. In RE Mayer (Ed.), *The Cambridge handbook of multimedia learning* (pp. 147–158). New York: Cambridge University Press.

Mayer, RE, & Chandler, P. (2001). When learning is just a click away: does simple user interaction foster deeper understanding of multimedia messages? *Journal of Educational Psychology, 93*, 390–397.

Mayer, RE, & Moreno, R. (1998). A split-attention effect in multimedia learning: evidence for dual processing systems in working memory. *Journal of Educational Psychology, 90*(2), 312–20.

Mayer, RE, & Moreno, R. (2003). Nine ways to reduce cognitive load in multimedia learning. *Educational Psychologist, 38*, 43–52.

Mayer, RE, Heiser, J, & Lonn, S. (2001). Cognitive constraints on multimedia learning: when presenting more material results in less learning. *Journal of Educational Psychology, 93*, 187–198.

McDonald, JH. (2014). *Handbook of biological statistics*. Baltimore, MD: Sparky House.

Miller, WL, Baker, RS, Labrum, MJ, Petsche, K, Wagner, AZ (2015). Automated detection of proactive remediation by teachers in Reasoning Mind classrooms. *Proceedings of the FifthConference on Learning Analytics and Knowledge. 290-294. New York, NY: ACM.*

Moreno, R, & Mayer, RE. (1999). Cognitive principles of multimedia learning: the role of modality and contiguity. *Journal of Educational Psychology, 91*, 358–368.

Moreno, R, Mayer, RE, Spires, H, & Lester, J. (2001). The case for social agency in computer-based teaching: do students learn more deeply when they interact with animated pedagogical agents? *Cognition and Instruction, 19*, 177–214.

Ocumpaugh, J, Baker, RS, & Rodrigo, MMT. (2015). *Baker Rodrigo Ocumpaugh Monitoring Protocol (BROMP) 2.0 Technical and Training Manual. Technical Report.* New York, NY: EdLab. Manila, Philippines: Ateneo Laboratory for the Learning Sciences. http://www.columbia.edu/~rsb2162/BROMP.pdf. Accessed 24 March 2015.

Paquette, L, Baker, RS, Sao Pedro, MA, Gobert, JD, Rossi, L, Nakama, A, & Kauffman-Rogoff, Z. (2014). Sensor-free affect detection for a simulation-based science inquiry learning environment. In S Trausan-Matu, KE Boyer, M Crosby, & K Panourgia (Eds.), *Intelligent tutoring systems* (pp. 1–10). Switzerland: Springer International Publishing.

Pardos, ZA, Baker, RS, San Pedro, M, Gowda, SM, & Gowda, SM. (2014). Affective states and state tests: investigating how affect and engagement during the school year predict end-of-year learning outcomes. *Journal of Learning Analytics, 1*(1), 107–128.

Pasolunghi, MC, Cornoldi, C, & Liberto, S. (1999). Working memory and intrusions of irrelevant information in a group of specific poor problem solvers. *Memory & Cognition, 27*(5), 779–790.

Rodrigo, MMT, Baker, RSJd, D'Mello, S, Gonzalez, MCT, Lagud, MCV, Lim, SAL, Macapanpan, AF, Pascua, SAMS, Santillano, JQ, Sugay, JO, Tep, S, Viehland, NJB (2008). Comparing learners' affect while using an intelligent tutoring systems and a simulation problem solving game. *Proceedings of the 9th International Conference on Intelligent Tutoring Systems,* 40-49. Berlin, Germany: Springer Berlin Heidelberg.

Sabourin, J, Rowe, JP, Mott, BW, & Lester, JC. (2011). When off-task is on-task: the affective role of off-task behavior in narrative-centered learning environments. In G Biswas, S Bull, J Kay, & A Mitrovic (Eds.), *Artificial intelligence in education* (pp. 534–536). Germany: Springer Berlin Heidelberg.

San Pedro, MOZ, Baker, RS, Bowers, AJ, Heffernan, NT (2013). Predicting college enrollment from student interaction with an intelligent tutoring system in middle school. *Proceedings of the 6th International Conference on Educational Data Mining,* 177-184. Memphis, TN: International Educational Data Mining Society.

San Pedro, MOZ, Baker, RSJ, Gowda, SM, & Heffernan, NT. (2013b). Towards an understanding of affect and knowledge from student interaction with an intelligent tutoring system. In HC Lane, K Yacef, J Mostow, & P Pavlik (Eds.), *Artificial intelligence in education* (pp. 41–50). Germany: Springer Berlin Heidelberg.

San Pedro, MOZ, Ocumpaugh, JL, Baker, RS, Heffernan, NT (2014). Predicting STEM and non-STEM college major enrollment from middle school interaction with mathematics educational software. *Proceedings of the 7th International Conference on Educational Data Mining,* 276-279. Memphis, TN: International Educational Data Mining Society.

van Merriënboer, JJG, & Sweller, J. (2005). Cognitive load theory and complex learning: recent developments and future directions. *Educational Psychology Review, 17*(2), 147–177.

Waxman, HC & Houston, WR (2012). Evaluation of the 2010-2011 Reasoning Mind Program in Beaumont ISD. http://www.reasoningmind.org/wp-content/uploads/2013/11/2010-20111_Beaumont_ISD_Independent_Evaluation.pdf. Accessed 25 March 2015.

7

The effects of using exploratory computerized environments in grades 1 to 8 mathematics

Andrzej Sokolowski[1*], Yeping Li[2†] and Victor Willson[3†]

Abstract

Background: The process of problem solving is difficult for students; thus, mathematics educators have made multiple attempts to seek ways of making this process more accessible to learners. The purpose of this study was to examine the effect size statistic of utilizing exploratory computerized environments (ECEs) to support the process of word problem solving and exploration in grades 1 to 8 mathematics using meta-analysis.

Results: The findings of 24 experimental pretest and posttest studies (24 primary effect sizes) published in peer-reviewed journals between January 1, 2000, and December 31, 2013, revealed that exploratory computerized environments produced a moderate effect size (effect size (ES) = 0.60, SE = 0.03) when compared to traditional methods of instruction. A 95% confidence interval around the overall mean - C_{lower} = 0.53 and C_{upper} = 0.66 - indicated nonzero population effect and relative precision. A moderator analysis revealed differences among the effects on student achievement between traditional problem solving approaches and ECEs, favoring the latter.

Conclusions: The findings highlight the importance of providing students with opportunities to explore applications of mathematics concepts in classroom especially these supported by computers. A discussion of these findings and their potential impact on improving students' mathematical problem-solving skills, along with implications for further research, follows.

Keywords: Meta-analysis; Problem solving; Explorations; Computers; Student achievement; Grade 1 to 8 mathematics

Background

Advancement in the capabilities of varied technologies has meant that problem solving has become a domain of particular interest. While researchers have examined the use and impact of computers on presenting the content of word problems to learners (e.g., Gerofsky 2004), comparatively little research has focused on learners' use of computers to explore the relations between given problem's variables in the attempt to mathematize and solve it. Despite a wide range of interest in improving students' problem-solving skills, the rate of progress in this domain has not been satisfactory (Forster 2006; Kim & Hannafin 2011). It is still common that 'In typical elementary schools worldwide, the teaching of early arithmetic is predominantly focused on computational proficiency' (Greer et al. 2007, p. 97).

High interactivity of contemporary software that allows for dynamically representing problem contents are not utilized fully in mathematics classrooms yet and 'The *royal road* to the educational use of computers, software and communication technology within mathematics teaching and learning is still to be discovered, if it ever exists' (Laborde & Sträßer 2010, p. 125). Although more elements of explorations, such as measurement and data analysis, have received substantial attention in the newly developed common core standards (Porter et al. 2011), the process of inquiry organization in mathematics classes is not widely researched. Modern technology provides multiple opportunities for applying mathematical structures to quantify system changes (Arthur & Nance 2007; Pead et al. 2007). Moreover 'what technology has done is to return, after an absence of maybe a hundred or

* Correspondence: asokolowski@neo.tamu.edu
†Equal contributors
[1]Department of Mathematics and Science, Lone Star College, Tomball, TX 77375, USA
Full list of author information is available at the end of the article

two hundred years, return mathematics back into the full spectrum of science' (Pollak 2007, p. 117).

It is hypothesized that by enriching the process of solving word problem by employing phases such as analysis, model formulation, and model verification, applications of mathematics in real-world settings will be more accessible to students. Consequently, the shift from procedural to conceptual teaching methods in mathematics, advocated by research (e.g., Hiebert 2013), might be initiated. Exploratory computerized environments (ECEs), focusing on supporting mathematical explorations and problem solving, share many commonalities with scientific discovery. Although problem solving can integrate scientific methods, this idea remains absent in the current research. As in science classes, digital technology has been proven to help students with problem-solving techniques (e.g., see Reid et al. 2003; Stern et al. 2008); searching for ways to induce congruent ideas in a mathematics classroom appears to be a promising endeavor.

The role of technologies in mathematics teaching and learning

As emphasis in teaching of mathematics is no longer placed on the knowledge of rules and calculation routines, but on building up mathematical competences such as problem-solving, modeling, and concept formation, this shift of emphasis can be significantly promoted by the use of computers (Hußmann 2007). Technology accessed both offline and online, encompasses a large range of devices, such as calculators, laptops, desktop computers, and interactive whiteboards, as well as a substantial range of software applications, such as graphing devices, data editors, spreadsheets, and dynamic geometry. Technology supporting computations and representations (e.g., geometric figures, graphs of functions, or animations) provides interactive tools and makes key relations for mathematical understanding more transparent and tangible. Several studies (Grouws & Cebulla 2000; Wander & Pierce 2009) suggest that students who develop a mathematical conceptual understanding develop the skills of knowledge transfer that enable them to perform successfully on mathematics applications. Furthermore, technologies enable complex computations and dynamic modeling that lead to more experimental forms of teaching and learning mathematics (Joyce et al. 2009; Li & Li 2009; Passey 2012).

Learning using technology posits certain challenges for software programmers. They must consider what needs to be maintained as visible and how to present the key ideas in learning sequence that will engage and challenge the learners (Bos 2009). It is unlikely that technology *per se* will affect mathematical development in any significant way; instead, what might signify viable effects is how the technology is designed to support learning and how the mathematics tools within the technology connect with the learners. Passey (2012) formulated several domains in which technology can affect teaching and learning of mathematics: (a) devices, ranging from interactive whiteboards, to desktop computers, to iPods and iPhones; (b) learning activities, ranging from multiple-choice test to interactive videos; (c) the pedagogy embedded, ranging from knowledge acquisition, to finding specific values; (d) the learning settings and interactions, ranging from the teacher and learner alone, to learners in a group or community; and (e) the type of assessment measures used to identify the impact of a specific program on students' learning.

Explorations and problem solving in mathematics

This section summarizes the advantages of utilizing technology, focusing on its use to enhance students' competencies in explorations and problem solving. According to the National Council of Teachers of Mathematics (National Council of Teachers of Mathematics NCTM 2000), 'Technology is essential in learning mathematics' (p. 3). Applying technology to enhance students' problem-solving skills is an ultimate area of interest. A problem's setup and information component expressed in word format are often difficult for students to comprehend, analyze, and solve (Ngu et al. 2014). Such presented problems also have a low motivational factor, which consequently affects the degree to which a learner engages in the solution process. The advancement of multimedia technology has opened up new possibilities for dynamically expressing a problem's contents and extending its analysis. The process can now be externalized and amplified through digital constructions, showing more explicit properties and structures that were previously silent. Several researchers (e.g., Chen 2010; Merrill & Gilbert 2008) have found that students' word-problem-solving skills can be significantly enhanced through the integration of computer technologies.

Explorations

Exploration is defined as the act of searching with the purpose of discovery of information or resources (Kuhn 2007). Explorations give students the opportunity to appreciate applications of mathematical tools in real-life situations (Remillard & Bryans 2004). Explorations can take many forms, ranging from analyzing observed phenomena to undertaking more abstract, open-ended investigations. English and Watters (2005) found that young children are capable of exploring situations beyond those involving simple processes of counts and measures. Furthermore, researchers (e.g., English 2004; Lai & White 2012) have recommended that children receive more exposure to situations where they explore informal notions or where they quantify information, transform quantities, and deal with quantities that cannot be observed. Flum and Kaplan (2006) claimed that explorations engage the learner with the environment through definite actions of gathering and investigating information. By inducing the use of terms that are central to scientific inquiry, like *observe, identify,* and *analyze* (Slough & Rupley 2010), explorations promote the transfer of knowledge, problem-solving skills, and scientific reasoning (Kuhn 2007).

Schwarz and White (2005) advocated that learning about the nature of scientific models and engaging learners in the process of creating and testing models should be a central focus of science education. It is hypothesized that by enriching mathematics curriculum via elements of such inquiry, students' problem-solving skills can be strengthened. These shifts, however, posit certain challenges. At the elementary school level, manipulatives or their interactive replicates have been extensively used to help build conceptual understanding of abstract ideas (Jitendra et al., 2007) and research (Kieran & Hillel 1990; Reimer & Moyer 2005) has proven their positive impact on students' mathematics achievement. Since manipulatives are restricted to geometrical objects, their exploratory character is limited compared to explorations, which provide a far richer context for inducing and practicing more sophisticated mathematical ideas, for instance, the concept of rate of change. Viewed through this lens, interactive exploratory learning environments dominate the previously applied drill-and-practice computer applications, and their use in mathematics has gained momentum over the past decades (Neves et al. 2011). The process of explorations usually concludes with a formulation of a mathematical model. As such, multifaceted cognitive goals are achieved by learners while they undertake such activities. Bleich et al. (2006) concluded that such activities expand students' views of mathematics by integrating mathematics with other disciplines, especially sciences, and engage students in the process of mathematization of real phenomena.

Word problems and problem solving

Situations carrying open questions that challenge learners intellectually (Blum & Niss 1991) are called *word problems* or *story problems.* The general structure of word problems is centered on three components: (a) a setup component, which provides the content (for instance, the place or story problem); (b) an information component, which provides data from which to derive a mathematical model; and (c) a question component, which is the main task directed to the solver (Gerofsky 2004). A setup component of a word problem can be externalized by a static diagram, short video, computer simulation, or physical demonstration. With the exception of static diagrams, all of these means, though not yet commonly used in mathematics classes (Kim & Hannafin 2011), assist with the visualization of problem scenarios and thus help with identifying patterns and formulating their symbolic description. Word problem solving is one area of mathematics that is particularly difficult because it requires students to analyze content, transfer it into mathematical representations, and map it into mathematical structures. Therefore, it requires not only a retrieval of a particular problem-solving model from learners' long-term memory but also the need to create a novel solution (Zheng et al. 2011).

While word problems are often considered closed tasks that usually involve simplistic responses, problem solving and explorations gravitate toward mathematical modeling that require students to analyze a given situation, build model, and verify the model before applying it. A major contribution to the field of problem solving was made by Polya (1957), who codified four stages of the process: understanding the problem, devising a plan, carrying out the plan, and looking back. Bransford and Stein (1984) extended Polya's approach by developing a five-stage problem-solving model that encompassed identifying the problem, defining goals, exploring possible stages, anticipating outcomes, and looking back and learning. Among these phases, the phase of exploration, which leads the solver to a model formulation and validation, is of the highest importance (Arthur & Nance 2007). Once the model is validated, it can be used for forecasts, decisions, or actions determined by the problem-question component. Francisco and Maher (2005) suggested that the stage of exploration or modeling must exist in the problem-solving process for authentic mathematical problem solving to occur. A similar conclusion was previously reached by Gravemeijer and Doorman (1999), who claimed that 'the role of context problems and of symbolizing and modeling are tightly interwoven' (p. 112). The forms of the mathematical models depend on the problem content. At the elementary and middle school levels, they are often externalized by geometrical objects, ratios, and proportions (National Council of Teachers of Mathematics NCTM 2000). Over the past 30 years, the domain on teaching and learning mathematics applications has undergone modifications reflecting research advancements in the area, one of which is a change in the instructional approach to problem solving: from teaching problem solving, to teaching *via* problem solving (Lester et al. 1994). Some of the main elements of teaching via problem solving include (a) providing students with enough information to let them establish the background of the problem, (b) encouraging students to make generalizations about the rules or concepts, and (c) reducing teachers' role to providing guidance during the solution process (Evan & Lappan 1994). Yimer and Ellerton (2009) proposed an inclusion of a prelude phase, called *engagement,* whose role is to increase students' motivation and, consequently, their success rate. According to Kim & Hannafin (2011), these stages represent integral elements of contemporary problem-solving methods.

While technologies' engaging factors in improving student motivation have been often researched (e.g., see Lewis et al. 1998; Niss et al. 2007), their interactive features that enable the learner to hypothesize, make predictions, and verify those predictions have not yet been meta-analyzed at the elementary and middle school levels. This study sought to examine these areas and identify moderators that contribute to increasing effects on students' learning. As a result of this undertaking, we hope to formulate suggestions for a learning environment that will advance students' analytic skills and consequently improve the use of technological tools as a means of explorations in mathematics classes.

Synthesis of findings of prior meta-analytic research

The study of problem-solving methods in the domain of mathematics education has been frequently undertaken by researchers and has especially influenced mathematical practices during the past 30 years (Santos-Trigo 2007). Tall (1986) provided an insightful analysis on how computers can be used for testing mathematical concepts, claiming that 'computer programs can show not only examples of concepts, but also, through dynamic actions, they can show examples of mathematical processes' (p. 5). He questioned the formal approaches to mathematical representations used in textbooks, calling them inaccessible to students, and suggested instead using computer programs to visualize the dynamics of the processes.

Computer programs used to support problem solving were one of the moderators in a meta-analysis on methods of instructional improvement in algebra undertaken by Rakes et al. (2010). Using 82 relevant studies from 1968 through 2008, these researchers extracted five categories, of which two contained technology and computers as a medium supporting instruction and learning. Contrasting procedural and conceptual understanding of mathematics ideas, these scholars found that conceptual understanding as a separate construct, appearing initially in research in 1985, produced the highest effect size when enhanced by computer programs. The timeline of this finding corresponded with the emergence of mathematical explorations, which also exemplify mathematics conceptual understanding. In addition, Rakes et al. (2010) found that technology tools including calculators, computer programs, and java applets produced a moderate 0.30 effect size when compared to traditional methods of instruction. Another systematic review of computer technology use and its effects on K-12 students' learning in mathematics classes between 1990 and 2006 was undertaken by Li and Ma (2010). Analyzing the effects of tutorials, communication media, exploratory environments, tools, and programming language, they concluded that exploratory environments produced the highest (ES = 1.32) learning effect size. Li and Ma did not compute the effects of computer technology on mathematics cognitive domains and type of learning objectives; instead they suggested the need for another review focusing on 'the nature of the use of technology' (p. 235) on student achievement. Yet problems of implementation of pieces of (educational) software, learning environments, and use of communication technology are far from being solved (Laborde & Sträßer 2010), and many of the problems relate to improvement of students' problem-solving skills by the use of educational software. Artzt and Armour-Thomas (1992) reported that students' difficulties with problem solving are often attributed to their failure to initiate active monitoring and regulation of their own cognitive processes. Though several potential ways of improving students' initiation of active monitoring have already been researched (e.g., see Grouws & Cebulla 2000; Kapa 2007), in this study, we sought to uncover moderators that had been silent in the previous research. We were especially interested in learning whether extending the exploration stage of the solution process and guiding students through the phases of scientific inquiry could materialize as a construct worthy of investigation. The effect of such organized support might reduce the working memory needs and consequently free students from being overwhelmed at the start. Hart (1996) reported that students find word problems difficult because they lack motivation; thus, presenting word problems in an engaging format might increase learners' motivation factor and drive them to solve the problems. Furthermore, providing some guidance during the solution process might improve their productivity and decision-making (Stillman & Galbraith 1998). However, Blum and Niss (1991) cautioned that providing guidance in the form of ready-made software in applied problem solving may put an unintentional emphasis on routine and recipe-like procedures that neglect essential phases, such as critically analyzing and comparing models. Thus, closely examining how this concern is resolved in newly developed mathematics software was an additional focus of this meta-analysis.

Prior literature has provided many insightful conclusions about the effectiveness of exploratory computer programs on mathematics students' achievement. However, it has also led to many questions on how the content delivery methods or problem-solving settings presented by computer programs will yield the highest learning effect sizes.

Methods

A literature review can take several venues, for example: narrative, quantitative, or meta-analytic. This study took the form of the latter, using the systematic approach proposed by Glass (1976), called *meta-analysis*, which can further be described as an analysis of the analyses. A statistical meta-analysis integrates empirical studies, investigating the same outcome described as a mean effect size statistic. Meta-analytic techniques were selected for this study because they provide tools to assess effect size considering a pool of studies as a set of outputs collected within prescribed criteria. There are two main advantages of such investigations: (a) a large number of studies that vary substantially can be integrated, and (b) the integration is not influenced by the interpretation or use of the findings by the reviewers (Gijbels et al. 2005). Meta-analysis allows also for conducting a subgroup moderator analysis that provides tools of identifying factors that affect the magnitude of mean effect. A subsequent moderator analysis is anticipated to be employed in this study to answer additional research questions.

Key term descriptions

Treatment/instrumentation

The treatment for the study was defined as an exploratory environment that was digitally delivered and displayed on a computer screen or iPod that students used to formulate and mathematize patterns or solve problems. An exploratory learning can be defined as a medium that engages the learner with the environment through the definite actions of gathering and investigating information (Flum & Kaplan 2006) and formulating a general pattern or finding a unique solution. The treatment can include specific software, such as Frizbi Mathematics 4, SimCalcMathWorlds, NeoGeo, or Dynamic Geometry Environment (DGE). For the purpose of identifying which type of treatment produces higher effect sizes, treatments were further classified as being focused on either explorations or problem solving.

Explorations The purpose of explorations is to have students experiment with models and search for underlying structures. An example of such would be having students investigate the properties of polygons through the underlying principles of congruency and similarity.

Problem solving The main component of problem solving is asking the learner to find a specific numerical solution (Gerofsky 2004). Problem solving in this meta-analysis encompassed process associated with solving word problems, story problems, or statement problems that involve developing mathematical concepts and solving mathematical equations to find a specific numerical value.

Outcome variable of the research

The outcome variable whose overall effect size was sought in this meta-analysis was student achievement, defined as scores on solving various mathematical tasks or problems embedded in various mathematical structures, such as equations, ratios, proportions, and formulas, and measured by students' performance on standardized or researcher- or teacher-developed tests expressed numerically as a ratio or percent. Student achievement scores were further expressed as effect size computed using mean posttest scores of experimental and control groups and coupled standard deviation using Hedges (1992) formula:

$$g = \frac{\bar{x}_1 - \bar{x}_2}{s^*}, \text{ where}$$

$\bar{x}_1$ represents the posttest mean score of the treatment group

$\bar{x}_2$ represents the posttest mean score of the control group

s^* represents pooled standard deviation.

Research questions

The research questions reflected the study purpose and they were dichotomized into two groups: main and supplementary. The main research question was the following:

- What is the magnitude and direction of the effect size of using computerized exploratory environments to support the process of problem solving and explorations when compared to conventional learning methods?

As the main question led to computing the overall effect size of using ECEs, additional questions were formulated to enrich the study objective:

- Are the effect sizes of student achievement dependent on grade level?
- Are the effect sizes of student achievement different when problem solving is contrasted with exploration?
- Are the effect sizes of student achievement dependent on mathematics content domain?
- How does the type of instructional support (teacher guided or computer based) affect student achievement when computers are used?

While the answer to the main question was assessed via interpretation of the magnitude and direction of the computed mean effect size statistic, the answers to the additional research questions were based on applied subgroup moderator analysis and interpretation of the results.

Data collection criteria and procedures

Several criteria for literature inclusion in this study were established before the search was initiated. Despite the fact that computer programs as a medium supporting learning were introduced into education several decades ago (Joyce et al. 2009), a rapid increase in this field occurred around the year 2000, which was selected as the initial timeframe for the search. Thus, this synthesis intended to analyze and summarize the research published between January 1, 2000, and December 31, 2013, on using computerized programs to support student explorations in elementary and middle school mathematics classes in either public or private schools. The minimum sample size established in this meta-analysis was ten participants. The study included only experimental research that provided pretest-posttest mean scores, standard deviation (SD), *F*-ratios, *t*-statistics, or other quantifications necessary to compute the mean effect size. As treatment groups used computerized exploratory environments, the only control groups considered were those provided with traditional instruction, meaning use of traditional teacher-centered methods, where the students are given problems to work and when they seek help when needed as described by Pilli and Aksu (2013). This reduced the confounding of effects due to hybrid treatments.

Publication bias that is a threat to any research attempting to use the published literature (Hedges 1992) was addressed by creating funnel plot for the accumulated studies and by applying Rosenthal fail-safe *N* test and computing the fail-safe number (Rosenthal 1979). The test addressing so-called *file drawer problem* estimates the number of unpublished studies required to refute significant meta-analytic means.

Studies investigating the effects of applying exploratory computerized environments and satisfying the above conditions were identified through a search of databases of ERIC, Educational Full Text (Wilson), Professional Development Collection, ProQuest Educational Journals, as well as Science Direct, and Google Scholar. The search encompassed studies conducted globally but published in English language. Due to anticipated high range of variation of sampling methods and study-level variance that produce additional source of random influence (Cooper 2010), a random-effect model is anticipated to be used to calculate the mean effect size.

Key terms were selected by the authors from the literature pertaining this study's theoretical background and prior research. In the process of extracting the relevant literature, the following queries were used: [('explorations' OR 'problem solving' OR 'control of variables') AND ('students' achievement' OR 'elementary' OR 'middle school' OR 'computers')], [('simulations' AND 'mathematics')], and ['exploratory environment' AND 'mathematics']. The strings were arranged in a way that allowed maximizing the search engine capabilities. Thus, for example, explorations were disjoined from problem solving but both were combined with student achievement and various grade levels. Respectively, simulations and exploratory environments were joined with mathematics. This search returned 238 articles, out of which 14 satisfied the criteria discussed above.

In order to expand the pool, a further search, including PsycINFO and PsychARTICLES, was undertaken with broader conceptual definitions including synonyms. For instance, [('dynamic investigations' OR 'techniques of problem solving', OR 'computerized animations') AND ('learning' OR 'student achievement')]. These modifications, which allowed for the adjustment of the contexts and strengthening of the relevance of the literature (Cooper 2010), returned 107 studies. The additional search extracted a number of studies that, although very informative (e.g., Chen & Liu 2007; Eysink et al. 2009; Harter & Ku 2008), could not be included in this meta-analysis because computers were used in both the control and experimental groups. After further scrutiny, the pool was enhanced by 11 additional studies. Combing all search, the pool contained 25 primary studies and 25 corresponding effect sizes.

The adherence of the pool to established research criteria was supported by a double scrutiny process at the initial and the concluding stages of the selection process. Any discrepancies were resolved.

Coding features

The coding process was conducted in a two-phase mode reflecting the two-stage analysis. During the first stage, general characteristics of the studies, such as research authors, sample sizes, study dates, research design type, and pretest-posttest scores, were extracted to describe the study features. During the second phase, additional scrutiny took place to more accurately reflect on the stated research questions and seek moderators that might influence the strength of the effect sizes. The majority of the coding features, including study authors, study publication date, locale, and research design type, were extracted to support the study validity. The formulation of other coding, including grade level, instrumentation, and learning type, was enacted to apply moderator analysis that would lead to answering the supplemental research questions.

Descriptive parameters

Descriptive parameters encompassed the following: the grade level of the group under investigation, the locale where the study was conducted, the sample size representing the number of participants in experimental and control groups, the date of the study publication, and the time span of the research expressed in a common week metric.

Inferential parameters

Posttest mean scores of experimental and control groups and their corresponding standard deviations were extracted to compute study effect sizes. If these were not provided, *F*-ratios or *t*-statistics were recorded. Although most of the studies reported more than one effect size, for example, Kong (2007) and Guven (2012), who also reported on students' change of attitude toward computers, this study focused only on student achievement, thus reporting one effect size per study.

The research authors

A complete list of authors whose studies were selected was compiled in Table 1. As the analysis of the study progressed, each research study was labeled only by the first author and the year of research conduct.

Publication bias

All studies included in this meta-analysis were peer reviewed and published as journal articles; thus, no additional category in the summaries was created to distinguish the publication mode of the studies. We also examined the authorship and author group membership as a consideration of a possible publication bias in certain studies being over-represented, yet no publication bias was found. Publication bias was quantified and justified through using Rosenthal fail-safe N test and by creating and examining a funnel plot.

Group assignment

This categorization was supported by the way the research participants were assigned to treatment and control groups, as defined by Shadish et al. (2002). During the coding process, two main categories emerged: (a) randomized, where the participants were randomly selected and assigned to the treatment or control group, and (b) quasi-experimental, where the participants were assigned by the researchers.

Type of research design

Only experimental studies that provided pretest-posttest means or other statistic parameters representing the means were utilized in this study.

Type of instructional support

Two subcategories were identified to classify and evaluate the effects of the type of instructional support: (a) teacher-guided support, where the teacher served as a source of providing support during student explorations or problem solving, or (b) computer-based support,

Table 1 General characteristics of the studies' features

Authors	Date	Locale	RD	SS	Grade level	RTL (in wks)	Treatment approach	IS
Pilli & Aksu	2013	Cyprus	R	55	4th	12	EX	TG
Kong	2007	Hong Kong	QE	72	4th	5	EX	TG
Hwang & Hu	2013	Taiwan	R	58	5th	8	PS	CB
Lai & White	2012	USA	QE	12	6th & 7th	1	EX	CB
Chang, Sung, & Lin	2006	Taiwan	QE	132	5th	6	PS	TG
Erbas & Yenmez	2011	Turkey	QE	134	6th	2	EX	TG
Roschelle et al.	2010	USA	R	1621	7th	40	EX	CB
Roschelle et al.	2010	USA	R	825	8th	80	EX	CB
Kapa	2007	Israel	R	107	8th	8	PS	CB
Papadopoulos & Dagdilelis	2008	Greece	QE	98	5th & 6th	4	PS	TG
Eid	2005	Kuwait	QE	62	5th	1	PS	CB
Huang, Liu, & Chang	2012	Taiwan	QE	28	2nd & 3rd	1	PS	CB
Lan, Sung, Tan, Lin, & Chang	2010	Taiwan	R	28	4th	4	PS	CB
Van Loon-Hillen, van Gog, & Brand-Gruwel	2012	Netherlands	QE	45	4th	3	PS	CB
Guven	2012	Turkey	QE	68	8th	40	EX	CB
Chen & Liu	2007	Taiwan	QE	165	4th	4	PS	TG
Ku & Sullivan	2002	Taiwan	QE	136	4th	1	PS	CB
Suh & Moyer-Packenham	2007	USA	QE	36	3rd	1	PS	CB
Panaoura	2012	Cyprus	QE	255	5th	8	PS	CB
Kanive et al.	2013	USA	R	90	4th & 5th	1	EX	CB
Shin et al.	2013	USA	R	41	2nd	5	EX	CB
Hwang et al.	2010	Taiwan	QE	56	6th	1	EX	CB
Kesan at al.	2013	Turkey	R	42	7th	2	EX	TG
Cakir & Simsek	2010	Turkey	R	90	7th	2	PS	TG

R, randomized; QE, quasi-experimental; RD, research design; EX, explorations; SS, sample size; RTL, research time length; wks, weeks; CB, computer based; TG, teacher guided; PS, problem solving; IS, Instructional Support.

where the primary source of support was provided by the software and was available on the computer screen. In both of these settings, the medium of learning was digitally delivered by the computer.

Length of treatment

Three main categories were established for this moderator: short - 2 weeks or less; intermediate - between 2 and 5 weeks inclusively; and long - more than 5 weeks.

We were initially interested in examining the magnitude of the exploratory learning environments on improving students' problem-solving skills, specifically focusing on analyzing the effects of scientific inquiry; however, we encountered limited research findings for extracting such features. Thus, the effect of scientific empirical methods on building theoretical mathematical models could not be investigated to the scale it was intended. The objective of the research was then augmented to focus on comparing traditional methods of teaching problem solving and explorations to ones using digital technology as a medium for such.

Results and discussion

Homogeneity verification and summary of data characteristics

The data analysis in this study was initially performed using SPSS 21 with verification of homogeneity of the study pool as suggested by Hedges (1992). A standardized mean difference effect size was calculated using posttest means on experimental and control groups. The individual effect sizes were then weighted, indicated by ES in this study, and an overall weighted mean effect size of the study pool was calculated. In studies including multiple independent subgroups (e.g., separate data is presented for girls and boys in the experimental and control condition), first summary statistics for both conditions was recreated, and then this data was used to calculate the effect size. If different learning methods were assessed within the same study, the effects were not combined but instead the type of learning method that best matched the study's goals and research question was selected.

The homogeneity statistics (Q_T = 117.78, with d_f = 23, $p < 0.01$) showed that the set of effect sizes varied statistically significantly. This finding further supports the adoption of a random-effect model for the data analysis. If the Q_T had not been statistically significant, a fixed-effect model would have been adopted for the analysis. In order to detect potential bias due to underrepresentation of studies with small subject samples, a funnel plot was generated (see Figure 1). The funnel plot visualizes the position of the individual effect sizes, the mean effect size, as well as the confidence intervals for each study around the computed mean of the pool with 95th percentile confidence interval around the mean. Due to a high range of studies populations, the magnitudes of the populations were converted to a logarithmic scale.

The visual inspection of the funnel plot (see Figure 1) shows that the results from smaller sample size studies are more widely spread around the mean than the studies with larger sample size studies which according to

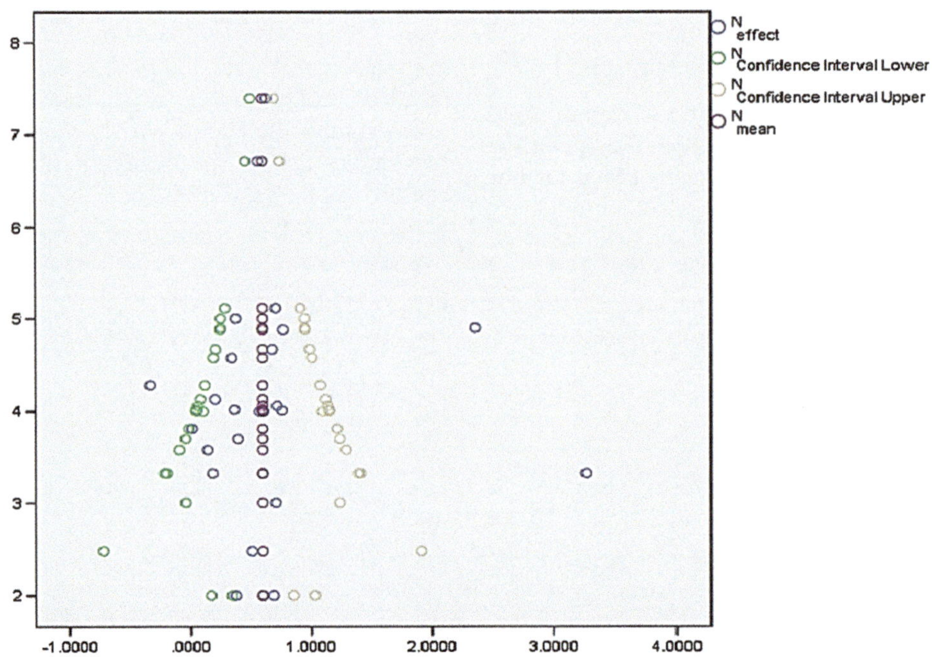

Figure 1 Funnel plot for the data.

Rothstein et al. (2006) minimizes the existence of publication bias in this meta-analysis. The funnel plot also showed some of the means located outside of the area of the funnel graph (see Figure 1), indicating a lack of homogeneity of distributions within the pool, which was also depicted by the significant p value ($p < 0.01$). As the main purpose of a meta-analysis is to compute overall effect size (Willson 1983), this deficiency did not undermine the validity of the calculated mean effect; rather, it explicated the characteristics of the studies, revealing that some of them, or their linear combinations, came from different distributions. For instance, Figure 1 illustrates three labeled studies - one by Kong (2007), labeled as 1; another by Erbas and Yenmez (2011), labeled as 2; and a third by Huang et al. (2012), labeled as 3 - whose means fell outside of the funnel graph. While Kong (2007) investigated the effects of digitally presented explorations on fouth grader understanding of fraction operations, Erbas and Yenmez (2011) investigated the effects of digitally presented explorations on sixth grader geometry concept understanding, and Huang et al. (2012) investigated the effects of digital explorations on second grader problem solving skills. These studies do not have specific common features though. Due to their complex study designs and valuable research findings, all of them were included in this meta-analysis, and thus all contributed through their weighted effect sizes to the overall effect size.

Table 1 summarizes the extracted general characteristics of the studies. The studies were further aggregated into classes to reflect the objectives of the research questions.

The calculated confidence intervals (CIs) for each study effect size (ES) consist of a range of values that act as good estimates of the ES of an unknown population. The selected 95% level indicates the probability that the CI captures this true population ES given a distribution of sample. It is to note that an ES of 17 of the studies (68%) placed within 95% CI, indicating their high precision. The duration of experimental treatment usually lasted for one unit lesson (45 min) with an average application frequency of twice a week. The majority of the studies (14, or 56%) were conducted quasi-experimentally, while the remaining ten (44%) were randomized. The study duration was expressed in a common (weeks) metric scale, although some of the studies reported the duration in months or by semesters. The highest sample size of 1,621 students was reported for a study conducted by Roschelle et al. (2010), and the lowest sample size of 12 participants was reported by Lai and White (2012). While analyzing the studies from a grade-level point of view, students whose primary level was grade 4 (28%) dominated the pool. Since this study focused on gathering research on exploratory environments provided by computer programs or the Internet, the examined studies were aggregated by their focus on supporting either problem solving or explorations in mathematics. For example, the study conducted by Lai and White (2012) was classified as an exploration because students explored the space and constructed shapes without constraints, and then provided their definitions for the various quadrilaterals. Thus, the explorations led them to formulate general patterns and descriptions. Similarly, a study by Kong (2007) was also classified as an exploration because it used a general partitioning model to have students explore the subject of common fractions and fraction operations. In contrast, problem-solving studies, such as the one conducted by Kapa (2007), followed the traditional four stages of problem solving: (1) understanding the problem, (2) making a plan, (3) executing the plan and thus finding a unique solution, and (4) reviewing the solution. The study-highlighted characteristics were further aggregated into subgroups (see Table 2) and corresponding effect sizes were computed.

Descriptive analysis

The analysis of the data was organized deductively. It began with a synthesis of the general features of the studies, furnished by a descriptive analysis, and then moved to an examination of the differences of the effect sizes mediated by the type of instrumentation, cognitive domain, study duration, grade level, and content domain.

The research pool encompassed 4,256 elementary and middle school students. The average sample size was 112 participants. Applied descriptive analysis provided information about the frequencies of the studies per year (see Figure 2) and the locale distribution where the studies were conducted (see Figure 3).

The majority of the studies (17, or 71%) were conducted within the past 5 years, which indicates a growing interest is using ECEs to support the learning of mathematics. In terms of research locale, Taiwan dominated the pool with seven studies (29%), followed by the United States with five studies (21%). The distributions show that applying and investigating the effects of ECEs in mathematics classrooms has accumulated a global interest.

Inferential analysis

Quantitative inferential analysis was performed on the primary studies to find individual weighted effect size and the mean weighted effect size of the study pool. The mean effect size for the 24 primary studies (24 effect sizes) was reported to have a magnitude of 0.60 (SE = 0.03) and a positive direction, which according to Lipsey and Wilson (2001) can be classified as of a medium size. A 95% confidence interval around the overall mean - $C_{lower} = 0.53$ and $C_{upper} = 0.66$ - supported its statistical significance and its relative precision as defined by Hunter and Schmidt (1990). When applied to school practice, it indicated that the score of an average student in the experimental

Table 2 Effect sizes of using ECEs in grades 1 to 8 mathematics

Study (first author)	ES	SE	95% CI		Reliability of measure	Program used, research findings, research specifications
			Lower	Upper		
Pilli (2013)	0.76	0.24	0.05	1.09	Researcher developed, Cronbach's $\alpha = 0.9$	Used Frizbi Mathematics 4. Explored arithmetic operations
Kong (2007)	−0.33	0.27	0.12	1.15	Teacher developed	Used Graphical Partitioning Model (GPM). Fraction operations were explored. GPM has a potential for promoting collaborative learning
Hwang (2013)	0.72	0.59	0.07	1.93	Researcher developed	Used virtual manipulative and 3D objects. Investigated the effect of peer learning
Lai (2012)	0.51	0.18	0.71	0.97	California Mathematics Standard Test	Used NeoGeo. Interactive environment helped make the applications meaningful. Investigated a peer effect
Chang (2006)	0.77	0.18	0.26	0.96	Researcher developed	Used schemata-developed problem solving. Provided teacher guidance to support phases of problem solving
Erbas (2011)	2.36	0.05	0.26	0.71	Researcher developed	Used DGE. Dynamic environment contextualized scenarios well
Roschelle (2010)	0.63	0.07	0.51	0.75	Researcher developed	Used SimCalcMathWorlds. Explored the concepts of change
Kapa (2007)	0.68	0.20	0.20	1.00	Ministry of Education guided	Used three-step problem-solving and open-ended scenarios
Papadopoulos (2008)	0.34	0.21	0.22	1.02	Researcher developed	Used computers to help explore hypotheses and verify the solutions
Eid (2005)	0.20	0.16	0.19	0.92	Standardized	Contrasted students' performance using computerized scenarios and traditional representations
Huang (2012)	3.27	0.26	0.29	1.13	Researcher designed	Used onscreen presented solutions to walk students through the course of thinking
Lan (2010)	0.18	0.40	0.09	0.42	CEA assessment	Used Group Scribbles (GS) platform that enhances collaboration. Developed stages of problem solving
Van Loon-Hillen (2012)	−0.01	0.39	0.20	1.40	Researcher developed	Worked examples to help with following procedures
Guven (2012)	0.61	0.32	0.19	1.22	Researcher developed	Used dynamic geometry software (DGS). Developed four stages of difficulty: recognition, analysis, deductive, and rigorous
Chen (2010)	0.71	0.34	0.01	1.30	Teacher developed	Incorporated personal contexts that helped students relate mathematics concepts with their experience
Ku (2002)	0.23	0.18	0.26	0.96	Teacher developed	Used personalized context to help students with mathematics concept understanding
Suh (2007)	0.14	0.34	0.09	1.30	Researcher developed	Incorporated principle of balance scale to model linear equations
Panaoura (2012)	0.37	0.13	0.34	0.85	Researcher developed	Developed program that divided problem into stages that focused the students' attention of cognitive processes
Kanive (2013)	0.36	0.27	0.05	1.14	Researcher developed	Computer program provides intermediate feedback
Shin (2013)	0.39	0.31	−0.04	1.23	Researcher developed	Computer program provided a game-like environment
Hwang (2010)	0.57	0.27	0.03	1.14	Teacher developed	Used computer programs to provide students with tasks descriptions
Kesan (2013)	0.71	0.32	−0.04	1.25	Researcher developed	Used Sketchpad geometry software
Cakir (2010)	0.69	0.22	0.17	1.03	Used PISA test bank	Used computer program to personalized and scaffold tasks

ES, effect size; SE, standard error; PISA, Program for International Student Assessment; DGE, Dynamic Geometry Environment.

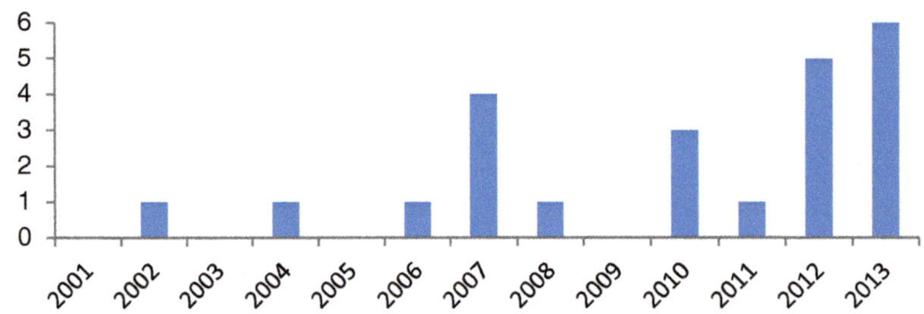

Figure 2 Distribution of studies per date of publication.

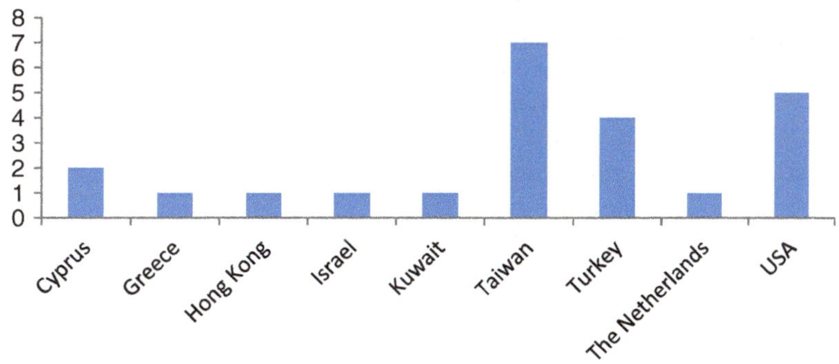

Figure 3 Distribution of studies per locale.

groups, who learned using ECEs, was 0.60 of standard deviation above the score of an average student in the control groups, who was taught using traditional methods of instruction. In order to quantify publication bias, Rosenthal's fail-safe procedure was used. The test has showed that an additional 480 unpublished null-effect studies would be required to bring the p level beyond the 0.05 threshold of significance. Further calculations show that only 130 unpublished research papers are needed for this study to nullify the mean of 0.6 below 0.05 level. Combining the results of both tests, the inspection of the funnel plot (see Figure 1) and procedure of fail-safe, we claim that the publication bias has minimal effects of the mean effect size calculations in this study. Further examination of the computed effect size and incorporation of the U_3 effect size matrix (Cooper 2010) led to the conclusion that the average pupil who learned mathematical structures using exploratory environments scored higher on unit tests than 70% of students who learned the same concepts using traditional textbook materials. It can thus be deduced that using exploratory environments as a medium of support in the teaching of mathematics has a significant impact on students' mathematics concept understanding when compared to conventional methods of teaching. Table 2 provides a summary of the individual effect sizes of the meta-analyzed studies along with their confidence intervals. The table also contains qualitative research findings, the computer programs used as the instruments, and the reliability of measures used to compute the individual mean scores, expressed by indicating whether the test was researcher developed or standardized. Where it was available, Cronbach's alpha (α) was also listed, along with additional information provided by the primary researchers that distinguish the given study within the pool.

The majority of the studies (16, or 84%) used researcher- or teacher-developed evaluation instruments, and only one (Pilli & Aksu 2013) reported a Cronbach's α coefficient of reliability measure. In addition, the majority of the studies (17, or 89%) reported positive effect sizes when an exploratory environment was used as a medium of learning. Only two studies - one conducted by Van Loon-Hillen et al. (2012) and one conducted by Kong (2007) - reported negative effect sizes favoring traditional instruction, illustrating that exploratory environments cannot replace good teaching and that some concepts, like operations on fractions (Kong 2007), require the instructor to deliver the concept and its stages and to suggest ways of overcoming obstacles that students may face. Exploratory environments seemed to produce high effect sizes in cases where students applied already-learned mathematics concepts in new situations (e.g., Chang et al., 2006; Guven, 2012; Roschelle et al., 2010) but not when students simultaneously explored new concepts and applied them. The highest effect size on explorations was reported by Erbas and Yenmez (2011; ES = 2.36), who examined the effect of open-ended geometry investigations, and the highest effect size on problem solving was noted by Huang and colleagues (2012; ES = 3.27), who investigated the effect of embedded support during the process of problem solving. Although an influx of onscreen instructional support might work well in many classroom settings, we believe that the elements of mathematical explorations induced in the study by Erbas and Yenmez (2011) more accurately supported the objectives of this study.

Possible moderators and analysis of their effects

Just as a mean effect size provides certain evidence for potential duplications of the study findings, subgroup analysis allows for uncovering moderators that optimize the effect. Since student mathematical achievement was the main construct under investigation, during the process of moderator formulation, attention was directed toward formulating and extracting the study features that could affect achievement when ECEs were utilized. We anticipated that through identifying such features, an optimum learning environment would emerge. By analyzing the settings of the primary research, a set of five moderators was identified: grade level, instrumentation, treatment duration, content domain, and type of learning setting. This categorization resulted in 12 subgroups whose effects were individually computed. The moderator analyses were performed for random-effects model because this meta-analysis sought also to reveal the relative effectiveness of ECE due to formulated moderators, and hence it did not assume that the effect size will be the same for all studies. The computations of effect sizes followed Cooper (2010), who suggested giving more weight to effect sizes with larger sample populations (w = inverse of the variance in the effect calculations). Along with calculating subgroup effects, corresponding confidence intervals and standard errors were also computed. Table 3 displays the effect sizes according to the formulated moderators and the subgroups. In order to provide a common metric for the subgroup effect magnitude comparisons, the effect sizes were weighted by the sample sizes. Although we realized that the effects of using ECEs might be strongly influenced by the degree of interactivity of the educational programs used and the applied scaffolding necessary to have students assimilate tasks presented in contexts, such extractions were not feasible due to the limited information provided in this regard by the primary researchers.

All of the magnitudes of the calculated effect sizes place within their confidence intervals, which proves the significance of the effect sizes and their relative precision (Hunter & Schmidt, 1990). Furthermore, considering, for example, teacher-guided support during explorations (ES = 0.75), one can conclude that the practitioners using such an approach can be 95% confident that the effect size of students' achievement will be 60% to 93% higher than when compared to traditional level of instruction. The categorization into subgroups and the descriptive analysis provided a more insightful picture about the effects of ECEs on the achievement of students in grades 1 to 8 mathematics classes and helped answer the research questions of this study, as discussed next.

Table 3 Summary of subgroups' weighted effect sizes

Moderator and subgroups	*N*	ES	SE	95% CI	
				Lower	Upper
Grade level					
Lower elementary: 1 through 3	3	0.61	0.03	0.54	0.67
Upper elementary: 4 to 5	12	0.41	0.07	0.27	0.54
Middle school: 6 to 8	9	0.65	0.04	0.57	0.73
Instrumentation					
Problem solving	12	0.54	0.07	0.41	0.67
Explorations	12	0.62	0.03	0.54	0.69
Treatment duration					
Short	8	0.47	0.14	0.11	0.74
Intermediate	9	0.63	0.09	0.45	0.81
Long	7	0.62	0.04	0.55	0.70
Content domain					
Geometry	9	0.67	0.22	−0.07	0.79
Arithmetic and algebra	15	0.61	0.03	0.43	0.56
Type of instructional support					
Teacher guided	8	0.75	0.08	0.59	0.92
Computer based	16	0.56	0.04	0.49	0.63

N, sample size; ES, effect size; SE, standard error.

Are the effect sizes of student achievement dependent on grade level?

A block of *grade level* was created to answer this question. Following NCTM (2000), three subgroup levels were formulated: lower elementary, which included grades 1 to 3; upper elementary, which included grades 4 and 5; and middle school, which encompassed grades 6 to 8. The computed effect size showed differences across grade levels, with middle school producing the highest effect size (ES = 0.65), which according to Lipsey and Wilson (2001) can be classified as moderate followed by lower elementary school (ES = 0.61) and upper elementary (ES = 0.41). It is inferred that this result can be attributed to the fact that students at the middle school level often use manipulatives to support their mathematics concept understanding (e.g., see Jitendra et al., 2007); thus, these students' transition to ECEs occurs more spontaneously, resulting in the highest score gain. The effect sizes in the other grades also showed a moderate magnitude.

Are the effect sizes of student achievement different when problem solving is compared to exploration?

The moderator category of *instrumentation* was used to conclude whether ECEs affect student achievement differently through supporting problem solving or exploration. As explorations have often led students to pattern formulations (e.g., see Panaoura, 2012; Suh & Moyer-Packenham, 2007), problem solving was usually constructed within defined stages, leading students toward finding numerical answers or unique solutions to the stated problems (e.g., see Chen & Liu, 2007; Hwang & Hu, 2013). When contrasted with problem solving, learning supported by explorations produced a higher effect size of ES = 0.62 (as opposed to ES = 0.54 for problem solving). This finding generated several conjectures. As the process of explorations resonates better with students' natural curiosity (Stokoe, 2012) and their prior experiences, working on explorations might ignite a higher student's motivation level, thus their higher achievement. Despite the fact that efforts to help students understand the solution process are multidimensional, ranging from creating schemas (Kapa, 2007) to inducing personalization (Chen & Liu,

2007; Ku & Sullivan, 2002), attempts at helping students learn the process of problem solving by embedding explorations in some of the transitioning stages are rare. With exceptions of researches conducted by Roschelle et al. (2010) and Panaoura (2012), an inquiry process is not emphasized in the accumulated pool of studies on problem solving despite a strong support by other researchers (e.g., see English, 2004). The current research on problem solving gravitates toward creating and examining the effects of cognitive support or showing worked-out solutions that students can follow (e.g., see Van Loon-Hillen et al., 2012). As illustrated by the computed effect sizes, all of these attempts seem to produce desirable positive results; however, by concentrating on simplifying or following the mechanics of the problem-solving process, the meaning of the context embedded in the problems is diminished. The question that arises here is How to convert word problems to explorations? Bonotto (2007) suggested 'Change the type of activity aimed at creating interplay between the real world and mathematics towards more realistic and less stereotyped problem situations' (p. 86) and 'change classroom culture by establishing new classroom socio-mathematical norms' (p. 86). (Greer et al. 2007) proposed to 'Valorize forms of answer other than single, exact numerical answers' (p. 92).

Are the effect sizes dependent on the mathematics content domain?

Two mathematics content domains dominated in this study pool: geometry and algebra. Geometry, traditionally supported by visualization, showed a higher effect size (ES = 0.67) compared to algebra (ES = 0.61). As geometric objects can also be easily externalized by their real embodiments, more effort should be placed on contextualization and visualization of other, more abstract mathematical structures such as functions. Teaching algebraic structures via exploratory environments is being practiced and researched, yet embodying algebraic structures by context-driven scenarios seems to be a challenge, which is reflected by locating only eight (33%) such studies.

How does the type of instructional support (teacher guided or computer based) affect student achievement when computers are used?

There were two main categories of instructional support provided to the students in the study pool: computer-based support displayed on the computer screen or teacher-centered support provided by the instructor. Computer-based instructional support dominated the study pool (16, or 67%) compared to teacher-based instruction (8, or 33%). When compared by learning effects, teacher-centered support produced a higher effect (ES = 0.75) than computer-based support (ES = 0.56). This result signifies the importance of the teacher's role in developing students' understanding of mathematics structures and helping them apply the structures to solve problems, and it corresponds with Li and Li's (2009) finding who claimed that 'teacher transfers the knowledge development and justification responsibilities to students' (p. 275). A particular instance that needs further investigation is transitioning from verifying to explaining (Hähkiöniemi & Leppäaho, 2012). Merchant et al. (2014) claimed that 'It is essential that teachers are made knowledgeable about the features and situations that make feedback effective' (p. 37).

Programmed tips are important and readily available to students, yet the expertise, encouragement, and support from a live person appear to have a higher impact on students' learning. Further research contrasting learning effect sizes by using as a moderator, for example, the frequency of seeking help available on the computer screen versus frequency of seeking help from the teacher along with quality of answers sought, would likely shed more light on the cause of the differences.

In addition to analyzing the effects of moderators that reflected the research questions, the effect of treatment length was also computed. The analysis showed that the treatment of length between 2 and 5 weeks, called *intermediate* herein, produced the highest effect size of (ES = 0.63). A similar conclusion was reached in a meta-analysis by Xin et al. (2005), who also proved that longer treatment results in higher student achievement. The student needs to be acquainted with the mechanics of the new learning medium; thus, it is important that the first contact and experience with an ECE be absorbed into a learner's working memory. It is hypothesized that longer and more frequent exposure to the new environment allows a higher focus on task-driven objectives related to the content analysis, which consequently results in better context understanding and higher learning effects. However, as Guven (2012) and Roschelle et al. (2010) found, there is an achievement saturation level, which perhaps suggests that in order to further increase learning effects, ECEs need to mediate with other factors, not necessarily related to content knowledge, for instance different forms of analysis, synthesis, or evaluation as suggested by Anderson and Krathwohl (2001).

When linking the subgroups with the highest learning effects, it appears that month-long geometry explorations in grades 1 to 3 mathematics classes, guided by the teacher, would produce the highest learning effects.

Conclusions

While this study found a moderate positive effect size (ES = 0.59) associated with ECE, this finding does not diminish the importance of good teaching. Several studies (Christmann et al. 1997; Clark, 1994; Povey & Ransom,

2000) found that using computers purely as a method of instruction does not improve students' mathematics understanding. Hence, although computers have been used in mathematics classrooms for several decades now, the question regarding to what extent they can impact the teaching and learning of mathematics seems to be open for further investigations. This meta-analysis of up-to-date literature allowed for formulations of some inferences based on implementations of technology; however, many new questions emerged, such as the following: How do exploratory environments help students with the transfer of mathematics concepts to new situations? How can we assure that the methods of quantitative scientific modeling that students apply in their science classes are coherent with the ones used in mathematics, and vice versa? Mathematics provides tools for phenomena quantifications; thus, unifications of the techniques of modeling seem to benefit the transition of knowledge between mathematics and science and consequently affect the learners' perception of mathematics as a subject with a high applicability range. Will such unification prompt students to increase their engagement in mathematics? More detailed studies in these domains are worthy of consideration, and the availability of ECEs will be very helpful in organizing such studies.

The impact of ECEs on students' problem-solving techniques

Problem-solving techniques are developed on the basis of understanding the context through identifying the principles of the system's behavior. However, it is a highly intertwined process that might include verbal and syntactic processing, special representation storage and retrieval in short- and long-term memory, algorithmic learning, and its most complex element - conceptual understanding (Goldin, 1992). Computerized programs offering a basis for investigation offer a great potential for improving conceptual understanding of problems; however, this study shows that this area is not yet fully explored, and taking full advantage of such learning environments to examine their impact on student achievement is a possible extension of this undertaking. More specifically, enriching the problem analysis through explorations to focus learners' attention more on the underpinning principles emerges as a possible objective of such studies. Higher student achievement on explorations (ES = 0.62), compared to problem solving (ES = 0.54), encourages designs of more comprehensive research about inducing an exploratory approach to problem solving also to solving standard textbook problems as opposed to current schemata-driven methods. Would giving students more ownership in exploring a given system's behavior, hypothesizing a solution, testing, and proving or disproving their hypothesis be a possible moderator affecting learning? Will these types of activities help solidify a notion and belief in the power of mathematics as sense-making subject? There also seems to be more work needed to evaluate how learners link mathematics concepts with principles embedded in given context and how they initiate applications of the procedures that they select. 'Only an analysis of the instrument, i.e., the interaction of the artifact and the utilization schemes of its users (teachers and students), the analysis of its *instrumental genesis* will help in the implementation of computers, software and communication technology in the mathematics classroom' (Laborde and Sträßer 2010, p. 131).

Limitations and suggestions for future research

This meta-analytic research has certain limitations, primarily because this study could not be conducted in an experimental fashion where ECEs constituted instrumentation provided by computer programs and a direct contrast between two different modes of learning - digital and traditional - were exploited. Furthermore, the limited count of studies available to be meta-analyzed affected the study generalizability. Although sensitivity to smaller sample sizes was restored by the process of weighing, the impact of the mean effect would validate the replication of the findings more significantly by being computed over a larger study pool.

The other factor affecting validity of the computed effect sizes is the high span of interactivity of the software used in the primary studies and their exploratory nature, ranging from linear equation exploration supported by an interactive balance scale (Suh & Moyer-Packenham, 2007) to investigation of rate of change supported by the SimCalcMathWorlds program (Roschelle et al. 2010). A metric for incorporating this moderator to effect size calculations could have been furnished by evaluating the designs of the interventions through the lens of the *multimedia principles* defined by Clark and Mayer (2011). This task, however, was not possible to accomplish due to the lack of the software detailed descriptions.

The validity of the research would have been higher if the calculated homogeneity statistics were not statistically significant. In this meta-analysis, $Q_T = 117.78$, with $d_f = 23$, $p < 0.01$), which implied a random-effect model for the data analysis instead of a more precise fixed-effect model.

Another factor limiting the study findings involves the widely varied student assessment methods, ranging from traditional multiple-choice questions mostly locally developed to new assessment techniques such as standardized-based assessments. Although one of the studies (Pilli & Aksu, 2013) reported a Cronbach's alpha reliability coefficient, most did not, thereby decreasing the reliability of the measuring instrument. The degree of diversity further extends due to obvious differences in mathematics curricula, objectives, and expectation levels in the nine countries whose research studies were represented herein. Even though control groups in the extracted pool of studies were taught traditionally, the term *traditional teaching* might have been interpreted differently depending on the country. For example, Lan et al. (2010)) defined traditional instruction as being without the support of technological devices, whereas Papadopoulos and Dagdilelis (2008) defined traditional teaching as a paper-and-pencil environment. Both descriptions imply that technology was not being used, but the treatment applied in the control groups might have varied in terms of degree of representations and method used, or teacher qualifications, which potentially could have mediated with the control groups' posttest scores. We concluded, however, that these fluctuations did not affect the overall effect size in a manner that would question the validity of the computed overall effect size.

Though at first we intended to examine the effects of embedded scientific inquiry methods in exploratory environments on students' problem-solving skills, we encountered a limited number of research studies addressing this domain. Thus, we modified the study focus. We realized that exploratory environments used in both types of interventions - explorations and problem solving - contained, to a certain degree, some elements of scientific inquiry and affected students' problem-solving skills, not just students' problem-solving performance as measured by testing. Further studies focusing primarily on the effects of inducing scientific inquiry processes in mathematical modeling and problem solving would serve to extend this paper. Technology has encouraged researchers to consider not only how to best adapt tools to the learning of mathematics but also how to adapt the content of mathematics in light of new, tool-rich possibilities to enable learners to perform tasks that would not previously have been possible (Hoyles & Noss, 2009). The task of explorations seems to provide basis for inducing such adaptations.

This meta-analysis, to a certain extent, exposed the focus of the existing primary studies on the effects of exploratory environments on problem solving in mathematics education. We advocate for searching and formulating more constructs to quantify students' problem-solving techniques with ECEs as a medium of context.

Competing interests

The authors declare that they have no competing interests.

Authors' contribution

AS was conducted research as part of his dissertation. YL and VW co-chairman of the research dissertation.

Author details

[1]Department of Mathematics and Science, Lone Star College, Tomball, TX 77375, USA. [2]College of Education and Human Development, Department of Teaching Learning and Culture, Texas A&M University, College Station, TX 77843-4225, USA. [3]College of Education and Human Development, Department of Educational Psychology, Texas A&M University, College Station, TX 77843-4225, USA.

References

Anderson, L, & Krathwohl, DA. (2001). *Taxonomy for learning, teaching and assessing: a revision of Bloom's Taxonomy of Educational Objectives*. New York, NY: Longman.

Arthur, JD, & Nance, RE. (2007). Investigating the use of software requirements and engineering techniques in simulation modeling. *Journal of Simulation, 1*(3), 159–174.

Artzt, AF, & Armour-Thomas, E. (1992). Development of a cognitive-metacognitive framework for protocol analysis of mathematical problem solving in small groups. *Cognition and Instruction, 9*(2), 137–175.

Bleich, L, Ledford, S, Hawley, C, Polly, D, & Orrill, C. (2006). An analysis of the use of graphical representation in participants' solutions. *The Mathematics Educator, 16*(1), 22–34.

Blum, W, & Niss, M. (1991). Applied mathematical problem solving, modeling, applications, and links to other subjects: state trends and issues in mathematics instruction. *Educational Studies in Mathematics, 22*(1), 37–68.

Bonotto, C. (2007). How to replace word problems with activities of realistic mathematical modelling. In W Blum, P Galbraith, HW Henn, & M Niss (Eds.), *Modelling and applications in mathematics education: the 14th ICMI Study* (pp. 45–56). New York, NY: Springer.

Bos, B. (2009). Virtual mathematics objects with pedagogical, mathematical, and cognitive fidelity. *Computers in Human Behavior, 25*(2), 521–528.

Bransford, JD, & Stein, BS. (1984). *The ideal problem solver. A guide for improving thinking, learning, and creativity*. New York, NY: Freeman.

Cakir, O, & Simsek, N. (2010). A comparative analysis of the effects of computer and paper-based personalization on student achievement. *Computers & Education, 55*(4), 1524–1531.

Chang, KE, Sung, YT, & Lin, SF. (2006). Computer-assisted learning for mathematical problem solving. *Computers & Education, 46*(2), 140–151.

Chen, CH. (2010). Promoting college students' knowledge acquisition and ill-structured problem solving: Web-based integration and procedure prompts. *Computers & Education, 55*(1), 292–303.

Chen, CJ, & Liu, PL. (2007). Personalized computer-assisted mathematics problem-solving program and its impact on Taiwanese students. *Journal of Computers in Mathematics and Science Teaching, 26*(2), 105–121.

Christmann, E, Badgett, J, & Lucking, R. (1997). Microcomputer-based computer-assisted instruction within differing subject areas: a statistical deduction. *Journal of Educational Computing Research, 16*(3), 281–296.

Clark, RE. (1994). Media will never influence learning. *Educational Technology Research and Development, 42*(2), 21–29.

Clark, RC, & Mayer, RE. (2011). *e-Learning and the science of instruction: proven guidelines for consumers and designers of multimedia learning*. San Francisco, CA: Pfeiffer.

Cooper, H. (2010). *Research synthesis and meta-analysis* (4th ed.). Thousand Oaks, CA: Sage.

Eid, GK. (2005). An investigation into the effects and factors influencing computer-based online mathematics problem-solving in primary schools. *Journal of Educational Technology Systems, 33*(3), 223–240.

English, L. (2004). Mathematical modeling in the primary school. In *Mathematics education for the third millennium: towards 2010 (Proceedings of the 27th Annual Conference of the Mathematics Education Research Group of Australasia* (Vol. 1, pp. 207–214). Sydney, Australia: MERGA.

English, LD, & Watters, JJ. (2005). Mathematical modeling in the early school years. *Mathematics Education Research Journal, 16*(3), 58–79.

Erbas, AK, & Yenmez, AA. (2011). The effect of inquiry-based explorations in a dynamic geometry environment on sixth grade students' achievements in polygons. *Computers & Education, 57*(4), 2462–2475.

Evan, R, & Lappan, G. (1994). Constructing meaningful understanding of mathematics content. In D Aichele & A Coxford (Eds.), *Professional development for teachers of mathematics* (pp. 128–143). Reston, VA: NCTM.

Eysink, TH, de Jong, T, Berthold, K, Kolloffel, B, Opfermann, M, & Wouters, P. (2009). Learner performance in multimedia learning arrangements: an analysis across instructional approaches. *American Educational Research Journal, 46*(4), 1107–1149.

Flum, H, & Kaplan, A. (2006). Exploratory orientation as an educational goal. *Educational Psychologist, 4*(2), 99–110.

Forster, PA. (2006). Assessing technology-based approaches for teaching and learning mathematics. *International Journal of Mathematical Education in Science and Technology, 37*(2), 145–164.

Francisco, JM, & Maher, CA. (2005). Conditions for promoting reasoning in problem solving: insights from a longitudinal study. *The Journal of Mathematical Behavior, 24*(3), 361–372.

Gerofsky, S. (2004). *A man left Albuquerque heading east: word problem as genre in mathematics education* (Vol. 5). New York, NY: Peter Lang.

Gijbels, D, Dochy, F, Van den Bossche, P, & Segers, M. (2005). Effects of problem-based learning: a meta-analysis from the angle of assessment. *Review of Educational Research, 75*(1), 27–61.

Glass, GV. (1976). Primary, secondary, and meta-analysis of research. *Educational Researcher, 5*, 3–8.

Goldin, GA. (1992). Meta-analysis of problem-solving studies: a critical response. *Journal for Research in Mathematics Education, 23*(3), 274–283.

Gravemeijer, K, & Doorman, M. (1999). Context problems in realistic mathematics education: a calculus course as an example. *Educational Studies in Mathematics, 39*(1), 111–129.

Greer, B, Verschaffel, L, & Mukhopadhyay, S. (2007). Modelling for life: Mathematics and children's experience. In W Blum, P Galbraith, HW Henn, & M Niss (Eds.), *Modelling and applications in mathematics education: the 14th ICMI Study* (pp. 89–98). New York, NY: Springer.

Grouws, DA, & Cebulla, KJ. (2000). *Improving student achievement in mathematics*. Geneva, Switzerland: International Academy of Education.

Guven, B. (2012). Using dynamic geometry software to improve eighth grade students' understanding of transformation geometry. *Australasian Journal of Educational Technology, 28*(2), 364–382.

Hähkiöniemi, M, & Leppäaho, H. (2012). Prospective mathematics teachers' ways of guiding high school students in GeoGebra-supported inquiry tasks. *International Journal for Technology in Mathematics Education, 19*(2), 45–58.

Hart, JM. (1996). The effect of personalized word problems. *Teaching Children Mathematics, 2*(8), 504–505.

Harter, CA, & Ku, HY. (2008). The effects of spatial contiguity within computer-based instruction of group personalized two-step mathematics word problems. *Computers in Human Behavior, 24*(4), 1668–1685.

Hedges, LV. (1992). Meta-analysis. *Journal of Educational and Behavioral Statistics, 17*(4), 279–296.

Hiebert, J (Ed.). (2013). *Conceptual and procedural knowledge: the case of mathematics*. New York, NY: Routledge.

Hoyles, C, & Noss, R. (2009). The technological mediation of mathematics and its learning. *Human Development, 52*(2), 129–147.

Huang, TH, Liu, YC, & Chang, HC. (2012). Learning achievement in solving word-based mathematical questions through a computer-assisted learning system. *Educational Technology & Society, 15*(1), 248–259.

Hunter, JE, & Schmidt, FL. (1990). *Methods of meta-analysis: correcting error and bias in research findings*. Newbury Park, CA: Sage.

Hußmann, S. (2007). Building concepts and conceptions in technology-based open learning environments. In W Blum, P Galbraith, HW Henn, & M Niss (Eds.), *Modelling and applications in mathematics education: the 14th ICMI Study* (pp. 341–348). New York, NY: Springer.

Hwang, WY, & Hu, SS. (2013). Analysis of peer learning behaviors using multiple representations in virtual reality and their impacts on geometry problem solving. *Computers & Education, 62*, 308–319.

Hwang, GJ, Wu, PH, Zhuang, YY, & Huang, YM. (2013). Effects of the inquiry-based mobile learning model on the cognitive load and learning achievement of students. *Interactive Learning Environments, 21*(4), 338–354.

Jitendra, AK, Griffin, CC, Haria, P, Leh, J, Adams, A, & Kaduvettoor, A. (2007). A comparison of single and multiple strategy instruction on third-grade students' mathematical problem solving. *Journal of Educational Psychology, 99*(1), 115–127.

Joyce, B, Weil, M, & Calhoun, E. (2009). *Models of teaching* (8th ed.). Boston, MA: Pearson.

Kanive, R, Nelson, PM, Burns, MK, & Ysseldyke, J. (2014). Comparison of the effects of computer-based practice and conceptual understanding interventions on mathematics fact retention and generalization. *The Journal of Educational Research, 107*(2), 83–89.

Kapa, E. (2007). Transfer from structured to open-ended problem solving in a computerized metacognitive environment. *Learning and Instruction, 17*(6), 688–707.

Kesan, C, & Caliskan, S. (2013). The effect of learning geometry topics of 7th grade in primary education with dynamic Geometer's Sketchpad geometry software to success and retention. *Turkish Online Journal of Educational Technology-TOJET, 12*(1), 131–138.

Kieran, C, & Hillel, J. (1990). "It's tough when you have to make the triangles angle": insights from a computer-based geometry environment. *The Journal of Mathematical Behavior, 9*(2), 99–127.

Kim, MC, & Hannafin, MJ. (2011). Scaffolding problem solving in technology-enhanced learning environments (TELEs): bridging research and theory with practice. *Computers & Education, 56*(2), 403–417.

Kong, SC. (2007). The development of a cognitive tool for teaching and learning fractions in the mathematics classroom: a design-based study. *Computers & Education, 51*(2), 886–899.

Ku, HY, & Sullivan, HJ. (2002). Student performance and attitudes using personalized mathematics instruction. *Educational Technology Research and Development, 50*(1), 21–34.

Kuhn, D. (2007). Is direct instruction the answer to the right question? *Educational Psychologist, 42*(2), 109–114.

Laborde, C, & Sträßer, R. (2010). Place and use of new technology in the teaching of mathematics: ICMI activities in the past 25 years. *ZDM, 42*(1), 121–133.

Lai, K, & White, T. (2012). Exploring quadrilaterals in a small group computing environment. *Computers & Education, 59*(3), 963–973.

Lan, YJ, Sung, YT, Tan, NC, Lin, CP, & Chang, KE. (2010). Mobile-device-supported problem-based computational estimation instruction for elementary school students. *Educational Technology & Society, 13*(3), 55–69.

Lester, FK, Jr, Masingila, JO, Mau, ST, Lambdin, DV, dos Santon, VM, & Raymond, AM. (1994). Learning how to teach via problem solving. In D Aichele & A Coxford (Eds.), *Professional development for teachers of mathematics* (pp. 152–166). Reston, VA: NCTM.

Lewis, R, Stoney, S, & Wild, M. (1998). Motivation and interface design: maximizing learning opportunities. *Journal of Computer Assisted Learning, 14*(1), 40–50.

Li, Y, & Li, J. (2009). Mathematics classroom instruction excellence through the platform of teaching contests. *ZDM, 41*(3), 263–277.

Li, Q, & Ma, X. (2010). A meta-analysis of the effects of computer technology on school students' mathematics learning. *Educational Psychology Review, 22*(3), 215–243.

Lipsey, MW, & Wilson, DB. (2001). *Practical meta-analysis*. Thousand Oaks, CA: Sage.

Merchant, Z, Goetz, ET, Cifuentes, L, Keeney-Kennicutt, W, & Davis, TJ. (2014). Effectiveness of virtual reality-based instruction on students' learning outcomes in K-12 and higher education: a meta-analysis. *Computers & Education, 70*, 29–40.

Merrill, MD, & Gilbert, CG. (2008). Effective peer interaction in problem-centered instructional strategy. *Distance Education, 29*(2), 199–207.

National Council of Teachers of Mathematics (NCTM). (2000). Principles and standards for school mathematics. Reston, VA: NCTM.

Neves, RG, Silva, JC, & Teodoro, VD. (2011). Improving learning in science and mathematics with exploratory and interactive computational modeling. *Trends in Teaching and Learning of Mathematical Modeling, 1*(4), 331–339.

Ngu, BH, Yeung, AS, & Tobias, S. (2014). Cognitive load in percentage change problems: unitary, pictorial, and equation approaches to instruction. Instructional Science, 42(5), 685–713.

Niss, M, Blum, W, & Galbraith, P. (2007). Introduction. In W Blum, P Galbraith, HW Henn, & M Niss (Eds.), *Modelling and applications in mathematics education: the 14th ICMI Study* (pp. 3–33). New York, NY: Springer.

Panaoura, A. (2012). Improving problem solving ability in mathematics by using a mathematical model: a computerized approach. *Computers in Human Behavior, 28*(6), 2291–2297.

Papadopoulos, I, & Dagdilelis, V. (2008). Students' use of technological tools for verification purposes in geometry problem solving. *The Journal of Mathematical Behavior, 27*(4), 311–325.

Passey, D. (2012). Educational technologies and mathematics: signature pedagogies and learner impacts. *Computers in the Schools, 29*(1–2), 6–39.

Pead, D, Ralph, B, & Muller, E. (2007). Uses of technologies in learning mathematics through modelling. In W Blum, P Galbraith, HW Henn, & M Niss (Eds.), *Modelling and applications in mathematics education: the 14th ICMI Study* (pp. 309–318). New York, NY: Springer.

Pilli, O, & Aksu, M. (2013). The effects of computer-assisted instruction on the achievement, attitudes and retention of fourth grade mathematics students in North Cyprus. *Computers & Education, 62*, 62–71.

Pollak, H. (2007). Mathematical modelling—a conversation with Henry Pollak. In W Blum, P Galbraith, HW Henn, & M Niss (Eds.), *Modelling and applications in mathematics education: the 14th ICMI Study* (pp. 109–120). New York, NY: Springer.

Polya, G. (1957). *How to solve it*. Princeton, NJ: Lawrence Erlbaum.

Porter, A, McMaken, J, Hwang, J, & Yang, R. (2011). Assessing the common core standards: opportunities for improving measures of instruction. *Educational Researcher, 40*(4), 186–188.

Povey, H, & Ransom, M. (2000). Some undergraduate students' perceptions of using technology for mathematics: tales of resistance. *International Journal of Computers for Mathematical Learning, 5*(1), 47–63.

Rakes, CR, Valentine, JC, McGatha, MB, & Ronau, RN. (2010). Methods of instructional improvement in algebra: a systematic review and meta-analysis. *Review of Educational Research, 80*(3), 372–400.

Reid, DJ, Zhang, J, & Chen, Q. (2003). Supporting scientific discovery learning in a simulation environment. *Journal of Computer Assisted Learning, 19*, 9–20.

Reimer, K, & Moyer, PS. (2005). Third-graders learn about fractions using virtual manipulatives: a classroom study. *Journal of Computers in Mathematics and Science Teaching, 24*(1), 5–25.

Remillard, JT, & Bryans, MB. (2004). Teachers' orientations toward mathematics curriculum materials: implications for teacher learning. *Journal for Research in Mathematics Education, 35*(5), 352–388.

Roschelle, J, Shechtman, N, Tatar, D, Hegedus, S, Hopkins, B, Empson, S, & Gallagher, LP. (2010). Integration of technology, curriculum, and professional development for advancing middle school mathematics: three large-scale studies. *American Educational Research Journal, 47*(4), 833–878.

Rosenthal, R. (1979). The file drawer problem and tolerance for null results. *Psychological bulletin, 86*(3), 638.

Rothstein, HR, Sutton, AJ, & Borenstein, M. (2006). *Publication bias in meta-analysis: prevention, assessment and adjustments*. Chichester, UK: Wiley & Sons.

Santos-Trigo, M. (2007). Mathematical problem solving: an evolving research and practice domain. *Mathematics Education, 39*(5/6), 523–536.

Schwarz, CV, & White, BY. (2005). Metamodeling knowledge: developing students' understanding of scientific modeling. *Cognition and Instruction, 23*(2), 165–205.

Shadish, WR, Cook, TD, & Campbell, DT. (2002). *Experimental and quasi-experimental designs for generalized causal inference*. Belmont, CA: Wadsworth Cengage Learning.

Shin, N, Sutherland, LM, Norris, CA, & Soloway, E. (2012). Effects of game technology on elementary student learning in mathematics. *British journal of educational technology, 43*(4), 540–560.

Slough, SW, & Rupley, WH. (2010). Re-creating a recipe for science instructional programs: adding learning progressions, scaffolding, and a dash of reading variety. *School Science and Mathematics, 110*(7), 352–362.

Stern, L, Barnea, N, & Shauli, S. (2008). The effect of a computerized simulation on middle school students' understanding of the kinetic molecular theory. *Journal of Science Education and Technology, 17*(4), 305–315.

Stillman, GA, & Galbraith, PL. (1998). Applying mathematics with real-world connections: metacognitive characteristics of secondary students. *Educational Studies in Mathematics, 36*, 157–195.

Stokoe, R. (2012). Curiosity, a condition for learning. *The International Schools Journal, 32*(1), 63.

Suh, J, & Moyer-Packenham, P. (2007). Developing students' representational fluency using virtual and physical algebra balances. *Journal of Computers in Mathematics and Science Teaching, 26*(2), 155–173.

Tall, D. (1986). Using the computer as an environment for building and testing mathematical concepts: a tribute to Richard Skemp. In Papers in honor of Richard Skemp (pp. 21–36). Retrieved from http://homepages.warwick.ac.uk/staff/David.Tall/pdfs/dot1986h-computer-skemp.pdf

Van Loon-Hillen, N, van Gog, T, & Brand-Gruwel, S. (2012). Effects of worked examples in a primary school mathematics curriculum. *Interactive Learning Environments, 20*(1), 89–99.

Wander, R, & Pierce, R. (2009). Marina's Fish Shop: a mathematically- and technologically-rich lesson. *Australian Mathematics Teacher, 65*(2), 6.

Willson, VL. (1983). A meta-analysis of the relationship between science achievement and science attitude: kindergarten through college. *Journal of Research in Science Teaching, 20*(9), 839–850.

Xin, YP, Jitendra, AK, & Deatline-Buchman, A. (2005). Effects of mathematical word problem-solving instruction on middle school students with learning problems. *The Journal of Special Education, 39*(3), 181–192.

Yimer, A, & Ellerton, NF. (2009). A five-phase model for mathematical problem solving: identifying synergies in pre-service-teachers' metacognitive and cognitive actions. *ZDM, 42*, 245–261.

Zheng, X, Swanson, HL, & Marcoulides, GA. (2011). Working memory components as predictors of children's mathematical word problem solving. *Journal of Experimental Child Psychology, 110*(4), 481–498.

8

Teachers' perceptions of students' mathematical work while making conjectures: an examination of teacher discussions of an animated geometry classroom scenario

Wendy R Aaron[1] and Patricio G Herbst[2*]

Abstract

Background: This paper reports on a study examining teachers' perceptions of students they observed in an animated episode and who were engaged in the work of making conjectures in a geometry classroom. We examined eight conversations among subsets of 29 experienced geometry teachers with respect to how they described students and the mathematical work they perceived students to be engaged in.

Results: Across the study group conversations, participants described students in terms of the tasks' mathematical resources which students could understand or misunderstand and the tasks' material and social resources which they could use or misuse, but participants paid little attention to the operations that students might employ in the task or the goals that students were working toward in the task.

Conclusions: This study suggests that, when supporting students' work on conjecturing tasks, teachers focus on the tasks' resources which students use. This conjecture suggests in turn that in exchanging students' work on conjecturing tasks for claims that students have learned a bit of the geometry curriculum, teachers might deem that particular work valuable on account of the resources used.

Keywords: Geometry; Teachers' perceptions; Conjecturing; Mathematics education; Animation; Students; Task

Background

Across the world, mathematics education reform efforts and mathematics education researchers have recommended a focus on conjecturing and justification in school mathematics (Haggarty and Pepin, 2002; Jones and Fujita, 2013; Kilpatrick, Swafford, and Findell, 2001; Lannin et al., 2011; National Council of Teachers of Mathematics (NCTM), 2000; National Governors Association Center for Best Practices and Council of Chief State School Officers, 2010). As reform movements - like the Common Core State Standards for Mathematics (CCSSM) in the United States - take root, teachers face the challenge of incorporating conjecturing activities into their lessons in ways that build on students' capabilities and reflect fidelity to the discipline of mathematics.

A novel feature of the CCSSM is the eight Standards for Mathematical Practice added to mathematical content standards for each grade level and domain. One of those eight Standards for Mathematical Practice, Standard 3, specifically asks students to engage in conjecturing activities: Students are to construct viable arguments and critique the reasoning of others. To meet this standard, students are asked to 'make conjectures and build a logical progression of statements to explore the truth of their conjectures' (National Governors Association Center for Best Practices and Council of Chief State School Officers, 2010, p. 6). On the one hand, the explicit push for students to engage in producing and justifying conjectures is exciting because it encourages students to engage in authentic mathematical work (as described by Lakatos, 1976; and Thurston, 1994, among others). On

* Correspondence: pgherbst@umich.edu
[2]School of Education 610 East University Ave. University of Michigan, Ann Arbor, MI 48109-1259, USA
Full list of author information is available at the end of the article

the other hand, the push could be daunting if it further complicates the work of teaching, which is probable considering the complexity of the work expected from students and the expectation that teachers be responsive to students as they support students' conjecturing.

The study reported on here explores one of the sources of increased complexity of teachers' work as they support students to engage in making conjectures: What teachers perceive in students' work as they are engaged in making conjectures. Through understanding teachers' perceptions of students while they are engaged in making conjectures, we can gain insight into the work that teachers do to support students. These insights can be instrumental in supporting teachers to expand the types of reasoning that students engage in within the classroom.

We consider this research on teachers' perceptions of students' work in context as an important complement to existing and ongoing research on teachers' perception of students' identities that pays attention to their membership in communities (e.g., Clark et al., 2009) as well as to existing and ongoing work in educational psychology on teachers' perception of students' ability (e.g., Jussim, 1989). Indeed, in a key precursor of our study, Morine-Dershimer (1978-79) noted that 'teacher conception of pupils appear to be embedded in an instructional context' (p. 43).

This paper begins with a discussion of what conjecturing activities look like in schools and the impact that teachers' perceptions of students have on students' learning opportunities. We then introduce the conceptual framework of practical rationality and show how it can be useful for understanding the work that teachers do while supporting students in making conjectures. The Results section examines the ways that groups of teachers perceived students actions as those teachers saw students engaged in the work of making conjectures. We end by sharing a conjecture about how teachers' perception of students' work in conjecturing task might inform the exchange teachers need to make of students' work on conjecturing tasks for claims that students have learned a bit of the geometry curriculum.

Reasoned conjectures in classrooms and teachers' work

Research on student thinking shows that learners are capable of making reasoned and insightful conjectures (for examples, see Balacheff, 1988; Boero et al., 1999; Ellis, 2007a; 2007b; Herbst, 2006; Lee and Sriraman, 2011; Mariotti, 2006; Martin and Pirie, 2003; Mueller and Maher, 2009; Yerushalmy, 1987, 1993). This body of research provides a template for the types of conjecturing activities that students could engage in during instruction. For instance, Ellis (2007b) shows three primary categories of conjecturing activities enacted by learners: *relating* similar situations or objects, *searching* for relationships, procedures, patterns, or solutions, and *extending* patterns or relationships into more general structures. Yerushalmy (1987, 1993) decomposed students' work on conjecturing tasks into three conjecturing activities: developing and identifying categories for generalization, forming a coherent sample of instances, and inducing generality from a sample of instances.

The examples summarized above are a small sample of the range of work that has shown learners' capabilities with respect to conjecturing and reasoning activities. They illustrate in particular that conjecturing work, when it happens, calls for students to engage in cognitive operations. However, students do not always have the opportunity to create and express these reasoned and insightful conjectures in classrooms. Writing about geometry classrooms, Herbst and colleagues have described the teacher's management of 'making conjectures' as a special case of the instructional situation of *exploration* which is a student-centered alternative for the introduction of a new idea. Herbst (2010) notes that in a situation of exploration,

> the work to be done includes the students' free choosing among a range of material operations to apply on concrete (physical or pictorial) embodiments of the concept depending the tools available to them, their reading of the particular results of those operations, and the translation of those results into general statements made in the conceptual register. The reasoning that students could thus have the opportunity to engage in can be described as abductive, proceeding from particular to general (p. 42).

To further describe what making conjectures involves in the high school geometry classroom, we propose a set of instructional norms to underpin the interaction among teacher and students around conjectures (see Table 1).

As is the case with norms for any instructional situation, the statements in Table 1 represent our hypotheses of shared expectations of the teacher and students regarding students' mathematical work and the exchange value of that work; they do not represent standards for

Table 1 Instructional norms for 'making conjectures'

Instructional norms
1. The teacher provides students with diagrams of mathematical objects and tools to use in conjecturing and prompts students to come up with conjectures
2. The teacher expects students to generate conjectures that state properties about said objects
3. The teacher does not have expectations for the generality of students' conjectures
4. The teacher enables students' to share their conjecture with the class
5. The teacher oversees discussion of each conjecture

correctness or desirability we espouse. Rather, those statements represent what we hypothesize are the norms teacher and students recognize for the situation of 'making conjectures': Our laying out of such norms is meant, like any theoretical assumption in research, as a way to simplify a system under study so that further claims about that (simplified) system can be made. This means that proposing the norms themselves is not an end in itself but a means to further understand 'making conjectures.' One could ask at some point whether those norms are indeed recognized as such by high school geometry teachers (see Herbst, et al., 2013, for an example of how to instrument such verification) but the value of asking that verification question will be heightened if one could show first that the conjectured norms are useful; this paper is concerned with those norms only insofar as their usefulness to further understand 'making conjectures.'

From the list of instructional norms in Table 1, we can imagine how the work of 'making conjectures' might unfold in classrooms. The norms suggest that instructional work includes the teacher presenting a task that provides students with mathematical, material, and social resources and asks students to make a conjecture; those resources could include a diagram and tools to gather information from it, as well as some description of the concepts students are to work with and the request to make some conjectures. Students have time to work on the task, and this work may include both observing the diagram and observing how the diagram responds to actions the students may do on them, such as drawing in or measuring attributes. The teacher expects that students will be able to craft conjectures, which will be statements about the figure represented, but more than one conjecture may be possible for students to offer for a given diagram. The teacher also does not usually expect students to have a proof for their conjecture or an explanation detailing how they arrived at their conjecture. The teacher then chooses a student to share his conjecture with the class. After the student has shared his conjecture, the teacher oversees the discussion of the conjecture, either through sharing her own comments or by asking the class to share their comments. Once the conjecture has been discussed, the class moves on to discussing another conjecture or transitions to another activity (for example, to the proof of an endorsed conjecture).

The research mentioned above suggests that 'making conjectures' unfolds in classrooms in two distinct phases: (1) students work privately (individually or in groups) making conjectures and (2) the class publicly discusses those conjectures. Herbst (2010) also notes that in an exploration,

> There are engagement stakes, according to which it is important to involve students in actively doing something self directed in geometry. There are also content stakes that include new general statements about a generic instance of an abstract concept (p. 42).

That is, *a priori*, one can expect that an exploration is done so that students consider particular ideas, but one can also expect that the exploration is done so that students participate in mathematical activity. One question to ask about situations of conjecturing is whether and how those two goals can be pursued together and how those two goals frame the way teachers perceive students' work. The current study investigates how teachers perceive students' work within 'making conjectures' and how those perceptions could impact teachers' negotiation of the stakes of the activity in terms of engagement or content. Below, we discuss research that examines the connection between teachers' perceptions of students and how those perceptions impact the opportunities that students have to engage in mathematical work.

Impact of teachers' perceptions of students on students' opportunities to learn

Research on teachers' perceptions of students has been conceptualized around what individual teachers know, believe, or notice about individual students (Hill et al., 2008; Morine-Dershimer, 1978; Sherin et al., 2010). The study reported in this paper builds on prior work to investigate the categories that the mathematics teaching profession uses to describe students, as illustrated within conversations among a group of teachers.

The categories of students that groups of teachers use to describe and discuss their students inform the ways in which teachers' actions are contingent on the work they see their students engaging in. These categories reveal clues about the features of student activity that teachers respond to and the possibilities for student action that are supported by teachers (Horn, 2005, 2007). In particular, research has shown that groups of teachers who discuss their students in dynamic and flexible ways also provide increased opportunities for students to learn (Horn, 2005). By exploring the ways in which teachers talk about students' actions while they are making conjectures, we hope to uncover the aspects of students' work that teachers respond to and the opportunities to do mathematical work that teachers create for students.

Conceptual framework

The present inquiry is inscribed within efforts to describe the practical rationality of mathematics teaching - the categories of perception and appreciation that underpin the work of teaching mathematics. Teachers' perceptions of their students are part of that rationality; those perceptions are expected to inform the decisions teachers make in instruction (Herbst and Chazan, 2011a; Green, 1976). *Practical rationality* is a general expression that covers experiences, knowledge, perceptions, and judgments that are shared among teachers of similar courses of study, such as algebra, geometry, or calculus. Practical rationality points to teaching knowledge as not limited to being rational in the sense of goal oriented or correct but also rational as sensible, adapted to the demands of the work that teachers do. This is consistent with the way in which Kahneman (2002) has described rationality as bounded to the works of two cognitive systems, a rational, explicit, and slower one, and an adaptive, tacit, and faster one. In our case, we are interested not so much on individuals' rationality but on the rationality of the professional collective for which we hypothesize some actions to be warranted on deliberate application of principles and reasons while others on the custom of replicating past patterns of interaction. This view of rationality allows for tensions, contradictions, and inconsistencies to exist in teachers' actions and decision-making and for research into that practical rationality to inquire on how teachers resolve them.

In particular, practical rationality is concerned with *categories of perception*, or how teachers perceive 'people, events, things, and ideas in the shared world of the classroom', and *categories of appreciation*, or 'the principles and qualities on which practitioners rely to establish an attitude toward people, events, things, or ideas' (Herbst and Chazan, 2011a, p. 430-1). The current study investigates teachers' categories of perception and appreciation related to students. That is, we are interested in the specific types of students that teachers perceive in the classroom and how they make sense of students' work in relation to the work of teaching.

We hypothesize that the set of categories of perception and appreciation that teachers use to describe their students is not a simple reflection of the types of students who populate their classroom. The categories reflect important features of the work of teaching and imply a social and moral order that is embedded in the work of teaching (see Bowker and Star, 1999, for a discussion of the social and moral order inherent in classification systems). By understanding the categories of perception and appreciation that teachers use in relation to their students, we learn about what teachers see as important in their work and how characteristics of student work are valued or not within the confines of that work. This in turn informs our understanding of instructional actions.

To understand classroom interactions we use a model based on the notion of a symbolic economy (Bourdieu, 1980, 1998) and a didactical contract (Brousseau, 1997). According to this model, teachers and students act as if they are managing a trade between accomplished classroom work and claims that the students have had an opportunity to learn a bit of the content at stake. The foundational hypothesis is that inside educational institutions, the teacher and her students enter into this economy because of their obligation to a didactical contract that brings students and teachers together to teach and learn mathematics. A didactical contract specifies what it means to teach and learn and what the content is that needs to be taught and learned.

Research on the use of specially designed tasks (e.g., Brousseau, 1997; Herbst, 2003) has shown that one way teachers exchange students' mathematical work for a claim on what students know is by negotiating with them how the didactical contract applies to the task when a task is enacted. This negotiation is particularly needed when the task is novel (Doyle, 1988): The negotiation may involve changes to the task itself or to what the task completion is taken to be evidence of. In the extreme, the task can be dramatically changed or its place as part of the course of studies can be severely alienated.

Another way in which the exchange between students' mathematical work and a teacher's claim on what they know is by framing such work as an instance of an *instructional situation* (Herbst, 2006; Herbst and Chazan, 2012). Instructional situations are recurrent patterns of activity that organize the actions of the students and teacher around mathematical objects. An instructional situation clusters tasks that are similar to each other in terms of what mathematical elements they contain, what actions they call forth from teacher and students, and what their completion is evidence of. In particular, tasks that are commonplace in a mathematics course, such as 'solve $2x - 1 = 3x + 4$' in algebra, do not often call for a negotiation of the task, since the word 'solve' and the existence of one variable both act as cues to conjure up what the student is supposed to do (Chazan and Lueke, 2009). In general, we hypothesize that these customary, recurrent patterns of activity, these instructional situations, make room for some canonical tasks saving teachers and students the need to negotiate how the contract applies for the task.

To conceptualize the work that students do in classrooms, we follow Doyle (1983, 1988) in using 'mathematical task' to describe self-contained segments of mathematical work that students do in classrooms. In developing his model of task, Doyle (1983) was interested in accounting for the curriculum from the students' perspective; accordingly, he described tasks as consisting of the *goal* that students are working toward, the *resources* (these could be mathematical, material, or social) that they have available to pursue those goals, the *operations* (mental or physical) that they enact to move toward their goal, and the value of the completed work with respect to an *accountability system* (particularly the grades students could get from completing the task; for an example of how students might value their work on tasks, see Aaron and Herbst, 2011). In our case, as the interest is in tasks from the teacher's perspective, the fourth element of accountability is expressed in terms of the currency the teacher manages, namely the knowledge at stake - hence the notion of instructional exchange noted above.

A goal for a task could be the construction of a conjecture. That is the case in a lesson about the angle bisectors problem, which we used to inquire on teachers' perceptions of students. The goal of the task was for students to make a conjecture about the angle bisectors of a quadrilateral: After reminding students what happens with angle bisectors of a triangle, the teacher asks 'what can one say about the angle bisectors of a quadrilateral'. In the angle bisectors problem, operations could include the drawing of quadrilaterals and their angle bisectors and observing whether the angle bisectors of those quadrilaterals meet at a point or make some other configuration. The resources could include the diagrams, prior knowledge about the definition of angle bisector, knowledge of the fact that angle bisectors of a triangle meet at a point, or time to work independently on the task.

The study reported on here informs the question of how teachers could draw on the classroom accountability system in order to exchange students' work on conjecturing tasks for claims that they have learned some bit of the geometry curriculum. We see this as a critical question related to teachers' increased responsibility to integrate conjecturing into what they are responsible for teaching. Without a clear sense of the value of students' mathematical work on conjecturing, teachers may (understandably) marginalize or exclude this work from their instruction. To inform this question, we examine how teachers perceive students' work on conjecturing tasks; such examination can provide grounds for hypotheses about how teachers could allocate value to this work. We ask the following research questions:

- What perceptions of students do teachers draw upon while observing students working independently to make conjectures?
  - What *resources* do teachers perceive students using?
  - What *operations* do teachers perceive students deploying?
  - What *goals* do teachers perceive students working toward?
- What perceptions of students do teachers draw upon while orchestrating the sharing and discussing of conjectures?
  - What *resources* do teachers perceive students using?
  - What *operations* do teachers perceive students deploying?
  - What *goals* do teachers perceive students working toward?

In thinking about teachers' perceptions of students, we hypothesize that when teachers talk about their students within the context of instruction, they describe their students in terms that can be understood to relate to the task; and that teachers might talk about their students differently depending if students are engaged in working independently to make conjectures or if students are engaged in sharing and discussing conjectures. Insights gained from these research questions will be used to inform the question of how teachers manage the exchange of students' work on conjecturing tasks for claims that students have learned a bit of the geometry curriculum. In the following section, we describe the data and analytic method that was used in the current study to inform these research questions.

Methods

The current section describes the data and analytic method used in this study. The phenomenon we are after is the collective resources that professionals who teach geometry use when observing students' work on conjecturing tasks - we elicited that data by listening to groups of teachers who were prompted to talk by a representation of instructional practice (Herbst and Chazan, 2011b) in which students were making and discussing conjectures. A representation of practice was used to create a context in which participants' discussion about students' work could be concrete. While methodologically the use of a specific classroom scenario poses questions of construct validity, we see this as a first step in exploring the sort of perceptions of students' work that teachers have; obviously, this exploration could use being followed by other studies that confront teachers with a variety of representations of students' conjecturing work.

The representation of teaching used was an animation of a classroom scenario, which had been rendered using nondescript cartoon characters with voice over. The use of an animation helped focus participants' discussion on the actions happening in the lesson (hence on the universe that contains students' mathematical work) without encouraging assumptions about the larger social context or histories of the individuals involved. Prior research (Herbst and Kosko, 2014) has shown that animations are just as good as video records in eliciting teachers' tacit knowledge of practice; we have used these representations in other studies (e.g., Herbst et al., 2011a; Weiss and Herbst, in press) where they have provided context for participants' conversations about practice and helped elicit other categories of perception and appreciation.

Our examination of group conversations among experienced geometry teachers about an animated classroom scenario used tools from systemic functional linguistics (Halliday, 1994; Martin and Rose, 2003). Our analysis identified the descriptions of students that teachers constructed during their conversations around the conjecturing task shown in the animation and resulted in a list of descriptions of students that are relevant to aspects of the conjecturing task.

Data

The data presented here were collected over the course of two school years in study groups with experienced[a] geometry teachers. Participants served students from a diverse group of schools including urban, suburban, and rural schools. Each year, two groups of five to twenty teachers met for 3 h once per month. Study group sessions around animated classroom scenarios were aimed at uncovering the practical rationality of geometry teaching; in particular, the animated classrooms scenarios were designed and employed to elicit from teachers' recognition of instructional norms that guide their work with students and mathematics content in classrooms.

In the study group sessions, participants watched and responded to animated classroom scenarios[b] in conversations with fellow participants and members of the research team. See Figure 1 for a still image from an animated classroom scenario. The animated classrooms scenarios were designed to provide enough detail about the scenario so they would evoke from teachers' relational and temporal demands of teaching while also being lean enough so they would allow for teachers to project the demands of their own teaching context (Aaron and Herbst, 2007). Participants also engaged in other activities related to the animated scenarios, like working on mathematical tasks, looking at student work, and reading and writing scripts for classroom scenarios.

The sessions were video and audio recorded and then transcribed and indexed for analysis. To index the data corpus, sessions were divided into *intervals* based on changes in the activity structure of the session (Herbst et al., 2011b; see also Lemke, 1990). An interval is a continuous length of time during a study group session in which participants are engaged in a particular activity or conversation. Herbst et al. (2011b) define it thus, '[a] n interval consists of segments of group interaction that participants construct as units of conversation by way of employing a combination of... organizational features' (p. 231). Organizational features include who the active participants are, the division of labor in the conversation, the labels that participants use to describe the theme being discussed, and length of interval (intervals are normally on the order of 2 to 8 min). The parsing of sessions according to these features resulted in intervals that cover the timeline of the session and overlap at their boundaries.

The data for this study consist of all the intervals in which the participants discussed one particular animated scenario, The Square (the plot of The Square is outlined below). The Square was watched in eight sessions, which are divided into of 368 intervals. During those sessions, The Square was discussed in 119 intervals[c]. In the remainder of the intervals, participants were discussing other animated scenarios, responding to prompts not related to any animated scenario, discussing logistics, or taking breaks.

Description of the animated scenario The Square

The animated scenario used in the study groups, The Square, shows a geometry class working on several

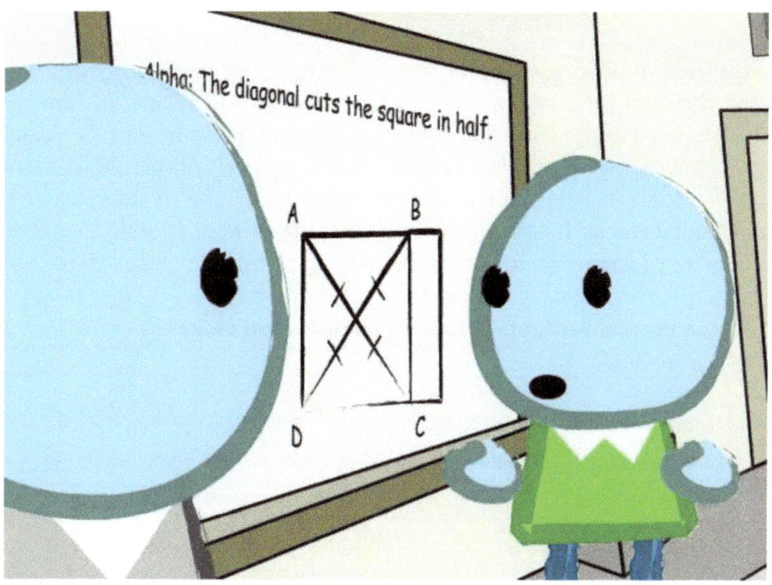

Figure 1 A student contributing to a discussion of a conjecture in the animation The Square". © The Regents of the University of Michigan, all rights reserved, used with permission.

different, but related, mathematical tasks. In this study, we examine the first few tasks, which are framed as an example of 'making conjectures.' These segments of the animated scenario elicited conversations among the participants that contained descriptions of students related to instructional work around conjecturing tasks.

The animated episode begins with the teacher giving the class the angle bisectors of a quadrilateral problem, as noted above. The teacher then says to the class 'I'll give you some time to make conjectures and then we will see if we can prove some of those conjectures'. After some time, a student, Alpha, shares a conjecture about diagonals of a square; the teacher evaluates the conjecture by reminding the class that the task is about angle bisectors; the teacher asks the class if diagonals and bisectors are the same thing; another student, Gamma, further evaluates Alpha's conjecture by illustrating that diagonals and angle bisectors are different using the case of a rectangle; and in light of Gamma's counter-example, the class reformulates Alpha's conjecture to be that the angle bisectors of a square meet at a point. The episode ends with the class attempting to prove the reformulated conjecture.

In the Results section, we share the descriptions of students that came from participants' conversations around the portions of the episode when the class was engaged in 'making conjectures'. In the following section, we describe how the data were analyzed.

Analysis of data

To analyze the data of study group conversation, we made use of systemic functional linguistics. Systemic functional linguistics (SFL) is a theory of language as a social semiotic system, developed originally by Michael Halliday (Halliday and Matthiessen, 2004). SFL looks closely at the word choices that individuals deploy in order to construct meaning through language, and it is founded on the idea that language provides organized resources to make various kinds of meaning: ideational, interpersonal, and textual. We look in particular at the ideational meta-function of language and how individuals construct the participants, processes, and context that populate discourse (Lemke, 2012). The transcripts of intervals were first coded using elements from participant analysis and cohesion chains (Halliday, 1994; Martin and Rose, 2003). Participant analysis focuses on the people and things that take part in the actions described in the conversation. Cohesion chains trace how actors and objects are represented across the conversation. These analyses provided information about how the teachers' use of words and phrases represented their perceptions of students.

Categories of perception of students were coded in the transcript whenever participants described either an animated student from The Square, a real student from their own classroom, or a hypothetical student[d] in relation to 'making conjectures'. When participants described any of these, the coding scheme recorded both the description that the participant gave and any additional information that participants gave about the student, like actions that the student performs, challenges they present for the teacher, etc. Each description was coded with respect to the dimension of the task (resource, operation, or goal) and the phase of 'making conjectures;' working independently to make conjectures, or sharing and discussing students' conjectures, that the description related to.

The methods described above allow for analysis of participants' perceptions of students and for relating descriptions of students used in discussions among teachers to how teacher perceive their students. Below, we collect the descriptions of students who teachers perceived as being relevant to the teacher's work of supporting students in making conjectures.

Results

Below, we provide examples of the ways that participants in study groups described students while discussing instructional decisions in the context of the animated classroom episode, The Square. (see Table 2 for a summary of perceptions of students.) The descriptions of students in the results are grouped by the phase of 'making of conjectures' that the described students were engaged in. We first report on how the students were

Table 2 Focal students while the teacher facilitates work on conjecturing tasks

Phase of activity	*Focal students*	*# Descriptions across # intervals*
Making conjectures	• Students who misuse task resources	10/7
	• Students who would benefit from the use of additional resources	8/6
	• Students who might encounter difficulty making a conjecture	21/16
Sharing and discussing conjectures	• Students who share their conjecture at the board	5/4
	• Students who have trouble making sense of their peers' conjectures	11/7
	• Students who used their peers' conjectures to better understand their own conjecture	3/3

described with respect to working independently to make conjectures; then we report on how students were described with respect to sharing and discussing conjectures. Over the 119 intervals that were coded for perceptions of students, 58 descriptions of students emerged across 36 intervals. Thirty-nine descriptions were related to working independently to make a conjecture, and 19 descriptions were related to sharing and discussing a conjecture.

Perceptions of students related to working independently to make a conjecture

The animation The Square gave participants a context to discuss students' independent work making a conjecture. While students are working on crafting a conjecture, the teacher has the opportunity to guide and observe each dimension of the task; namely, the resources that students use, the operations that students perform, and the goals that students work toward. Below are descriptions of students from the participants' discussion of how students work on the conjecturing task. In the data, we see that the majority of participants' descriptions of students related to working on the task can be placed into three categories: students who misuse task resources, students who would benefit from the use of additional resources, and students who might be unsuccessful in making a conjecture.

Students who misuse task resources

When participants described students working on the conjecturing task, we see evidence that they perceived students in light of students' misuse of task resources, in particular, angle bisectors and diagonals. Students were described as misusing task resources ten times across seven intervals. One participant, Tina, expected that students' confusion around angle bisectors and diagonals was inevitable. She said, 'I think that confusion would've been there, no matter what. When you say angle bisectors, half the class is going to [think] diagonals anyway' (TMW111506, 40, 1115). Another participant, Denise, said that if she insisted to her students that diagonals and angle bisectors are different, her students would look at their diagram of a square and respond, 'No, you don't know what you're talking about because they are the same' (TMW111506, 48, 1326). In the quotes, we see the participants anticipating that students will conflate the resources of the task.

Students who would benefit from the use of additional resources

We also see evidence in the data to support the claim that the participants perceived students in terms of additional task resources that would improve students' success with making conjectures. Across six intervals, participants provided eight descriptions of students related to additional resources aimed at improving students' work on making conjectures. Participants saw that the animated teacher could have provided the class with a worksheet that contained several examples of one type of quadrilateral, several different quadrilaterals, or a hierarchical list of the quadrilaterals (Jillian, TMW111506, 30, 830; Jillian, TM W111506, 30, 832; James, ThEMaT081905, 9, 142). Raina suggested that students could have worked with a partner. She said, 'maybe [Alpha's] got the kid that he's sitting next to that he's working with and they come up with this idea together' (TMT110706, 17, 206). Lucille recommended that students could have use technological support. She said, 'I think some kids like the computers or the calculators' (ESP091305, 4, 45). Thus, additional resources like worksheets that structured students' work, provided diagrams of quadrilaterals, partners for students to share their thinking with, or extra tools were suggested as things that students could use.

Students who might encounter difficulty making a conjecture

In the study group data, participants described students who they expected might encounter difficulty as the class worked toward making conjectures. In 16 intervals, there are 21 instances of participants describing how students might be unsuccessful in arriving at a conjecture. Tina said, 'I'll have kids who'll draw a square three times in a row. "Well, draw something different than a square"... Other kids who have done, maybe done three different ones, you might just say, "Good job", you know, "Keep going" you know, "Draw some conclusions"' (TMW111506, 13, 359). Tabitha indicated which students would have needed help, 'I'd probably start with the kids who are sitting there, either talking to their neighbor or staring at the wall and say, "alright, well, draw something with four sides. Draw in angle bisectors. Draw something else with four sides"' (TMW111506, 12, 327). Participants perceived that students might be unsuccessful for a variety of reasons, including oversimplifying the problem by not making use of the range of useful resources or operations or not being able to formulate a plan or enter into the work.

Looking across these categories of students that participants described with respect to working independently to make conjectures, we see that participants are primarily concerned with ensuring that students understand the resources of the task, such as diagonals and angle bisectors, and that students will know what operations they can deploy with those resources. We see evidence that participants perceive students in terms of their successful use of appropriate resources and operations, but we do not see evidence that participants attend to the goal of the task, the conjecture that students are working toward. In particular, students were not differentiated in terms of what conjecture they could come up with. Rather, participants appeared to accept any conjecture students might come up with as long as resources had been used appropriately.

Perceptions of students related to sharing and discussing students' conjectures

The animation The Square also gave students a context to respond to how a class might discuss students' conjectures. While students are sharing and discussing their conjectures, the teacher has the opportunity to choose which students share conjectures, which conjectures get shared, and how students interact with each other's conjectures. Below are descriptions of students from the participants' comments on how students share and discuss conjectures. In the data, we see that the majority of participants' descriptions of students related to sharing and discussing conjectures can be placed into three categories: students who share their conjecture with the class, students who have trouble making sense of their peer's conjecture, and students who use their peers' conjectures to better understand their own conjecture.

Students who share their conjecture at the board

Participants' discussed students sharing their conjectures using only five descriptions across four intervals. Despite the critical impact that the choice of which student shares and which conjecture is shared can have on the class' discussion, we do not have much evidence about how participants perceive students who are engaged in this work. Megan said that she would call on the student who explored an interesting case, 'The minute I was done with [Alpha's conjecture], I would've picked [the student with a conjecture about a kite]' (TMT110706, 13, 123). Denise saw the reasonableness of recording several conjectures with the hope that collectively they would lead to an interesting conclusion, 'I think they were trying to just put all the points up there so you can come up with one big point' (TMW111506, 37, 985). Across the data, participants described students in relation to the quadrilateral that they used as a basis for their conjecture and in relation to the number of students who would have their conjecture shared. One could imagine that participants would describe students in terms of the content of their conjecture or the process that students used to arrive at their conjecture; however, this is not apparent in our data.

Students who have trouble making sense of their peer's conjecture

The majority of participants' descriptions of students related to sharing conjectures reflect a concern that students in the class will have difficulty making sense of the conjecture that is shared. Participants describe students as having difficulty making sense of conjectures shared by others in 11 descriptions across seven intervals. As students shared conjectures that distinguished between diagonals and angle bisectors, Tina said that she would work to emphasize the distinction; she said, 'Because half the class is going be thinking "diagonal"' (TMW111506, 43, 1201). Melanie worried that students would have difficulty making sense of complicated diagrams that accompanied conjectures. She said,'There's a few [students] that would understand [the diagram] but it would lose the majority [of students]' (TMT110706, 55, 767). Some of participants' descriptions of students revisit the issue of misusing task resources, noting that confusion could prevent students from understanding the conjectures shared by their peers. Participants also describe students in relation to confusion that students might experience when confronted with a complicated diagram accompanying another student's conjecture. Both of these barriers to making sense of classmates' conjectures are tied to the resources that are used as the foundation of the conjectures being shared.

Students who used their peers' conjectures to better understand their own conjecture

In participants' descriptions of students related to sharing and discussing conjectures, we see evidence of the perception that students' discussion of their peers' conjectures can improve their understanding of their own conjectures. We see three descriptions of this type across three intervals. In response to a student who overgeneralized from the case of a square, Tina planned to ask a second student who made a conjecture about rectangles to share their conjecture to contradict the first student's claim. She said, 'And hopefully you'll have the kid who draws the rectangle [share their conjecture]' (TMW111506, 14, 395). We see evidence that participants expect that students could conclude that their conjecture was incorrect based on a peer's conjecture. The sharing and discussing of conjectures could support students in revising their conjectures without direct intervention from the teacher.

Looking across the three categories of students that participants describe with respect to sharing and discussing conjectures, we see evidence that participants attend to which students share their conjectures, how students are making sense of the conjectures shared by their classmates, and how students deepen their understanding of their own conjecture through discussing their classmates' conjectures. Interestingly, we again see participants describing more students in terms of the resources that they use to make conjectures and less description of students in terms of the conjectures that are shared or students' strategies for making conjectures.

The participants' comments highlighted above inform the question of how teachers perceive students as they are engaged in making conjectures. The descriptions of students were collected from conversations around the animated story, The Square; however, the ways in which participants described students are arguably relevant to teachers' work of supporting students in making conjectures in other geometric contexts. The comments that the animated episode elicits provide more than just information about participants' perception of the scenario presented in The Square; they can also be used to gain a deeper understanding of the categories of perception that guide teachers' work in classrooms. In the following section, we discuss the observations in terms of how teachers' perceptions of students shape students' work on making conjectures.

Discussion

From examining teachers' descriptions of students, we learn about the specific ways that students' work on conjecturing tasks is perceived by teachers and gain insight into how teachers manage the exchange of students' work on conjecturing tasks for claims that students have learned a bit of the geometry curriculum. In response to the first phase of work, working independently to make conjectures, teachers were concerned with the task resources that students use to make conjectures - in particular, teachers were concerned with how students misused task resources and what additional resources they might benefit from using. Additionally, teachers were concerned with the difficulties that students might encounter while working to make conjectures, such as not using the full range of resources and operations that they had available to them. In response to the second phase of work, sharing and discussing conjectures, we see teachers still attending to the resources that students are using (or misusing) with some attention to the operations that students perform. We see this through how teachers frame their concern with which students would share conjectures, how students would make sense of each other's conjectures, and how students would better understand their conjecture through discussing other students' conjectures.

As we look across teachers' descriptions of students with respect to the conjecturing task, it is striking that teachers describe students primarily in terms of the task resources, occasionally in terms of the task operations, and descriptions of students in terms of the task goal are absent. One can contrast that perception of students from what one might expect from other stakeholders. From the point of view of a mathematician, for example, the most important aspect of a conjecturing task might be the goal, the conjecture that results from the conjecturing activity, and how that conjecture expands the sphere of potential mathematical knowledge (Thurston, 1994). One could imagine that a mathematician would attend to the conjecture that students produced and how they worked toward or away from particular conjectures. In contrast, mathematics educators and learning scientists are likely to be cued into the task operations that students make use of when engaged in a task. Looking at the research on students' conjecturing, we see mathematics educators attending to the particular moves that students make while they are conjecturing, such as; relating similar situations or objects, searching for relationships, procedures, patterns, solutions, and extending patterns or relationships into more general structures (Ellis, 2007b) or developing and identifying categories for generalization, forming a coherent sample of instances and inducing generality from a sample of instances (Yerushalmy, 1987, 1993), and how these moves support students in successfully making conjectures.

Teachers' attention to the resources that students' use on conjecturing tasks may seem unlikely given what one might expect from mathematicians or mathematics educators; however, we see this attention consistent with teachers' obligations to value students' work in terms of the geometry curriculum. A principal component of the curriculum in high school geometry is knowledge of the mathematical concepts that students would be making conjectures about; quadrilaterals, angle bisectors, diagonals, etc. The specific operations that students perform during conjecturing tasks are not part of what the teacher is responsible for within the high school geometry curriculum. In terms of operations, teachers are responsible for supporting students in learning much broader categories of work, such as 'logical reasoning' or 'critical thinking.' Teachers hold themselves accountable to teach these broader operations during situations of 'doing proofs' when students are expected to work on proof tasks (Herbst and Brach, 2006). Within the 'doing proofs' situation students' work is exchanged for the claim that students have developed skill with specific operations, such as applying theorems and identifying giving information.

Herbst (2010) had described and illustrated how situations of exploration can be used to engage students in the introduction of new material. Clearly, conjecturing tasks could usher a class into a new theorem and some curricula have been developed to introduce geometric theorems through conjecturing (Serra, 1997). But new theorems are not necessarily introduced through engaging students in conjecturing tasks; quite often, they are merely installed by the teacher (Herbst et al., 2011b). Situations of geometric calculation (Hsu and Silver, 2014) or of doing proof (Herbst and Brach, 2006) are often used to create context for students to show they know those theorems. Situations of exploration seem however useful for teachers to ensure student participation and engagement; our data do show their concern with enabling and sustaining this participation.

Despite appearing as if teachers are not attending to important aspects of students' work on conjecturing tasks, we see that teachers' attention can be attributed to their responsibility in the didactical contract and the need to manage the exchange between students' work on conjecturing tasks and claims that some piece of the geometry curriculum has been taught and learned. We see evidence that teachers are attuned to the resources that students make use of while working on conjecturing tasks, and we can see that knowledge of these resources, such as mathematical objects and their definitions, are principal components of the geometry curriculum that high school geometry teachers see as exchanging for students' work on conjecturing tasks.

Conclusions

In this paper, we report on a study that looked at geometry teachers' perceptions of students while they are making conjectures. Scholars in educational psychology and in the growing area of mathematical identity have described students and teachers' perceptions of students in terms of enduring or emerging personal characteristics. For example, see work on students' open and closed understandings of mathematics (Boaler, 1998; 2002), growth and fixed mindsets (Dweck, 2006), grit (Duckworth et al., 2007; Tough, 2013), and classic work on multiple intelligences (Gardner, 1993). In contrast with those studies and following our earlier work (Aaron and Herbst, 2012) looking at students' in the context of the mathematical work they do, this study looks at teachers' perceptions of students within work environments, particularly within making conjectures. The generalizability of our findings is limited by the fact that we only looked at making conjectures, we relied on responses from a small number of practitioners to a particular scenario, and we analyzed these data qualitatively. In spite of those limitations, the findings suggest that in the context of conjecturing tasks, teachers perceive students primarily in terms of the resources that students use (and misuse) and in terms of their level of engagement. These perceptions can be attributed to the didactical contract of the high school geometry classroom and the pieces of the curriculum that teachers see as corresponding to students' work on conjecturing tasks.

As teachers frame conjecturing tasks as primarily about the resources that students use, we see that the operations that students use to make conjectures and the conjectures that students arrive at could be underspecified and undervalued in classrooms. As a result, 'making conjectures' could be seen as an ancillary activity. One way to increase the specificity and value of students' work on conjecturing tasks would be to increase and broaden the role that conjecturing plays in complying with the didactical contract in geometry. This might begin with policy changes, such as the inclusion of Standards for Mathematical Practice in the Common Core State Standards for mathematics. Further, conjecturing, including the specific operations that students engage in and the conjectures that they produce, would need to appear prominently in artifacts that shape teachers' vision of the curriculum, including textbooks and local and national assessments. This study speaks to the interplay between what students know and are able to do mathematically in classrooms and the impact that teachers' perceptions of students' work have on the mathematical opportunities that students have in classrooms.

Endnotes

[a]We considered teachers to be experienced if they had taught geometry for at least 3 years.

[b]Animated classroom scenarios created by this project, including the animated scenario used in this study, can be viewed online at www.lessonsketch.org.

[c]When quotes from the transcripts of sessions are displayed in the Results section, they are labeled with a parenthetical citation that contains the name of the session, the interval number within the session, and the transcript line number within the session. Session names identify each of the groups and preserve the dates when the sessions were held.

[d]Herbst (1998) discusses the *modal student* or 'a hypothetical person playing the role [of student] generalized across all students in the class' (p. 150).

Abbreviations

CCSSM: Core State Standards for Mathematics; NCTM: National Council of Teachers of Mathematics.

Competing interests

The authors declare that they have no competing interests.

Authors' contributions

WA contributed to the design of the animation, proposed this research project, performed the analysis of the discourse data, and drafted the manuscript. PH was the main designer of the animations and of the larger study to which this project contributed; PH contributed to the framing and final writing of the article. All authors read and approved the final manuscript.

Acknowledgments

The work reported here was part of the doctoral dissertation of the first author, done at author, done at the University of Michigan under the supervision of the second author. The work was done with the support of the U.S. National Science Foundation (NSF) grants ESI-0353285 to the second author. Writing was also supported by the NSF grant RF 229-227. All opinions are those of the authors and do not necessarily represent the views of the Foundation.

Author details

[1]College of Education 204E Furman Hall Oregon State University, Corvallis, OR 97330, USA. [2]School of Education 610 East University Ave. University of Michigan, Ann Arbor, MI 48109-1259, USA.

References

Aaron, W., & Herbst, P. (2007). *The use of animated sketches in constructing narratives of geometry teaching*. Chicago, IL: Paper presented at the Annual Meeting of AERA.

Aaron, W., & Herbst, P. (2011). An exploration of "studenting" in high school geometry classrooms. *Proceedings of the 33nd annual meeting of the North American Chapter of the International Group for the Psychology of Mathematics Education*. Reno, NV: University of Nevada, Reno.

Aaron, W. & Herbst, P. (2012). Teachers' and students' perceptions of classroom discussions. *Proceedings of the 34nd annual meeting of the North American Chapter of the International Group for the Psychology of Mathematics Education*. Kalamazoo, MI: Western Michigan University.

Balacheff, N. (1988). Aspects of proof in pupils' practice of school mathematics. In D Pimm (Ed.), *Mathematics, teachers and children* (pp. 216–235). London: Hodder & Stoughton.

Boaler, J. (1998). Open and closed mathematics: student experiences and understandings. *J Res Math Educ, 29*(1), 41–62.

Boaler, J. (2002). *Experiencing school mathematics: traditional and reform approaches to teaching and their impact on student learning*. Mahwah, NJ: Erlbaum.

Boero, P, Garuti, R, & Lemut, E. (1999). *About the generation of conditionality of statements and its links with proving (In Proceedings of the Conference of the International Group for the Psychology of Mathematics Education* (Vol. 100, p. 566)). Israel: Haifa.

Bourdieu, P. (1980). *The logic of practice*. Stanford, CA: Stanford University Press.

Bourdieu, P. (1998). *Practical reason: on the theory of action*. Stanford, CA: Stanford University Press.

Bowker, GC, & Star, SL. (1999). *Sorting things out: classification and its consequences*. Cambridge, MA: MIT Press.

Brousseau, G. (1997). *Theory of Didactical Situations in Mathematics: Didactique des mathématiques, 1970–1990. (N. Balacheff, M. Cooper, R. Sutherland, & V. Warfield, Eds. and Trans.)*. Dordrecht, The Netherlands: Kluwer.

Chazan, D, & Lueke, HM. (2009). Exploring tensions between disciplinary knowledge and school mathematics: implications for reasoning and proof in school mathematics. In D Stylianou, E Knuth, & M Blanton (Eds.), *Teaching and Learning Mathematics Proof Across the Grades* (pp. 21–39). Mahwah, NJ: Erlbaum.

Clark, LM, Johnson, W, & Chazan, D. (2009). Researching African American mathematics teachers of African American students: conceptual and methodological considerations. In DB Martin (Ed.), *Mathematics teaching, learning, and liberation in the lives of black children* (pp. 39–62). New York: Routledge.

Doyle, W. (1983). Academic work. *Rev Educ Res, 53*, 159–200.

Doyle, W. (1988). Work in mathematics classes: the context of students' thinking during instruction. *Educ Psychol, 23*(2), 167–180.

Duckworth, AL, Peterson, C, Matthews, MD, & Kelly, DR. (2007). Grit: perseverance and passion for long-term goals. *J Pers Soc Psychol, 92*(6), 1087. New York: Random House.

Dweck, C. (2006). Mindset: the new psychology of success. Random House LLC.

Ellis, AB. (2007a). Connections between generalizing and justifying: students' reasoning with linear relationships. *J Res Math Educ, 38*(3), 194–229.

Ellis, AB. (2007b). A taxonomy for categorizing generalizations: generalizing actions and reflection generalizations. *J Learn Sci, 16*(2), 221–262.

Gardner, H. (1993). *Frames of mind* (2nd ed.). New York: Basic Books.

Green, T. (1976). Teacher competence as practical rationality. *Educational Theory, 26*(3), 249–258.

Haggarty, L, & Pepin, B. (2002). An investigation of mathematics textbooks and their use in English, French and German classrooms: who gets an opportunity to learn what? *Br Educ Res J, 28*(4), 567–590.

Halliday, MAK. (1994). *An introduction to functional grammar*. London: E. Arnold.

Herbst, P. (1998). What works as proof in the mathematics class (Doctoral dissertation, University of Georgia, 1998). *Diss Abstr Int, 59*, 10A.

Herbst, P. (2003). Using novel tasks to teach mathematics: three tensions affecting the work of the teacher. *Am Educ Res J, 40*, 197–238.

Herbst, P. (2006). Teaching geometry with problems: negotiating instructional situations and mathematical tasks. *J Res Math Educ, 37*, 313–347.

Herbst, P. with González, G, Hsu, H Y, Chen, C, Weiss, M, and Hamlin, M. (2010). Instructional situations and students' opportunities to reason in the high school geometry class. Manuscript. Deep Blue at the University of Michigan, http://hdl.handle.net/2027.42/78372.

Herbst, P, Aaron, W, Dimmel, J, & Erickson, A. (2013). *Expanding students' involvement in proof problems: are geometry teachers willing to depart from the norm?* California April-May: Paper presented at the annual meeting of the American Educational Research Association San Francisco. 2013.

Herbst, P, & Brach, C. (2006). Proving and 'doing proofs' in high school geometry classes: what is 'it' that is going on for students and how do they make sense of it? *Cogn Instr, 24*, 73–122.

Herbst, P, Chazan, D, Chen, CL, Chieu, VM, & Weiss, M. (2011a). Using comics-based representations of teaching, and technology, to bring practice to teacher education courses. *ZDM: The International Journal on Mathematics Education, 43*(1), 91–103.

Herbst, P, & Chazan, D. (2011a). Research on practical rationality: studying the justification of actions in mathematics teaching. *The Mathematics Enthusiast, 8*(3), 405–462.

Herbst, P, & Chazan, D. (2011b). On creating and using representations of mathematics teaching in research and teacher development: introduction to this issue. *ZDM - The International Journal of Mathematics Education, 43*(1), 1–5.

Herbst, P, & Chazan, D. (2012). On the instructional triangle and sources of justification for actions in mathematics teaching. *ZDM: The International Journal on Mathematics Education, 44*(5), 601–612.

Herbst, P, & Kosko, K. (2014). Using representations of practice to elicit teachers' tacit knowledge of practice: a comparison of responses to animations and videos. *J Math Teach Educ, 17*(6), 515–537.

Herbst, P, Nachlieli, T, & Chazan, D. (2011b). Studying the practical rationality of mathematics teaching: what goes into "installing" a theorem in geometry? *Cogn Instr, 29*(2), 218–255.

Hill, HC, Ball, DL, & Schilling, SG. (2008). Unpacking pedagogical content knowledge: conceptualizing and measuring teachers' topic-specific knowledge of students. *J Math Educ, 39*(4), 372–400.

Horn, IS. (2005). Learning on the job: a situated account of teacher learning in high school mathematics departments. *Cogn Instr, 23*(2), 207–236.

Horn, IS. (2007). Fast kids, slow kids, lazy kids: framing the mismatch problem in mathematics teachers' conversations. *Journal of the earning Sciences, 16*(1), 37–79.

Hsu, H. Y. & Silver, E. (2014). Cognitive Complexity of Mathematics Instructional Tasks in a Taiwanese Classroom: An Examination of Task Sources. Journal for Research in Mathematics Education, 45(4), 460–496.

Jones, K, & Fujita, T. (2013). Interpretations of national curricula: the case of geometry in textbooks from England and Japan. *ZDM: The International Journal on Mathematics Education, 45*(5), 671–683.

Jussim, L. (1989). Teacher expectations: self-fulfilling prophecies, perceptual biases, and accuracy. *J Pers Soc Psychol, 57*(3), 469–480. 10.1037/0022-3514.57.3.469.

Kahneman, D. (2002). Maps of bounded rationality: a perspective on intuitive judgment and choice. *Nobel prize lecture, 8*, 351–401.

Kilpatrick, J, Swafford, J, & Findell, B (Eds.). (2001). *Adding it up: helping children learn mathematics*. Washington, DC: National Academy Press.

Lakatos, I. (1976). *Proofs and refutations: The logic of mathematical discovery (J. Worrall and E. Zahar, Eds.)*. Cambridge, UK: Cambridge University.

Lannin, J K, Ellis, A B & Elliott, R. (2011). Developing essential understanding of mathematical reasoning for teaching mathematics in prekindergarten-grade 8. Reston, VA: National Council of Teachers of Mathematics.

Lee, KH, & Sriraman, B. (2011). Conjecturing via reconceived classical analogy. *Educ Stud Math, 76*(2), 123–140.

Lemke, JL. (2012). Analyzing verbal data: principles, methods, and problems. In *Second International Handbook of Science Education* (pp. 1471–1484). Netherlands: Springer.

Lemke, JL. (1990). *Talking science: language, learning, and values*. Norwood, NJ: Ablex Publishing Corporation.

Mariotti, M. A. (2006). Proof and proving in mathematics education. In. A. Gutierrez & P. Boero (Eds),Handbook of research on the psychology of mathematics education: Past, present and future, (pp. 173–204). Rotterdam, The Netherlands: Sense.

Martin, L, & Pirie, S. (2003). Making images and noticing properties: the role of graphing software in mathematical generalisation. *Math Educ Res J, 15*(2), 171–186.

Martin, JR, & Rose, D. (2003). *Working with Discourse: meaning beyond the clause London: Continuum*.

Morine-Dershimer, G. (1978). How teachers "see" their pupils. *Educ Res Q, 1978–79*(3), 83–99.

Mueller, M, & Maher, C. (2009). Learning to reason in an informal math after-school program. *Math Educ Res J, 21*(3), 7–35.

National Council of Teachers of Mathematics (NCTM). (2000). *Principles and standards for school mathematics*. Reston, VA: Author.

National Governors Association Center for Best Practices and Council of Chief State School Officers. (2010). *Common core state standards for mathematics*. Washington, DC: Authors.

Serra, M. (1997). Discovering geometry: An investigative approach. Emeryville, CA: Key Curriculum Press.

Sherin, M, Jacobs, V, & Philipp, R (Eds.). (2010). *Mathematics teacher noticing: seeing through teachers' eyes*. New York: Routledge.

Thurston, W. (1994). On proof and progress in mathematics. *Bull Am Math Soc, 30*, 161–177.
Tough, P. (2012). How children succeed: grit, curiosity, and the hidden power of character. New York: Houghton Mifflin.
Weiss, M. and Herbst, P. (in press). Geometry teachers' mathematical sensibility: the role of theory-building and problem-solving in the secondary geometry course. *Educational Studies in Mathematics*.
Yerushalmy, M. (1987). *Introduction and generalization: an experiment in teaching and learning high school geometry (Doctoral Dissertation, Harvard University)*. Ann Arbor, MI: University Microfilms, Inc.
Yerushalmy, M. (1993). Generalization in geometry. In J. L. Schwartz, M. Yerushalmy, and B. Wilson (Eds), *The Geometric Supposer, what is it a case of?*, (pp. 57–84). Lawrence Erlbaum.

On understanding and improving the teaching of university Mathematics

Alan H. Schoenfeld[1*], Mike Thomas[2] and Bill Barton[2]

Abstract

Background: This paper reports on a professional development workshop in University level mathematics. The workshop was grounded in Schoenfeld's (How we think. A theory of goal-oriented decision-making and its educational applications, 2010) theoretical approach, emphasizing the roles of *R*esources (primarily, knowledge), *O*rientations (primarily, beliefs), and *G*oals (*R/O/Gs*) as factors in teachers' "in the moment" decision-making. Participants characterized their *R/O/Gs* prior to instruction, bringing for discussion videotapes of their instruction that raised issues for them about their *R/O/Gs* or the choices they made during teaching.

Results: For a surprisingly large percentage of these university mathematicians, the "mathematical correctness" of what they presented was a dominant consideration, to the point where it overshadowed other considerations.

Conclusion: This gives rise to a conjectural characterization of three somewhat overlapping classes of teachers (university mathematicians, expert teachers, and proficient teachers), with the suggestion that professional development might profitably differ in the ways that it is targeted to these three groups.

Introduction and overview

Truly expert teachers bring to their teaching at least two bodies of knowledge and beliefs. On the one hand, they have deep knowledge of the topics they teach—not "just" the main ideas, but a sense of how things fit together, ideas about what is important and generative, and ideas about what is essential to get right. On the other hand, they have a rich sense of students and learning—of what students are likely to understand or misunderstand and what to do about that, and about which examples will be memorable and will help to communicate the key ideas.[1] In the expert teacher (of a particular area; expertise is context-specific, of course), these two areas of knowledge blend together seamlessly and synergistically, producing pedagogical decisions that are both true to the content and pedagogically well guided.

This set of considerations is represented, in generic form, by Fig. 1.

All teachers draw upon mathematical and pedagogical considerations to varying degrees as they teach. What one can imagine is that for any particular teacher, mathematical knowledge and considerations, and pedagogical knowledge and considerations, may be more or less rich and one or the other may dominate in the teacher's decision-making. This paper suggests that university mathematicians' in-the-moment decision-making is significantly shaped by their mathematical knowledge and considerations. It also suggests that a form of professional development that focuses on having teachers elaborate on content considerations, what they believe is central about student learning, and their goals for instruction, can serve as a mechanism for productive reflections on teaching.

In what follows, we discuss three groups of teachers: (a) expert teachers (ETs), like those described by Ma (2010), whom we can think of as having a deep understanding of the content and pedagogy *of particular subject matter*, (b) university mathematicians (UM), who bring great strength of and commitment to subject matter knowledge in their teaching, and (c) proficient teachers (PT), who blend some skills and understandings from the two boxes in the middle of Fig. 1.

In the first, theoretical section of this paper, we argue that each of these three groups has distinctive characteristics that shape their in-class decision-making—characteristics that are documented in the section "Aspects of The University Mathematician's Practice". The underlying

* Correspondence: alans@berkeley.edu
[1]School of Education, University of California, EMST, Tolman Hall # 1670, Berkeley, CA 94720-1670, USA
Full list of author information is available at the end of the article

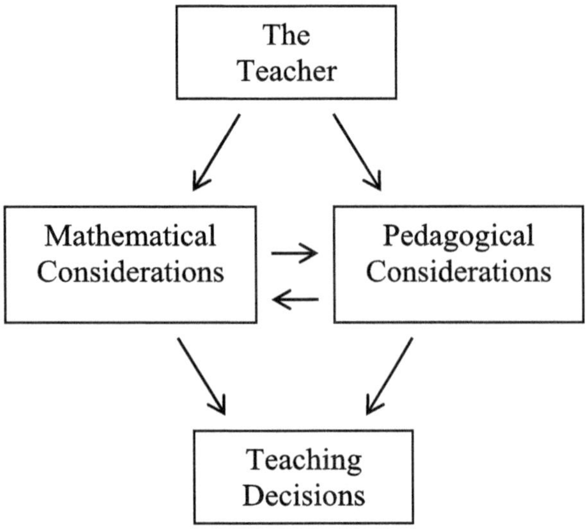

Fig. 1 A generic frame for teachers' decisions

theoretical approach for this characterization is Schoenfeld's (2010) theory of teachers' decision-making. That theoretical perspective served as the basis for a series of pedagogical development efforts with university mathematics faculty. In those efforts, which are described in the section "The professional development model" of this paper, the core constructs in the theory—a teacher's *R*esources (primarily knowledge), *O*rientations (such as beliefs) and *G*oals, or *R*/*O*/*G*—sometimes became the explicit focus of conversations about, and reflections upon, the faculty's teaching. As part of the professional development, observations, round table discussions and interviews with those faculty took place in the context of a supportive professional community. Ongoing conversations revealed an interesting commonality in the mathematician's orientations—what we call "effectively non-negotiable" aspects of their beliefs and orientations.

In total, this paper offers three novel contributions: a crisp framing of mathematics teachers' decision-making as suggested in Fig. 1, a discussion of how the *R*/*O*/*G* can serve as the foundation for the pedagogical development of university faculty (section "The professional development model"), and a description of how certain aspects of their content understandings—specifically, that the mathematics they teach must be nailed down irrefutably—appear to be core to the mathematicians' pedagogy (sections "Theoretical backdrop and assertions" and "Aspects of The University Mathematician's Practice").

Background

Theoretical backdrop and assertions

Research into teaching in schools has received wide attention, but the literature characterizing the practice of university lecturers is much sparser (Speer et al. 2010), and hence, much less is known about the effectiveness of UM pedagogical approaches. A key component of developing teaching practice is deciding where to focus attention (Russ et al. 2011). Speer (2008), following teacher education practice, suggests a focus on small, but meaningful, aspects of practice, especially those related to in-the-moment lecture decisions of academic staff. One such aspect that can repay attention is an analysis of the questions used in teaching practice. In this regard, Rowland (2000) observes that the style and format of the questions used by lecturers can profoundly influence students' conceptions of what mathematics is about and how it is conducted. Hence, an analysis of the different types of questions that UMs consider important, and the reasons for asking them, can lead to the enrichment of students' understanding and appreciation of mathematics. In addition, Barton and Paterson (2009) showed the positive value to practice when teachers work on areas of their practice they have personally identified as of concern. We sought to consider these principles the present study.

There are studies, often involving both mathematics educators and UMs, that have explored the teaching of UMs in lectures (Gueudet 2015; Gueudet et al. 2014; Jaworski et al. 2009; Lew et al. 2014; Nardi 2008; Nardi et al. 2005; Petropoulou et al. 2011; Thomas 2012) and in tutorials (Mali et al. 2014). The typical "chalk and talk" lecture has been shown to be alive and well (Lew et al. 2014), and it has been suggested that the recognition of teaching intentions, goals, and actions, and the identification of teaching tools, can provide the start of a "tool box" for improving teaching (Nardi et al. 2005). Two studies that focussed on UMs' teaching goals (Jaworski et al. 2009; Thomas 2012) employed theoretical constructs that focus on the student-centered nature of teaching. These are the *spectrum of pedagogical awareness*, which captures the degree to which teachers consciously engage with didactical issues to design teaching that engages students, and *the teaching triad* that identifies sensitivity toward students. One strategy to enhance student construction of meaning observed by Petropoulou et al. (2011) is a lecturer's use of well-chosen examples to illustrate critical characteristics of concepts. Other studies have focussed on lecturer's use of resources (Gueudet 2015; Gueudet et al. 2014), applying a documentational framework to analyze teacher involvement with sets of resources in goal-oriented activity, but without considering how this shapes practice. The issue of practice is crucial for us, in particular how UMs might gain relevant insights into teaching processes in order to develop their teaching (Jaworski et al. 2015).

In order to characterize practice-oriented professional development, we adopt the theory of decision-making described in Schoenfeld (2010). The core idea is that it is possible not only to understand but also to model a teacher's decisions by examining three fundamental factors:

- His/her *Resources*—primarily knowledge, but also including, for example, the technology in the classroom (Things are different with and without computers, clickers, etc.)
- His/her *Orientations* to the domain—in essence, what he or she considers important
- His/her *Goals* for the teaching interaction—in essence, what he or she is trying to achieve

In practice, a teacher or lecturer[2] uses their orientations to establish teaching goals, both before and during a lesson or lecture. The orientations are also used to adjust to the class situation and to activate relevant knowledge. Then, decisions consistent with the goals are made, consciously or unconsciously, about the directions to pursue and the resources to use. Such in-the-moment decisions are crucial since they affect how successful the teacher will be in attaining the goals they set (Schoenfeld 2010). Modeling teachers' decision-making is not our intention here—rather, we seek practical applications of the theory, aimed at understanding and improving teaching. The question is whether a focus on a teacher's *R*esources, *O*rientations, and *G*oals (*R*/*O*/*G*s) can be a productive mechanism for engaging teachers in rich conversations about their practices and, one hopes, enhancing their teaching thereby.

Our suggestion, based on data presented in the section "Aspects of the university mathematician's practice" is that for many UMs, some of the mathematical considerations in Fig. 1 are so strong as to be in effect non-negotiable—that, in essence, instruction will not proceed unless the instructor is convinced that the mathematics being discussed is absolutely correct. We suggest that there are parallel but different considerations for the highly qualified ET, for whom deeply connected content understandings at the relevant grade levels, including understandings of what students tend to understand and have difficulty with (a.k.a. pedagogical content knowledge; see Schoenfeld (2006) and Shulman (1986, 1987)), play the driving role with regard to mathematical considerations. In both of these cases (UM and ET, which are not necessarily mutually exclusive), subject matter considerations play a powerful role in framing the ways in which the teacher considers what is essential about the mathematics that will be learned by the student. (Note, however, that these concerns can be different for the two groups.) Given this perspective, "audience" or pedagogical considerations come after content considerations—the question being, "Given what the teacher deems to be important about the mathematics, what portion of that mathematics is right for this student audience, and how does the teacher feel students should interact with it?" As described below (and speaking in generalities, of course), considerations are different for the third category, PT.

On the differences between ET, UM, and PT

Both the expert teacher and the university mathematician have a particular kind of subject matter expertise—but these differ in kind, although they are overlapping. Perhaps the best known description of expert teaching is Ma's (2010) description of Chinese teachers who have "Profound Understanding" of the content they teach—at a level relevant to their teaching. One of Ma's examples is the topic of fractions (rational numbers) and operations on them.

On the one hand, there is the formal definition of rational number, which we take from Wikipedia:

(A) "The rational numbers can be formally defined as the equivalence classes of the quotient set $(\mathbf{Z} \times (\mathbf{Z} \setminus \{0\})) / \sim$, where the Cartesian product $\mathbf{Z} \times (\mathbf{Z} \setminus \{0\})$ is the set of all ordered pairs (m,n) where m and n are integers, n is not zero $(n \neq 0)$, and "$\sim$" is the equivalence relation defined by $(m_1,n_1) \sim (m_2,n_2)$ if, and only if, $m_1n_2 - m_2n_1 = 0$."

On the other hand, consider the following problem, taken from Ma (2010):

(B) Imagine that you are teaching division with fractions. To make this meaningful for kids, something that many teachers try to do is relate mathematics to other things. Sometimes they try to come up with real-world situations or story-problems to show the application of some particular piece of content. What would you say would be a good story or model for $1\frac{3}{4} \div \frac{1}{2}$?

The definition in (A) is "home turf" for mathematicians, who read it easily; but they might struggle to come up with 3 or 4 different stories to model different conceptions of $1\frac{3}{4} \div \frac{1}{2}$, the simple division in (B). In contrast, the expert teachers interviewed by Ma had no difficulty producing a range of stories that represent division by fractions—but many if not most would find the definition in (A) utterly incomprehensible. The point of this example is that the teachers Ma studied were *expert teachers of fractions*—they could run rings around university mathematicians when working with children because they had broader knowledge of the mathematics at the level of engagement with children, and of children's understandings, even though the university mathematicians' knowledge of the mathematics of rational numbers is much more advanced (and abstract). That is, the ET knows a great deal about the students and content that is relevant for teaching that content effectively and in a deep way, at that particular level—but he or she may not have significant understanding of the content beyond that level.

At the secondary level, the PT would be the one who can, for example, explain the various equations for a line—the point-slope formula, two-intercept formula, slope-intercept formula, and so on, and show students how to use them. The expert secondary teacher would have examples at hand, tailored to what he or she knows of student understandings and misconceptions—but, he or she would also know that students tend to see the formulas as separate "rules" to be memorized and used when one encounters a particular situation (e.g., "when I have a point and know the slope, I use the point-slope formula"). Thus, ET also stresses the fact that *any* two pieces of information about a line enable one to determine the equation, that the formulas can be derived from each other, and that one can be flexible in deriving equations because of that fact. UM knows this, of course—and some UMs are ETs—but in general, a UM may or may not be aware of the student tendency to think of the different formulas as being fundamentally unrelated, or think to take explicit steps to correct that misunderstanding. The same can be said about more advanced topics as well. (For an example of an ET at the university level, consider George Pòlya's teaching in the film "let us teach guessing." Pòlya was, of course, a UM par excellence—and clearly an ET as well).

With this as a backdrop, we consider the three classes of teachers: UM, ET, and PT. We note that these classes can overlap, and that in particular, designations of expertise are tied to context: any teacher (UM or not) may be an ET in some content areas and a PT in others.

The UM

We introduce this section with a familiar anecdote characterizing the stereotypical mathematician. The mathematician is lecturing about a topic. He writes a preliminary lemma on the board and then says "This result is trivial to prove." At that point, he stops, pausing pensively. After a few minutes, he says "Excuse me" and leaves the room. Ten minutes later, he returns and says "Yes, it *is* trivial, so let's move on," continuing the lecture from where he had left off.

Putting aside the question of how we use "trivial" as a community, we wish to focus on what is essential in this anecdote: *understanding the underlying mathematics is a necessary condition for the mathematician to continue.* Part of what makes us mathematicians is the understanding that claims must be justified and justifiable: if we make a claim in an instructional context, we must be able to back it up. This is part of the mathematician's belief system. (That is, it is a core pedagogical orientation of the university mathematician).

In schematic form (and, obviously, generalizing and simplifying[3]), one can represent the perspective of the university mathematicians as in Fig. 2:

In short, no matter what group the UM is interacting with, that mathematician will need to feel that the mathematics is "under control." When it is, he or she can turn to the question of which mathematics is appropriate for the given audience and the appropriate form(s) of pedagogy for that group. As evidence of this phenomenon, in the section "Aspects of the university mathematician's practice," we provide examples of faculty who "stop cold" in lecture to make sure the mathematics is right—and then decide which mathematics to present to students. (Specifically, one lecturer considers sweeping details "under the rug" for a particular beginning undergraduate class, but another will make sure that his students in a beginning graduate class see the gory detail, and his struggles with it, because those students are being initiated into the world of the serious mathematician).

The ET

Consider now an expert secondary teacher, corresponding to the elementary teachers described by Ma (2010). This teacher may not have anywhere near the mathematician's knowledge of the formal mathematics—indeed, it is most unlikely that he or she would. At the same time, he or she has a kind of knowledge that UM may not – a knowledge of examples and connections that enrich the mathematics at the level of instruction and that are suited to help students develop (the beginnings of) a similarly deep understanding. As noted, an elementary school ET working on division of fractions may well have a large number of stories that represent models of

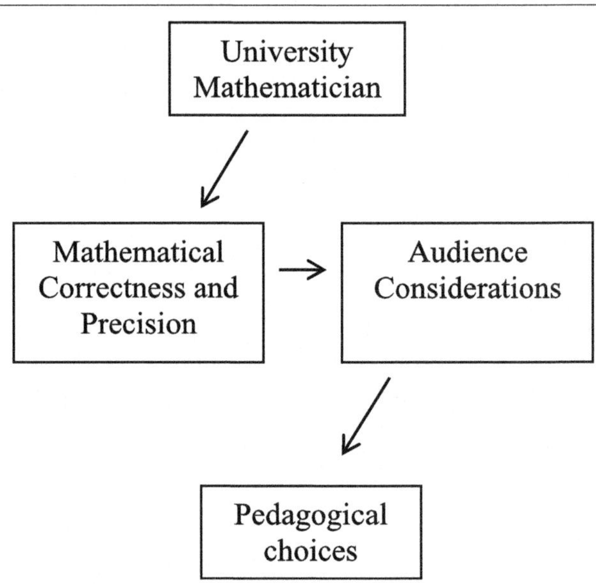

Fig. 2 A frame for characterizing UM's decision-making

division and know contexts that would help students understand them; he or she may have ways of explaining certain rules (e.g., why it makes sense to invert the denominator and multiply by it when taking the quotient of two fractions) that are mathematically correct and that extend far beyond UM's repertoire (which includes formal ways to prove that inverting the denominator and multiplying by it is correct, but may not include explanations that are accessible to children). Similarly, the secondary ET would have a large set of contextual examples of derivatives of a function of one variable and ways of explaining limits and the limiting process. This knowledge in general has been referred to as "mathematical knowledge for teaching" or MKT (Ball et al. 2005; Ball et al. 2008; Hill and Ball 2004); the expert version of MKT was called "Profound Understanding of Fundamental Mathematics" (PUFM) by Ma (2010).

In consequence, the left-hand side of Fig. 1 looks different for expert teachers than it does for mathematicians. The mathematical considerations are of richness and connectedness, often at the grade or "horizontal" level, rather than mathematical depth (the "vertical" level). Of course, ETs will also consider requirements of the succeeding grade levels in their teaching.

Pedagogical considerations may differ as well. Like the mathematician, the expert teacher takes audience considerations into account—"This subset of what I know is appropriate for these students." In addition, he or she has a repertoire of knowledge and techniques designed to "meet students where they are" and lead them into the richness of the mathematics.[4] Thus, the version of Fig. 1 that describes expert teachers looks like Fig. 3.

The PT

In a sense, the generic frame in Fig. 1 characterizes the proficient, but non-mathematician, non-expert teacher. For the most part, all of us, in instruction, have a certain "comfort zone"—the content about which we feel comfortable and about which are willing to go out on a limb. When we move outside that comfort zone, we tend to be more careful, and more wary—indeed, unless we are particularly adventurous, we may avoid opportunities to venture into such territory. The same is true of our pedagogy: we tend to operate within our pedagogical comfort zone, unless circumstances force us outside of it (as in the case of the mathematicians undergoing professional development in this study, who were deliberately considering new pedagogies). Hence, Fig. 1 can be modified as in Fig. 4.

From our perspective, the challenge for professional development is to find ways to help all teachers move toward both broader and deeper mathematical development (expanding their mathematical comfort zones) and to broaden and connect their pedagogical repertoires to work with that mathematical content and their growing understanding of students as learners (expanding their pedagogical comfort zones).

Methods

The professional development model

In this section, we give an account of our approach to constructing a professional development model that has the discussion of *R/O/G*s by university mathematicians as a core strategy, and how it evolved into a project to test it in practice. In the third section, we

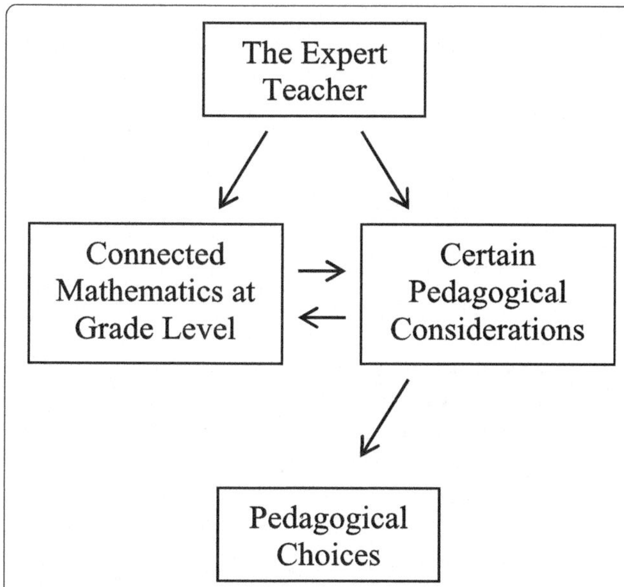

Fig. 3 A frame for characterizing ET's decision-making

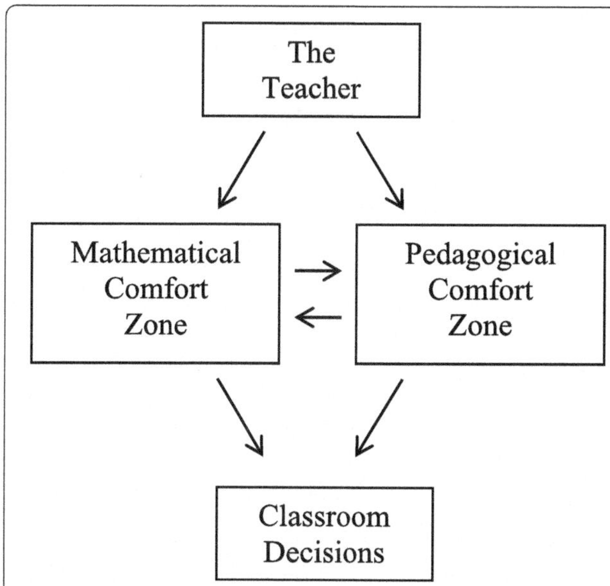

Fig. 4 A frame for characterizing teachers' decision-making in general

provide data from an implementation of the professional development model to substantiate the claims made above.

We were guided in our search for a suitable professional development model for university mathematicians to ask whether we could use what is known about secondary teaching and its development to guide us at the tertiary level. There were, at that time, few theoretical studies of university mathematics teaching (Speer et al. 2010), a substantial amount of published opinion, and many studies that explored particular approaches. For example, Bergsten (2007) considered what constitutes the notion of quality in undergraduate mathematics teaching, concluding that in addition to mathematical exposition the factors "Teacher Immediacy" (including personal language, use of gestures and humor) and "General Criteria" (such as orchestration of subject matter teaching, cognitive activation of learners, and effective learner-oriented classroom management) are critical for high-quality teaching.

We believe that mathematics teaching at university has a distinctive character, with unique characteristics, challenges, and joys (Barton 2011; Schuck and Pereira 2011) although we acknowledge that there is much to be learned from generic studies of tertiary teaching (e.g., O'Neill et al. 2005).

For example, Kember and Kwan (2000) argue that in general, university lecturers tend to adopt either content- or learning-centered approaches to teaching (the former reflecting a focus on the content or material to be taught, the latter focusing on the learning of their students). They conclude that "Fundamental changes to the quality of teaching and learning may only result from changes to conceptions of teaching." (ibid, p. 489)—that is, that a significant change in pedagogy must come from reflection on the underlying focus of pedagogy, and an evolving view of what that focus should be. Another aspect, revealed in research on tertiary teaching in general, is that lecturers value collaborative learning in professional development, including discussions with peers (Ferman 2002). It was against this background that we looked for opportunities to develop a theory- and research-based approach to mathematics lecturer development in a systematic, collaborative manner.

In order to support university mathematicians with appropriate pedagogical professional development, we considered it important to incorporate Schoenfeld's (2010) theoretical framework characterizing decision-making, as outlined in the section "Theoretical backdrop and assertions". Our hypothesis was that any development process needed to assist mathematicians to be aware of the foundation of the mathematics/pedagogy dialectic that would likely occur in their practice and simultaneously, through a shift toward a more student-centered conception of teaching, build a desire for a change of practice.

During previous applications of Schoenfeld's *R*/*O*/*G* framework to detailed analysis of teacher decision-making (Schoenfeld 2008), the researcher had inferred the teacher *R*/*O*/*G* from classroom video. Our intention was to place the *R*/*O*/*G* within the attention of the lecturer as a potential catalyst for developmental discussion. Originally, we intended that the lecturer would write a version of their *R*/*O*/*G* before a lecture and would then review it afterwards, considering how it played out in practice and whether they met their goals. However, in practice, this sometimes changed, as we document below.

The development process

In any professional development (PD) model, it is important to have certain key components in place. If the group is to function in a collaborative manner, where a culture of enquiring conversation is developed (Rowland 2000), then its composition is crucial (Ferman 2002). Engaging in collaborative inquiry into, and critical reflection on, the process of teaching practice, is what makes the collective a community of inquiry (Kane et al. 2004; Wells 1999; Jaworski 2003). It was important to us to construct a group where, as part of the process of co-learning (Wagner 1997; Jaworski 2001), each member was likely to be supportive of the endeavor, and each other, *and* be willing and able to provide supportive feedback in a non-judgmental manner. This consideration came to the fore in constructing a group. This occurred when the four mathematics education researchers from Auckland University's mathematics department instigating the study approached four university research mathematician colleagues who they thought would be interested to join the research, in order to form a group of eight. All four, Sandy, Simon, Abi, and Mark (pseudonyms), immediately agreed to be part of the PD research. Three of them are applied mathematicians and one a pure mathematician. The research questions for the group, focused on PD, were

- How can Schoenfeld's resources, orientation and goals (*R*/*O*/*G*) framework be adapted to support lecturer professional development?
- Can an effective lecturing professional development strategy be built around peer discussion of lecturer *R*/*O*/*Gs* matched against videoed lecturing practice?

In the initial meeting of all eight participants, an overview of the project was discussed, along with the level of individual involvement required. One of the mathematics educators then presented the idea of *R*/*O*/*G*s, and their role in the project and a two-page summary of these ideas was given to each member of the group. This included the complexity of the dynamic relationship between knowledge, orientations, and goals and their role in setting priorities in decision-making. Following this meeting, one of the mathematics educators circulated an example of his *R/O/G* for a second year lecture and this was considered. The next two meetings covered the timetable of meetings and lecture videoing along with practical project details such as who would do what and when. This included the need for one member of the group to operate the video to record the lecture and another to act as a note-taking observer. By the fourth meeting, 2 months after the first, there were two lecture videos ready to discuss.

Lecturers were encouraged to structure their *R/O/G* using three sections, resources, orientations, and goals. Prior to each lecture, the lecturer wrote a *R/O/G* comprising their view of the task ahead, what they considered important, their goals for the lecture, and how they thought they would accomplish them and emailed these to the rest of the group. It became clear that in writing their *R/O/G*s, lecturers were often able to articulate their goals more clearly than their orientations. Example of goals were

- to survey those topics in number theory that are most traditionally taught at masters level. [Simon]
- to define continued fractions, to show how to compute them, and to prove some basic theoretical results. [Simon]
- to show students that interesting, unexpected things happen to the solution as the parameter changes. [Sandy]
- to show how easy it is to discover these things by using MATLAB. [Sandy]
- for the students to appreciate the appearance of Fibonacci numbers in nature. [Abi]
- to keep all the students engaged throughout the lecture. [Abi]

However, we see that these goals are not all about the content delivery but include variables such as student discovery, interest, appreciation, and engagement. Further, some lecturers such as Abi did list orientations. She said: I see this whole course partially as an exercise in "public understanding of mathematics," and Sandy's comments also record his beliefs, such as, "I hope that my slides, being based on the course-book, allow students to follow what is going on without the distraction of extensive note taking."

A second vital component in the PD model was that each person whose practice was under discussion should have complete control over all aspects of the process as it pertained to their involvement. Two members of the group chose not to be observed. In each meeting, the whole group sat around a table in a conference room to discuss the chosen segment. Each of the six who were observed chose the lectures they wanted video-recorded, and then, from a tape of the lecture, they chose a short segment (less than 5 min) they felt comfortable discussing with the group, which included some aspect of instruction they wanted to discuss. We were also able to ascertain why they chose that particular section to be viewed by the group. The focus on a written *R/O/G* prior to the lecture meant that sometimes the *R/O/G* was evident in the choice of section that we watched, as seen in Simon's comment.

> I think I disobey my *R/O/G* and then come back to it in some sense, so that's why I picked on this...I should be able to say it's a one line proof, you guys can see that but instead I sort of get a bit too carried away in the detail, it blows out of all proportion.

Similarly, Abi's reason for choosing one video segment suggests that she was made more aware of her orientations by the *R/O/G* emphasis. Here, she expresses her belief that while she can elicit student responses, she feels she could deal with them better and has set this as a new teaching goal.

> [I] picked this segment because I'd like to maybe get some ideas on how to better deal with student responses because I'm quite good at getting them to say stuff at me now but then I don't know what to do when they do.

Thus, the *R/O/G* was a good way to introduce the segment, enabling the lecturer to begin the discussion by orienting the group members to his/her beliefs about the content and the students, the goals for the lecture, and how well they thought it had gone. The meeting proceeded with a collective viewing of the videotape and then the lecturer was asked to comment on what had been seen. This led to a discussion of how the *R/O/G*s had played out in practice, with the lecturer playing a major role in shaping the discussion, which was facilitated by the group organizers. The lecturer sometimes looked for group reactions ("It felt right at the time but I looked at it and thought I'm not sure about that...so I just wanted reaction, whether you have reaction to that") and sometimes they wanted to discuss the unexpected route they had taken in a lecture ("Someone asks you about something and then you go off and follow a path that you never intended to follow I suppose. That's probably why I picked it...Usually, you worry about a misconception or unpacking something if it's going to cause you trouble later, do you know what I mean. If you can function perfectly well without it, if you said well this maturity will come and ability to understand it. So the amount of effort you put into explaining something is often the function of how much effort you'd have to put in to unexplain it later.") Interestingly, they mostly chose segments about which they felt somewhat uncomfortable about how things went—mathematics educators tended to choose segments where their mathematical knowledge might be questioned, and mathematics researchers tended to choose moments of pedagogical concern.[5] During the ensuing discussion, the mathematics educators would occasionally try to focus its direction using ideas from *R*/*O*/*G* theory. For example, in one meeting, the influence of the *R*/*O*/*G* on decision-making was highlighted, and the lecturer, Sandy, was able to recognize that this was applicable to his lecture.

> Maths educator: So these *R*/*O*/*G*s lead to the sort of routines that we're used to so if you get a wrong answer you have some sort of routine that you use to deal with that. We talked about this, what did you say, an internal conversation in your head in order to make that decision and only you know what that was, and why you made that decision but it's clear there was a decision to be made.

> Sandy: Yeah in fact my decision was based on the fact that I'd already spoken far longer than I'd planned to on the existing equation and it was time to actually go and do some problems which was supposed to be the rest of the lecture so I got onto that.

These discussions proceeded extremely well, with all members participating. Often, the content of the discussions moved considerably, ranging across pedagogical issues and mathematical topics.

After the meeting to discuss the video, each lecturer reviewed their written *R*/*O*/*G* on the basis of the discussion and the outcomes of the lecture, appending written comments about it to the *R*/*O*/*G*. An example that shows that Sandy had reflected on the relationship between orientations, goals and decisions, writing,

> I'm happy with the discussion that the DATUM group had about the video clip. The analysis of the clip is encouraging in that I gained a mathematics education perspective of the clip, which clarified in my own mind what I do when I teach. In particular, the model of teaching that [maths educator] presented in terms of a lecture being a set of goals influenced by a sequence of decisions was pertinent here. I certainly made a decision not to continue with an unexpected outcome on a graph in the first part of the lecture. Part of me wanted to address this at the time but I had already gone over time with this part of the lecture and had achieved the goals I desired.

Abi too thought about how she could improve the level of student engagement in her lecture and wrote this in her post-discussion comment on her *R*/*O*/*G*.

> One that has stuck in my mind particularly, which I will use next time, is to tell all the students that they must do the computations (on calculator, phone etc.), and that I'm going to pick people out to tell me what they got (since it's such an easy calculation to do). Then if wrong answers are given, since everyone will have done the calculations, they are more likely to speak up.

Each semester, the group had at least three 1-h meetings to discuss lecture segments, prompted by prior viewing of one or two excerpts and reading the *R*/*O*/*G*s. At these meetings, we sometimes looked at two video sections, taking half an hour for each. Overall, each of the six who were observed had at least two, and up to five, lectures discussed. Over 2 years, a total of 19 lectures were captured on video and 15 full meetings were held and transcriptions produced.

The data analysis focussed on the video of the chosen lecture segments, the transcription of the group discussion of these and the relationship between the decision points identified in the lecture segments, and the written and inferred *R*/*O*/*G*s. One pair of researchers independently looked through the transcripts of the videos and meetings coding elements that could be inferred as part of the *R*/*O*/*G* as well as segments that represented recurring features or ideas that we had previously identified as of interest based on the our theoretical framework (e.g., are orientations and goals involved in decision-making, and if so how?). During this process, we also encountered other areas of interest and these were also coded for later analysis. One of these emerging themes in the discussions was that related to mathematical constructs. For example, we saw the value that the applied UMs placed on recurrence relations, since it is usually what they work with, compared with the school emphasis on general formulas for a function. Following the coding, the two researchers met together and agreed on the classifications and assignments. The themes that emerged from this analysis were also followed up in the interviews.

Results and discussion

Aspects of the university mathematician's practice

In this section, we examine some of the data arising from the professional development process outlined above. Our purpose in this section is not to provide a systematic analysis of the data from the professional development sessions. Such work has been done elsewhere (see e.g., Paterson et al. 2011a, b; Paterson et al. 2011); it can serve as additional context for the present paper. Rather, our purpose is to present rather striking—but we believe, not unrepresentative—evidence from the discussions of university teaching in those professional development sessions that we believe casts light on the manner in which the in-lecture decision-making of a university mathematician proceeds. We suggest that what follows is representative of a particular belief structure held, to some degree, by many university mathematicians. Awareness of this aspect of university mathematicians' practice should be taken into account when designing professional development for the UM.

First, we consider the example of Simon, an experienced pure mathematician. We were able to identify a number of Simon's orientations—some he listed explicitly, others we inferred from transcripts of the group discussions and interviews with him. A number of these, given below, indicate his emphasis on the beauty and power of mathematics, and especially on the need for it to be correct.

O1: Mathematics needs to be correct. 'Oh, this is not really right, I don't like it not to be right.'

O2: Mathematical notation needs to be consistent and accurate. 'Right so the symbols h_j over k_j will from now on will mean precisely one of these things for the specific numbers I am interested in.'

O3: Lecture notes need to be correct and mathematically informative. 'My response after this exercise was to go away and fix the notes because they were broken' and 'it's a tricky one because the notes clearly weren't ideal because this whole thing was sort of hidden.'

O4: Some proofs are more interesting and important than others. 'The real reason I think it's a cool proof is the fact that you prove a more general result. It's one of these things that happens a lot in mathematics but you don't see it so much at the junior level.'

O5: To emphasise to students that the right theoretical tools and proof techniques can tame a mathematical problem.

O6: Students who are talented at mathematics can cope when a lecturer dwells on the finer points in mathematics. 'There is also a confidence that the students can cope with – if I go off on my own little journey the students will have the tools to deal with that ... Whereas in another class you would be worried that if I'd lost them after 15 minutes then that's it.'

O7: Traditional lecturing by dictating notes is error prone.

These orientations gave rise to a number of goals, some of which he wrote in his *R*/*O*/*G* before the lecture, and others we were able to infer, which again emphasize mathematics, especially the importance and need for correctness of proofs in mathematics and how enjoyable they can be.

G1: to help students to understand the theory and do proofs

G2: to provide good general preparation for post-graduate study in number theory

G3: to increase the students' mathematical maturity
G4: to give exposure to different proof techniques

G5: the most important theoretical part is to state and prove correctness of the recurrence formulae for computing the convergents

G6: 'I hope to give a flavour for just how neat this proof is.'

G7: to engage with the mathematics for its own sake, 'it's fun.'

G8: to ensure that the mathematics he does is 'right,' part of his role as a lecturer

G9: to use notation that is consistent

G10: to induct students into thinking and behaving like mathematicians

In one of his lectures, Simon introduced a group of fourth year students to continued fractions as part of a course he describes as "...designed to be good general preparation for post-grad study in number theory." This lecture on continued fractions had a number of clear aims, as recorded in Simon's pre-lecture *R*/*O*/*G*:

To define continued fractions, to show how to compute them, and to prove some basic theoretical results. The most important theoretical part is to state and prove correctness of the recurrence formulas for computing the convergents. This proof works by studying a more general problem (real coefficients). I hope to give a flavor for just how neat this proof is – it is an example of how in mathematics it is sometimes easier to prove a more general result. This fact relates to one of the themes of the course: emphasizing to the students how the right theoretical tools and proof techniques can tame a mathematical problem.

Since he considered the students to be very able, this allowed him to consider taking a "detour" during the lecture. Commenting on a proof of the recurrence formulae, he said "Last year there was not the same ability so I went through the proof much more lightly with them. It wasn't necessary to dwell on this particular issue of the more general result." He had originally assumed that he would simply say "Just do it" when the need for this proof arose this time. However, in the moment, the need to "get it right" and a perceived need (G10) to induct these students into the mathematician's practices won the day. This goal of Simon is in agreement with the contention of Artigue et al. (2007) that learning at this level is often seen as enculturation into advanced mathematical practices and of Ben-Zvi and Arcavi (2001) that making meaning in mathematics is about doing mathematics, which also involves socialization into its culture and values. In the event—in the middle of this proof of the recurrence formulae—he suddenly realised that there was a "notational conundrum" about to rear its head, and he was faced with an unexpected decision. Here is what he says, taken from the transcript of the lecture:

1. So, by the inductive hypothesis, I know what this... It is some h_i over k_i.
2. I'm going to call it ... Did I give it a name? I didn't give it a name. It's just some h_i over k_i. But whatever that h_i over k_i is it apparently satisfies the recurrence formula.

At this point, he stood back, paused, and looked at the board. He was clearly making a decision about whether or not to untangle the notation. The lecture transcript continues:

3. Yeah, I mean this is *an* h_i over k_i but it's not *the* [italics added] h_i over k_i that I am really thinking of. This is a very subtle point.
4. Let's define h_i over ... Let's define h_j over k_j to be these things up to a_j where I have worked these out already all the way up to i ... This thing I have written down here is not the h_i over k_i in that notation because this end term is wrong.

In a later interview, he explained what he was thinking at this point, and the decision he faced.

> This is exactly the point where I suddenly realize that it is sort of not quite fitting how I was using those symbols previously. I was thinking ahead to where the proof was going and suddenly it becomes clear to me that there is a problem ahead but it's not clear to anyone else yet.
>
> This is the point where I have made a decision. I have somehow made a decision to somehow do it right. Oh this is not really right...at that point the whole world disappeared and it's just me and the mathematics.

The decision point is manifest here: a need for the mathematics to be clearly correct (see O1, O2 and O3) directed this university mathematician to make "a decision to somehow do it right." Only after the mathematics is correctly sorted out does he pay attention to his audience, a part of the whole world that had temporarily "disappeared". The later group's discussion of this episode, a central part of the professional development model, provided the opportunity for Simon to carry out what he called "a retrospective analysis of the situation." He chose this section of the lecture to review with the group. As his comments indicate, the UM stance regarding the importance of getting the mathematics exactly right was central in his decision-making.

> I think I disobey my *R/O/G* [6] and then come back to it in some sense, so that's why I picked on this. So I've said in my *R/O/G* that I assume the students are mature and independent and they're able to do things and I'm assuming the class is talented and so forth and that's all good. The proof itself is written as a sort of one line argument. I thought that I would unpack it in the lecture a little bit and I kind of got myself in a bit of a pickle because I realised somehow my notation was a bit confusing and then I sort of had this realization oh yeah that doesn't really make sense and then rather than go further and unpack it completely, so I'm disobeying my *R/O/G*, I should be able to say it's a one line proof, you guys can see that but instead I sort of get a bit too carried away in the detail, it blows out of all proportion. I realise that I've got a notation problem and I should really do more and I go back to my *R/O/G* saying these guys should be able to figure it out.
>
> I think I, if it was the *R/O/G* I would have said there's a detail here but you guys can work it out yourself because the *R/O/G* is saying they can be trusted to work out the details essentially and then I didn't. I really tried to. I thought no I'm going to labor the point.

When one of the group asked him during the discussion "How much were you being a mathematician in that moment, and how much were you being a teacher?", Simon replied:

> Yeah, I think it's much more the mathematician, because I think if I was concerned about the students you'd just do it like I've done it in the notes. You'd sweep it under

> the carpet and it would all proceed right. I think it's precisely being a mathematician and going mm... I want to make sure this is right, and so you make a big fuss out of something which is kind of...
>
> Yeah I mean it's half trying to decide exactly how the mathematics works out and half trying to decide how much detail to go on.

The transcript makes it clear that for Simon at this point, the need for the mathematics to be correct is non-negotiable; indeed, Simon later went back to the proof to be certain he had sorted out the details for the next time (O3). During his reflection, Simon makes the point that the audience comes second: "Yeah but after a while you begin to worry about the students."

A second lecturer

Sandy, the second lecturer whose data we discuss here is an applied mathematics researcher. The first of his lectures we describe is in a third year applied mathematics class on Laplace transforms. During the lecture, Sandy presents what he calls "a number of tricks" for calculating Laplace transforms and their inverses.

In his *R/O/G*, written prior to the lecture, one sees the conflict he perceives between what the student audience will want from him and his desire to "include proofs of results if I think that seeing the proof will help the students to understand the material." Because of timing, Sandy considered leaving out a central proof that day, although his final comments "I'll leave it until the end of the lecture or perhaps I'll prove it next time" indicate the importance of this mathematics to him. The timing of the proof could be left open but it was necessary to include it, as this excerpt from the *R/O/G* explains.

> However students have an assignment due tomorrow, so they'll also be expecting me to solve some problems from their problem sheet...I'll probably have to chop something out of the lecture in order to achieve this. The obvious choice is the proof of the convolution theorem. I try to include proofs of results if I think that seeing the proof will help the students to understand the material. This is only possible for proofs that aren't too lengthy and for which the students have the background knowledge to understand them. The convolution theorem is a good example of this – it makes use of switching the order of integration in a double integral. I'll leave it until the end of the lecture or perhaps I'll prove it next time.

Sandy explained why he chose a segment from the middle of the lecture where he made an in-the-moment decision to digress from his planned path and do the proof.

> I found it quite hard to choose a bit this time but this part, something unusual happened, well unusual in the sense that someone asks you about something and then you go off and follow a path that you never intended to follow I suppose. That's probably why I picked it.

The segment was related to a question response from a student. However, Sandy decided at that point to leave his plan and provide a proof.

> It was just that I felt that that's quite an important mathematical idea for them to understand and so that's why I went along that path.
>
> Yeah, I guess one of my guiding principles in teaching is that I should include proofs if I think it's going to help.

This was an unplanned, spur of the moment decision. Although considerations of how much time it would take did cross his mind, the need to have the mathematics clear won out:

> I didn't actually intend to do this of course but it's the thing that happened in the lecture but I guess it does actually apply to it... It's not entirely clear, there's a trick and you get to know the trick and it's basically always going to work and it could be effective, even in the absence of understanding.
>
> Yeah there was a bit of tension within me. I did that wondering if I had enough time to do everything else. I think to actually understand the material better they need to know this maths.

This case is not an example of "mathematics uber alles" as it seemed to be in the case of Simon, but it does indicate a strong driving force on the part of Sandy: understanding involves getting the mathematics right, and if possible, he wants students to see that (even if their use of "tricks" does get them the right answers).

In a second lecture with a second year applied mathematics class, Sandy was considering solutions of the logistic equation $x_m = qx_{m-1}(1 - x_{m-1})$ for various values of the parameter q. For a particular value of q, he displayed the graph using MATLAB and counted the troughs to obtain the period. The count of the period was 14, which is problematic —he knew that the correct value is 16, "...because the period doubles each time, so it goes from 2 to 4 to 8 to 16, so... and so on, so there's a theory that actually says the period has to double." He counted a second time, also obtaining 14. This discrepancy between 14 and 16 was unexpected: "I guess the thing that I was probably concerned about was um... observing something that I didn't expect and not being about to explain it immediately."

In the moment, Sandy had to decide whether or not to address what is, for him, a mathematical discrepancy. The result? In Sandy's words below, we see the tension. While "part of him" wanted to address it, audience considerations, the general mathematics class not requiring it and the fact that they had "grasped the concept [of the periodicity] quite well," caused him not to follow it up.

> Actually I would have liked to have pursued it a bit but we had already spent more than the allotted amount of time on this demonstration and I had shown them periodicity for shorter periods already so I think they had grasped the concept quite well so the fact that I didn't actually get a period of 16 bugged me a bit but not enough to ruin the rest of the lecture.
>
> I certainly made a decision not to continue with an unexpected outcome on a graph in the first part of the lecture. Part of me wanted to address this at the time but I had already gone over time with this part of the lecture and had achieved the goals I desired.

One of the later discussions afforded him the opportunity to reflect further on his stance as a mathematician. His comments show that while "of course the mathematics was important," an awareness of the audience needs and his primary teaching goals took priority in that moment.

> I think the teaching was actually more important than the, well of course the mathematics was important but to me, at that moment the teaching was more important I think. That was the main goal.

In this situation, with this particular audience, Sandy was happy with his decision and the way the lecture unfolded.

> I'm pretty happy with the way the lecture went. Students seemed interested, in our exploration of the logistic equation and participated in the exploration.
>
> The actual lecture itself went pretty well I was pleased with the demonstration um.. I think it was clear enough. The students were able to see what was going on.

Here again, mathematical correctness did not dominate for UM—but, it was a major issue and he revisited the unexpected outcome after the lecture to be sure he understood the mathematical basis of what happened.

A third lecturer

We have found that even when the level of the students has been taken into consideration by the UM, the need to have mathematical correctness and rigor first can tend to emerge (Paterson, Thomas, Postlethwaite, et al. 2011). In this example, we see the mathematician Abi altering her lecture, an introduction to the Fibonacci sequence, and the golden ratio for a general education first year course to provide more mathematical detail than she had initially planned. In designing the lecture, Abi used her PK to decide that these students do not need to know the mathematical details. Having introduced the students to the sequence through counting the whorls of pineapples and pinecones and providing the data to generate a table of the early Fibonacci numbers, she addresses the ratio between successive terms aiming to establish in the students' thinking that the limiting value for f_{n+1} divided by f_n is the golden ratio, ψ. After establishing by calculation that the value of $\frac{f_{n+1}}{f_n}$ oscillates about 1.6, or so, she says:

> OK suppose you want to compute what this number actually is.
>
> And it seems to be converging – and it does actually converge. [Uses the language of the UM]
>
> So you know that f_{n+1} is bigger than f_n so this is going to be a number that is bigger than 1.
>
> Right? Or equal to 1. [The UM's need for precision emerges]
>
> So ... If I am thinking about what this ratio becomes as n gets really, really big.
>
> So, for any specific n these 2 things are going to be different. Right?
>
> Because for one thing it was 1.6 and for the next one it was 1.625.
>
> So for any specific n it's going to be different. Right? But as n gets bigger and bigger and bigger these 2 things are going to get closer and closer together. Right? Yeh? [The formal idea of a limit is beyond what these students need]
>
> So if we imagine that we're at somewhere where n is really, really big these two things are going to be

really close together. OK? So let's call that thing in both cases, we are going to say this is approximately equal to this ψ, approximately equal to, and this is approximately equal to ψ as well. [The UM language of epsilon-delta is not here but the ideas are emerging]

As long as n is big enough. So we will assume that we are in a place where n is big enough then we can make these approximations. [An important qualifying statement for the UM]

Abi decided beforehand that there was no need to establish the limit ψ rigorously in this class. However, her language shows that, in the moment, there emerges the need to be mathematically explicit in her terminology and to add the necessary qualifiers and conditions that rigor requires to the general statements she is making. Examples include the use of language such as "converging" and qualifying the statement "bigger than one" with "or equal to". In addition, although the formal epsilon-delta approach is not employed, these ideas begin to emerge through words such as "getting closer and closer," "really close together," and "As long as n is big enough".

The rationale for this approach can be seen through Abi's response in a discussion: "So should you just ignore that corner [of important mathematics] and just hope that it's not noticed? But then is that bad because you've somehow told them something incorrect?" Here too, the importance of representing the mathematical ideas in a way that is faithful to the core (correct) mathematics is central. In a general education course, the assertion that the golden ratio occurs often in nature—and some nice pictorial demonstrations that illustrate that fact—might seem enough. However, this UM felt the need at least to reference the core mechanism of convergence.

Discussion

In this paper, we have described a general frame, represented schematically in Fig. 1, that we believe is capable of illuminating some of the reasons behind in-the-moment teaching/lecturing decisions. Underpinning this frame is a tacit consideration of the *R*/*O*/*G* of the individual; in particular, their beliefs about mathematics and pedagogy contribute to intensity of the links, represented by the arrows in Fig. 1. We have suggested that three key factors drive the decisions an instructor makes. These are the richness (depth, breadth, and connectivity) of their mathematical content knowledge (MCK), the extent of their pedagogical knowledge (PK), and the quality of the synergistic relationship between the two. In turn, the strength of these factors influences how much each of them is involved in the moment-to-moment decision-making process. In this regard, we have identified three general groups. First is the UM, where the MCK is deep and strong (reflecting, of course, a part of the UM's professional identity), but the PK may be relatively weaker,[7] and the synergy between them may not be so well developed. Second is the ET, whose MCK has strength and interconnectedness at the level of the mathematics he or she teaches, and is tightly coupled with high PCK. The vibrant synergy between them leads to excellent mathematical knowledge for teaching (Hill and Ball 2004).[8] Finally, there is the PT, who may have good MCK and PK along with a reasonable synergy between them.

This framework has been exemplified through three case studies of university mathematicians. In the first case, we saw that Simon's rich MCK was the driving force in his decision to make sure the mathematics was right—in order to attain his high priority goal of demonstrating the power that proof has to solve problems. For Simon, pedagogical considerations were activated second to confirm to him that the class both needed to cope with the details and was mathematically strong enough to do. Sandy was our second UM. In the first lecture discussed, Sandy's desire to make sure the mathematics was clear caused him to override the possibility that he had too much material for the lecture, resulting in a 5-min diversion from his planned lesson. In the second lecture, his rich MCK alerted him to a potential error and aroused his natural desire to require the mathematics to be correct. However, the synergy with his PK was sufficient to allow his primary lecture goals of demonstrating periodicity and the value of MATLAB as a tool to take precedence over a competing mathematical goal—to investigate further until it was evident to all that the mathematics was right. This student-centered decision was made to meet the needs of this particular class. The final case was that of Abi, who found it difficult to suppress the rigor of the mathematical details arising from the impetus of her strong MCK. However, her PK was quite well developed and the level of synergy between the two enabled her to keep the formal mathematics sufficiently in the background to accomplish her teaching goals for this class.

It stands to reason that professional development works best when it is well suited for those who receive it—meaning that it respects their values and gives them a significant role in shaping what happens. The value of the PD approach described in this paper for its intended audience, university mathematicians, can be seen in the comments of some of the UMs who took part. Simon speaks of the PD in these terms: "these activities are perfectly designed to be engaging and beneficial to the lecturers in the department." Similarly, Sandy expresses his view this way "This project is so good that I am still involved with it five years later." A third UM who was involved in the research speaks positively of the project in that it led to a "deeper and more sustained reflection on teaching practice." Further evidence of the effectiveness of the PD, its widespread adoption by the department that houses it, is discussed below. We hope that the detail given in the section "The development process" will support other departments in beginning to create such communities.

Before focusing on the implications of the work described here, we invoke a broad framing of learning environments that contextualizes what follows. Schoenfeld (2015) provided a characterization of the core dimensions of powerful adult learning environments. That framing is summarized in Fig. 5.

In broad terms, the PD described here can be seen to fit comfortably with the desiderata laid out in Fig. 5. The conceptualization of professionalism (dimension 1) employed in the PD is grounded in the literature on professional knowledge and decision-making. In beginning with and providing community discussions of the mathematicians' *R*/*O*/*G*s, and the problems of practice that the mathematicians bring to the group, the PD "meets the UMs where they are" and addresses the strengths and weaknesses of their particular practice; hence, it addresses dimensions 2 and 5 productively. Given that each participant has the opportunity to shape sessions devoted to his or her teaching, there is equitable access (dimension 3); and, precisely because the participants have the opportunity to shape the conversations around things that matter to them, there is significant room for agency (dimension 4). The comments above provide some evidence of the impact.

A number of implications for professional development (PD) programs follow from our assumptions. It should be clear, vis-à-vis "meeting teachers where they are," that all PD needs to take into account the mathematical and pedagogical orientations of the practitioner. Further, the framework suggests somewhat different emphases for the three populations, UM, ET, and PT.[9] To the degree that the UM is firmly grounded in the mathematics but perhaps less so in pedagogy, there should be a focus on key pedagogical understandings—but taking into account the mathematical context. These might include student-centered notions such as considering what the students currently understand, what the potential obstacles to furthering that understanding are, and what route through the ideas might be best to further their understanding. For the ET, PD might be best focused on the key mathematical understandings that help to complete the "big picture" of the mathematics under consideration. For example, how do the various algebraic formats of linear equations mentioned above relate to general methods for solving systems of linear equations, such as Gaussian elimination, that students will later experience? The expectation is that this enhanced mathematical awareness, in concert with the ET's pedagogical skills, result in enriched opportunities for students to see the "big picture." For the PT, the challenge is to enhance both mathematical and pedagogical understandings. For ideas about how to frame approaches to this challenge, see Schoenfeld (2014).

We propose that the insight into the influences on the pedagogical decisions of our three UMs is directly attributable to the model of PD employed in the study. This model provided an opportunity for the UMs to build an awareness of their *R*/*O*/*G*s and its role in their decision-making. Without this PD format, such information would probably have been less visible and the PD less productive. The PD used lecturer *R*/*O*/*G*s to initiate discussion of practice, doing so on an individual level (where the writing of the *R*/*O*/*G* helped raise lecturer awareness of orientations and goals) and in-group discussion (where all benefited from an explicit discussion of orientations and goals, leading to personal

Five Dimensions of Powerful Sites for Professional Growth

The Content (Professionalism)	Cognitive Demand (Room to Grow)	Equitable Access to Professional Growth	Agency, Authority, and Identity	Uses of Assessment
The extent to which the adults in the environment are supported in practices that build their capacity to create rich learning environments for their students.	*The extent to which adults at the site are coached and supported in ways that meet them where they are, and help them work on problems of practice that support their growth.*	*The extent to which support and accountability structures enfranchise all adults in the environment and help them grow.*	*The extent to which adults in the environment are supported in developing a sense of their own agency with respect to their growth and performance.*	*The extent to which accountability structures help teachers to identify strengths and weaknesses, and help to support professional growth.*

Fig. 5 Five dimensions of powerful adult learning environments (from Schoenfeld 2015, p. 165, with permission)

reflection). Sandy is typical of many UMs. He explained in his interview after the PD that other than a short course as a teaching assistant in the USA, he had received virtually no mathematics-specific pedagogical training. Since the practice of UMs involves what is in large measure a non-negotiable stance on making sure the mathematics is right, they want PD that focuses not only on key aspects of their practice but also takes into account the mathematics. Sandy stated that the model used here provided him with the best opportunity to reflect on his practice that he had ever experienced and he offered no suggestions for how it might be improved. He was keen to continue his involvement: "I've seen how useful it is and it would be great to get other people involved as well. I'm sure I could still get more out of it if I continued...I've got no objections to being videoed...Maybe once or twice a year I suppose, I've no objections to that. Especially if I try new things in my teaching." He also presented a paper on his experience at an international conference saying "I've enjoyed being involved in mathematics education for the first time, in fact even speaking at the conference [Volcanic Delta 2011, the Eighth Southern Hemisphere Conference on the Teaching and Learning of Undergraduate Mathematics and Statistics] was enjoyable because of the positive feedback that I got...I'll continue to do that I think at other conferences in the future."

To date, the PD model we have described (see Barton et al. 2014 for a full description) has proven successful, as evidenced by the comments and teaching practice of the UMs in the department. It has provided a method of opening up the theoretical and pedagogical knowledge of mathematics education to UMs in a manner that focuses on the UMs' orientations and goals and provides them with the means to achieve their goals. We perceive the key implementation principles to be as follows.

- Use a short (3–4 min) slice of the lecture video to focus group attention and provide a sufficient springboard for discussion.
- Allow the lecturer control over selection of the lecture to be videoed, the slice of chosen, and whether it is used.
- Develop a community of inquiry (we recommend six members) based on mutual trust.
- Community composition should be homogeneous with respect to a focus on a common discipline of interest but heterogeneous across a number of variables, such as: research field (UMs and mathematics educators); UM background (pure and applied, different perspectives were in evidence on some issues); years of experience; and seniority.
- The *R*/*O*/*G* framework is highly recommended. It was effective in developing and focusing the project and enhanced discussion.
- Encourage participants to develop awareness of their own teaching style and to use this as a catalyst for change.

(Based on Barton et al. 2014, pp. 160, 161)

There has been subsequent wider recognition in the university department where the PD model originated. The current Head of the Department stated "It has proved to be a most successful form of professional development, focusing on mathematics teaching, and the department has greatly benefited from this. [It] has reinvigorated the mathematics department's focus on quality teaching...I have appreciated the sustained and positive effect produced on the teaching culture and practice in the department over several years." Thus, the original structure of forming small heterogeneous groups comprising six to eight UMs and mathematics educators is now being employed with full departmental backing. Currently, there are two groups of six working together and all of the original UMs who participated (and were still in the department—one left for another institution) have been very happy to continue their involvement with the project, passing on their knowledge and experience to others. In addition, some who have more recently joined the program have been very happy to go on record (Paterson and Evans 2013) describing the positive benefits to their teaching of the PD they have received.

Endnotes

[1]There is a large literature on mathematics teachers' knowledge, heavily influenced by Shulman's (1986, 1987) introduction of the idea of "pedagogical content knowledge." See Schoenfeld (2006) for a review.

[2]Lecturers are more often called instructors in the USA.

[3]This may seem oversimplified almost to the point of caricature, but the evidence presented in the section "Aspects of The University Mathematician's Practice" of this paper suggests otherwise.

[4]We note that such repertoires are not universal. In some Asian nations, the primary mechanism for imparting information is lecturing—lecturing grounded in understandings of what causes students difficulty, what to build on, how to connect things, and so on. Expert primary and secondary teachers in English-speaking nations tend to use group work, student contributions, and such. Hence, there is no one model of "ideal" pedagogical considerations; "expertise" is culturally shaped, although student performance outcomes are the clear delineator of expert teaching.

[5]This speaks to the level of trust engendered in the community, which is an essential aspect of successful professional development.

[6]Initially, in line with the framework, we referred to Knowledge and hence *K*/*O*/*G*, rather than to Resources

and *R/O/G*. We have updated the transcription for consistency.

[7]We apologize if this seems to be a stereotype—but sometimes, there is truth behind stereotypes. Mathematicians are, in general, Ph.D.s; they are not necessarily extensively trained in pedagogy, though they may develop or be helped to develop deep pedagogical understandings. The three cases we presented are hardly enough to generalize from—but, they represented three out of the four UMs engaged in the PD; and, for what it's worth, the episodes described resonate with the authors' professional experience.

[8]Again, we note that expert teachers exist at all levels, from those expert elementary teachers described by Ma (2010) as having "profound understanding of fundamental mathematics" to university mathematicians like George Pólya. The categories overlap.

[9]It goes without saying that all PD should attend to both mathematical and pedagogical considerations. The point is that if different groups enter into PD with somewhat different orientations to both content and pedagogy, then PD should be responsive to those differences.

Competing interests

The authors declare that they have no competing interests.

Authors' contributions

All of the authors contributed to the conceptualization of the activity and report. BB, MT, and JP (see below) conducted the professional development sessions. AS, MT, and BB contributed to the writing. All authors read and approved the final manuscript.

Acknowledgements

This paper is dedicated to the memory of Judy Paterson, a valued colleague who contributed to the conceptualization and implementation of the professional development effort and who most unfortunately succumbed to cancer as the paper was being prepared.

Author details

[1]School of Education, University of California, EMST, Tolman Hall # 1670, Berkeley, CA 94720-1670, USA. [2]Department of Mathematics, The University of Auckland, Private Bag 92019, Auckland 1142, New Zealand.

References

Artigue, M, Batanero, C, & Kent, P (2007). Mathematics thinking and learning at post-secondary level. In F. K. Lester (Ed.), *The Second Handbook of Research on Mathematics Teaching and Learning* (pp. 1011–1049). Charlotte, NC: Information Age.

Ball, DL, Hill, HC, & Bass, H (2005). *Who knows mathematics well enough to teach third grade, and how can we decide? American Educator, Fall, 14-22 and 43-46.*

Ball, DL, Thames, MH, & Phelps, G (2008). Content knowledge for teaching: what makes it special? *Journal of Teacher Education, 59*(5), 389–407.

Barton, B (2011). Growing understanding of undergraduate mathematics: a good frame produces better tomatoes. *International Journal of Mathematical Education in Science and Technology, 42*(7), 963–973.

Barton, B, Oates, G, Paterson, J, & Thomas, MOJ (2014). A marriage of continuance: professional development for mathematics lecturers. *Mathematics Education Research Journal, 27*(2), 147–164. doi:10.1007/s13394-014-0134-7.

Barton, B, & Paterson, J (2009). Teachers Learning Mathematics: Professional development research. Wellington, New Zealand: Teaching and Learning Research Initiative.

Ben-Zvi, D, & Arcavi, A (2001). Junior high school students' construction of global views of data and data representations. *Educational Studies in Mathematics, 45*, 35–65.

Bergsten, C (2007). Investigating quality of undergraduate mathematics lectures. *Mathematics Education Research Journal, 19*(3), 48–72.

Ferman, T (2002). Academic professional development practice: what lecturers find valuable. *International Journal for Academic Development, 7*(2), 146–158. doi:10.1080/1360144032000071305.

Gueudet, G (2015). University teachers' resources and documentation work. *Paper presented at the CERME 9 Conference*, Prague, February, 2015. Downloaded from http://www.cerme9.org/products/twg14-under-construction/

Gueudet, G, Buteau, C, Mesa, V, & Misfeldt, M (2014). Instrumental and documentational approaches: from technology use to documentation systems in university mathematics education. *Research in Mathematics Education, 16*(2), 139–155.

Hill, H, & Ball, DL (2004). Learning mathematics for teaching: results from California's mathematics professional development institutes. *Journal for Research in Mathematics Education, 35*(5), 330–351.

Jaworski, B (2001). Developing mathematics teaching: teachers, teacher-educators and researchers as co-learners. In F.-L. Lin & T. J. Cooney (Eds.), *Making sense of mathematics teacher education* (pp. 295–320). Dordrecht: Kluwer.

Jaworski, B (2003). Research practice into/influencing mathematics teaching and learning development: towards a theoretical framework based on co-learning partnerships. *Educational Studies in Mathematics, 54*, 249–282.

Jaworski, B, Treffert-Thomas, S, & Bartsch, T (2009). Characterising the teaching of university mathematics: a case of linear algebra. In M. Tzekaki et al. (Eds.), *Proceedings of the 33rd Conference of the International Group for the Psychology of Mathematics Education* (Vol. 3, pp. 249–256). Thessaloniki, Greece: PME.

Jaworski, B, Mali, A, & Petropoulou, G (2015). Approaches to teaching mathematics and their relation to students' mathematical meaning making. In K. Beswick, T. Muir, & J. Wells (Eds.), *Proceedings of 39th Psychology of Mathematics Education Conference* (Vol. 3, pp. 97–104). Hobart, Australia: PME.

Kane, R, Sandretto, S, & Heath, C (2004). An investigation into excellent tertiary teaching: emphasising reflective practice. *Higher Education, 47*, 283–310.

Kember, D, & Kwan, K-P (2000). Lecturers' approaches to teaching and their relationship to conceptions of good teaching. *Instructional Science, 28*, 469–490.

Lew, K, Fukawa-Connelly, T, Mejia-Ramos, JP, & Weber, K (2014). Why advanced mathematics lectures often fail. In T. Fukawa-Connelly, G. Karakok, K. Keene, & M. Zandieh (Eds.), *Proceedings of the 17th Annual Conference on Research in Undergraduate Mathematics Education* (pp. 137–151). Denver, Colorado: SIGMAA-RUME.

Ma, L (2010). *Knowing and teaching elementary school mathematics: teachers' understanding of fundamental mathematics in China and the United States* (Anniversaryth ed.). New York: Routledge.

Mali, A, Biza, I, & Jaworski, B (2014). Characteristics of university mathematics teaching: use of generic examples in tutoring. In P. Liljedahl, S. Oesterle, C. Nico, & D. Allan (Eds.), *Proceedings of the 38th Conference of the Int. Group for the Psychology of Mathematics Education* (Vol. 4, pp. 161–168). Vancouver, Canada: PME.

Nardi, E (2008). *Amongst mathematicians: teaching and learning mathematics at university level*. New York, NY: Springer.

Nardi, N, Jaworski, B, & Hegedus, S (2005). A spectrum of pedagogical awareness for undergraduate mathematics: from tricks to techniques. *Journal for Research in Mathematics Education, 36*, 284–316.

O'Neill, G, Moore, S, & McMullin, B (Eds.). (2005). *Emerging issues in the practice of university learning and teaching* (pp. 27–36). Dublin: All Ireland Society for Higher Education (AISHE).

Paterson, J, & Evans, T (2013). Audience insights: feed forward in professional development. In D. King, B. Loch, & L. Rylands (Eds.), *Lighthouse Delta shining through the fog, The 9th Delta Conference* (pp. 132–140). Australia: Kiama.

Paterson, J, Thomas, MOJ, Postlethwaite, C, & Taylor, S (2011). The internal disciplinarian: who is in control? In Proceedings of the 14th Annual Conference on Research in Undergraduate Mathematics Education (Vol. 2, pp. 354–368). Portland, Oregon: RUME.

Paterson, J, Thomas, MOJ, & Taylor, S (2011a). Reaching decisions via internal dialogue: its role in a lecturer professional development model. In B. Ubuz (Ed.), Proceedings of the 35th Conference of the International Group for the Psychology of Mathematics Education (Vol. 3, pp. 353–360). Ankara, Turkey: PME.

Paterson, J, Thomas, MOJ, & Taylor, S (2011b). Decisions, decisions, decisions: what determines the path taken in lectures? *International Journal of Mathematical Education in Science and Technology, 42*(7), 985–996.

Petropoulou, G, Potari, D, & Zachariades, T (2011). Inquiring mathematics teaching at the university level. In. B. Ubuz (Ed), *Developing mathematical thinking* (Proceedings of the 35th conference of the International. Group for the Psychology of Mathematics Education), pp. 386–392. Ankara, Turkey: PME.

Rowland, S (2000). *The enquiring university teacher*. Philadelphia, PA: OU Press.

Russ, R, Sherin, B, & Sherin, M (2011) Images of Expertise in Mathematics Teaching. In Y. Li and G. Kaiser (Eds), Expertise in Mathematics Instruction, pp. 41–60. New York: Springer.

Schoenfeld, AH (2006). Mathematics teaching and learning. In P. A. Alexander & P. H. Winne (Eds.), *Handbook of Educational Psychology* (2nd ed., pp. 479–510). Mahwah, NJ: Erlbaum.

Schoenfeld, AH (2008). On modeling teachers' in-the-moment decision-making. In A. H. Schoenfeld (Ed.), *A study of teaching: Multiple lenses, multiple views (Journal for Research in Mathematics Education Monograph No. 14* (pp. 45–96). Reston: National Council of Teachers of Mathematics.

Schoenfeld, AH (2010). *How we think. A theory of goal-oriented decision making and its educational applications*. New York: Routledge.

Schoenfeld, AH (2014). What makes for powerful classrooms, and how can we support teachers in creating them? A story of research and practice, productively intertwined. *Educational Researcher, 43*(8), 404–412. doi:10.3102/0013189X1455.

Schoenfeld, AH (2015). Thoughts on scale. *ZDM Mathematics Education, 47*, 161–169. doi:10.1007/s11858-014-0662-3.

Schuck, S, & Pereira, P (2011). What counts in mathematics education? In S. Schuck & P. Pereira (Eds.), *What counts in teaching mathematics? Self study of teaching and teacher education practices* (Vol. 11, pp. 1–9). Dordrecht: Springer.

Shulman, LS (1986). Those who understand: knowledge growth in teaching. *Educational Researcher, 17*(1), 4–14.

Shulman, L (1987). Knowledge and teaching: foundations of the new reform. *Harvard Educational Review, 57*, 1–22.

Speer, NM (2008). Connecting beliefs and practices: a fine-grained analysis of a college mathematics teacher's collections of beliefs and their relationship to his instructional practices. *Cognition and Instruction, 26*(2), 218–267.

Speer, NM, Smith, JP, & Horvath, A (2010). Collegiate mathematics teaching: an unexamined practice. *Journal of Mathematical Behavior, 29*, 99–114.

Thomas, S (2012). *An activity theory analysis of linear algebra teaching within university mathematics* (Unpublished PhD thesis). UK: Loughborough University.

Wagner, J (1997). The unavoidable intervention of educational research: a framework for reconsidering research-practitioner cooperation. *Educational Researcher, 26*(7), 13–22.

Wells, G (1999). Dialogic inquiry: *Towards a sociological practice and theory of education*. Roskilde. Denmark: Roskilde University Centre.

10

Standards-based mathematics curricula and the promotion of quantitative literacy in elementary school

Jesse L. M. Wilkins

Abstract

Background: Prior research has shown that students taught using *Standards*-based mathematics curricula tend to outperform students on measures of mathematics achievement. However, little research has focused particularly on the promotion of student quantitative literacy (QLT). In this study, the potential influence of the *Investigations in Number, Data, and Space* curriculum on student quantitative literacy is investigated. Quantitative literacy is conceptualized as a hierarchical three-factor model comprising the interrelationship among a student's mathematical beliefs, disposition, and cognition. This theoretical model is validated with elementary-aged students and used to investigate whether students' quantitative literacy is related to the use of the *Investigations* curriculum.

Results: The hierarchical three-factor QLT model was found to have relatively good fit for the sample of elementary-aged students, and all inter-factor relationships were found to be consistent with the proposed theoretical model of the quantitative literacy construct. On average, students in the school district using a *Standards*-based mathematics curriculum had increased levels of quantitative literacy when compared to students in the district not using the curriculum or using it for less time.

Conclusions: Based on the findings of this study, the *Investigations* mathematics curriculum has potential to promote students' development of quantitative literacy in elementary school. Furthermore, the results of the study provide additional validation for the theoretical quantitative literacy construct modeled as a second-order factor comprising the interrelationship among a student's mathematical beliefs, mathematical disposition, and mathematical cognition.

Keywords: Quantitative literacy, *Standards*-based Mathematics curricula, Mathematical beliefs, Mathematical disposition

> The curriculum...should emphasize the mathematics processes and skills that support the quantitative literacy of students. (National Council of Teachers of Mathematics 2000, p. 16).

Background

Out of a call for reform in mathematics education (National Council of Teacher of Mathematics 1989; also see National Research Council 1989; American Association for the Advancement of Science 1990), the National Science Foundation funded several projects during the 1990s to develop mathematics curricula that were consistent with the standards outlined in the *Curriculum and Evaluation Standards for School Mathematics* (National Council of Teacher of Mathematics 1989) and later the *Principles and Standards for School Mathematics* (National Council of Teachers of Mathematics 2000). Research evaluating the impact of these curricula has consistently found that students who learn mathematics using these curricula outperform students who do not on measures of mathematics achievement, problem-solving, and reasoning (Post et al. 2008; Mokros 2003; Harris et al. 2001; McCaffrey et al. 2001; Reys et al. 2003; Senk and Thompson 2003; Thompson and Senk 2001; Riordan and Noyce 2001; Carroll 1997). However, most of these studies

Correspondence: wilkins@vt.edu
School of Education/Teaching and Learning, War Memorial Hall, RM 300C, Virginia Tech, 370 Drillfield Drive, Blacksburg, VA 24061, USA

focused primarily on measures of mathematics content and did not incorporate aspects of mathematical learning related to beliefs and attitudes. In other words, the impact of these curricula has not been evaluated directly for their impact on students' overall quantitative literacy (QLT).

The notion of quantitative literacy developed in the later part of the 20th century, also, out of a call for reform in mathematics education (American Association for the Advancement of Science 1990; National Council of Teacher of Mathematics 1989; National Research Council 1989; Cockcroft 1982; National Commission on Excellence in Education 1983). Although continued debate exists over what exactly constitutes a person's quantitative literacy, a review of the literature suggests that most would agree that it includes an everyday "walking around" knowledge of mathematics characterized by an ability to reason and think mathematically (Steen 1997, p. xvi; also see Cockcroft 1982; Steen 1999, 2001; National Council of Teacher of Mathematics 2000, 1989). However, different from mathematics, which is a discipline to be studied, quantitative literacy is a habit of mind that is further characterized by a person's beliefs about mathematics and their mathematical disposition (e.g., Wilkins, in press, 2010, 2000; Steen, 2001; National Council of Teachers of Mathematics 2000, 1989; Gal 1997; Atkins and Helms 1993; American Association for the Advancement of Science 1990). This expanded view of quantitative literacy embodies the mathematical goals for students advocated by the mathematics education reform begun in the later part of the 20th century (National Council of Teacher of Mathematics 1989, p. 5) and continuing into the 21st century (National Council of Teachers of Mathematics 2006, 2000; National Governors Association Center for Best Practices, Council of Chief State School Officers 2010).

In the USA, quantitative literacy is most often associated with upper secondary and post-secondary education as students prepare for adult citizenship (e.g., Gillman 2006a; Steen 2004; Madison and Steen 2003). However, before students reach secondary and post-secondary education, they are enculturated with beliefs and attitudes that shape the way they view and approach quantitative situations both in and out of school and in their current and future daily lives. For this reason, it is important to investigate potential influences on the early development of children's quantitative literacy. One such influence is the curriculum that is used in mathematics classrooms.

In this study, grounded in the notion of quantitative literacy outlined by Wilkins (in press, 2010), a measurement model of QLT is validated for a sample of elementary-aged students. This measurement model is then used to examine the level of quantitative literacy for these elementary-aged students as it relates to the use of a *Standards*-based mathematics curriculum (i.e., *Investigations in Number, Data and Space*, [Russell et al. 2004]).

Quantitative literacy

Based on earlier work to define quantitative literacy (e.g., Steen 2001; Wilkins 2000; Gal 1997; Dossey 1997), Wilkins (in press, 2010) conceptualized a theoretical framework and measurement model of quantitative literacy to include not only the cognitive aspects of quantitative literacy but also its affective components. Wilkins (in press, 2010) validated a three-factor model of quantitative literacy that incorporated the multiple aspects of quantitative literacy into one measure. Based on this framework, a person's quantitative literacy is characterized by the interrelationship among their (a) mathematical beliefs (b) mathematical disposition, and (c) mathematical cognition.

A person who is quantitatively literate tends to have beliefs about mathematics and statistics that are more humanistic in that they view quantitative information as accessible, interpretable, and producible by everyone, not just experts (Wilkins, in press, 2010, 2000; Steen 2001; Gal 1997). Hofer and Pintrich (1997; also see Hofer 2000) outlined personal epistemological beliefs into those related to the nature of knowledge and those related to the nature of knowing. Within these two categories, the nature of knowledge can be thought of in terms of the simplicity and certainty of knowledge, and the nature of knowing can be thought of in terms of the source and justification of knowledge. Wilkins (in press) used this framework to outline the views of mathematics that would be consistent or not consistent with a person who is quantitatively literate. A belief in the simplicity of mathematics would produce, for example, a view of mathematics as a set of predetermined facts and procedures as opposed to a network of interrelated concepts. A belief in the certainty of knowledge would produce a view of mathematics as static and known as opposed to constantly changing over time as new ideas are discovered. Source of knowledge relates to views about where mathematical knowledge originates from, externally or internally; for example, do mathematical ideas only come from textbooks, experts, or teachers or can they be created or re-created at some level by everyone? Justification of knowledge relates to how mathematical claims are warranted. For example, can mathematical ideas be justified by individuals or can they only be justified by experts, textbooks, or calculators? For a person who is quantitatively literate, mathematics is viewed more as a way of thinking and reasoning, as dynamic and open for discussion and new discoveries, instead of a static set of predetermined facts and formulas that are passed along in an authoritarian manner to be memorized.

A positive disposition toward mathematics would be characteristic of a person who is quantitatively literate

(Wilkins, in press, 2010, 2000; Steen 2001; National Council of Teachers of Mathematics 2000, 1989). In this case, a positive disposition would be characterized by a willingness to engage and persist in quantitative situations (Wilkins, in press, 2010). Grounded in the expectancy value theory of achievement motivation (Eccles et al. 1983), a quantitatively literate person would have increased expectations for success in quantitative situations, they would have an increased value in mathematics and statistics for its social utility and would have an increased level of intrinsic interest in quantitative situations (Wilkins, in press, 2010). A person's expectations for success with a given task and the values associated with the success of the task are related to how persistent a person is with that task (Eccles et al. 1983; Eccles and Wigfield 1995). This interrelationship among expectations and values becomes an essential component of a person's way of thinking and habit of mind, and thus, an important part of a person's quantitative literacy.

Mathematical cognition as it relates to quantitative literacy includes a functional knowledge of mathematics content—an ability to handle mathematics that one might find in everyday life; that is, mathematics necessary to balance a checkbook, shop for groceries, read a map or bus schedule, or read the newspaper. Such a facility with mathematics includes a breadth of knowledge as outlined, for example, by the National Council of Teachers of Mathematics (2000)—number and operations, geometry and measurement, data analysis, and algebra (see also Dossey 1997); or more generally an understanding of pattern, dimension, quantity, uncertainty, shape, and change (Steen 1990). Mathematical cognition further extends beyond content knowledge to include a person's ability to reason and think mathematically—to evaluate and synthesize information, make conjectures and draw logical conclusions, and apply knowledge to real-world problems and situations (Steen 2001; Wilkins 2000; National Council of Teachers of Mathematics 2000, 1989).

Purpose of study

This study has two interrelated purposes: (1) to create and validate a model of quantitative literacy for elementary-aged students and (2) to use this model to examine the relationship between student quantitative literacy and exposure to a *Standards*-based mathematics curriculum. In this study, quantitative literacy is modeled as a second-order factor that accounts for the interrelationship among three first-order factors (Wilkins, in press, 2010): a person's (a) mathematical beliefs, (b) mathematical dispositions, and (c) mathematical cognition. This theoretical model has been validated for secondary (Wilkins, 2010) and undergraduate (Wilkins, in press) students. The purpose of this study is to examine the construct validity of this hierarchical three-factor model of quantitative literacy for three cohorts of elementary-aged students. This model is then used to investigate whether elementary students, who are in a school district that has adopted and implemented a mathematics curriculum consistent with the goals of the National Council of Teachers of Mathematics (2000, 1989; cf. National Governors Association Center for Best Practices, Council of Chief State School Officers 2010), have increased quantitative literacy over students in the district not using the curriculum or for a shorter amount of time.

Methods

Data

This study involved 2490 fourth graders from one school district located in the southeastern USA. The sample was made up of three cohorts of students from three consecutive school years. Only students who were in the school district for at least two successive years (grades 3 and 4) were included in the study. The school district included 16 elementary schools.[1] The district had recently implemented the *Investigations in Number Data & Space* curriculum (Russell et al. 2004) in the elementary schools. The curriculum was implemented in shifts beginning with grades K-1 in school year 2000–2001, grades 2–3 in school year 2001–2002, and grades 4–5 in school year 2002–2003. Because of this implementation schedule, the first cohort of students was not involved with *Investigations*; the second cohort of students was involved with *Investigations* for 2 years, in grades 3 and 4; the third cohort of students was involved with *Investigations* for 4 years, in grades 1–4.

Teachers in the school district were provided with 153 h of professional development related to the implementation of the new curriculum during the summer prior to implementation and during the subsequent 2 years. Based on reports from the district mathematics supervisors, all schools used the *Investigations* curriculum but at differing levels of implementation.

The students in the first cohort ($n = 815$) were fourth graders in the school year 2001–2002 and were surveyed and tested in the spring of 2002, prior to the implementation of *Investigations* in the district. This sample was 49.2 % female and 50.8 % male. The sample was 80.6 % White, 13.4 % Black, and 6.0 % Other (Asian, Hispanic, American Indian). Of the sample, 18.7 % of the students received free or reduced lunch, with 0.6 % missing. The students in the second cohort ($n = 837$) were fourth graders in the school year 2002–2003 and were surveyed and tested in the spring of 2003, after implementation of *Investigations*. This sample was 48.7 % female and 51.3 % male. The sample was 80.5 % White, 11.9 % Black, and 7.5 % Other (Asian, Hispanic, American Indian). Of the sample, 19.0 % of the students received free or reduced lunch. The students in the third cohort

($n = 838$) were fourth graders in the school year 2003–2004 and were surveyed and tested, in the spring of 2004, also after implementation of *Investigations.* This sample was 48.8 % female and 51.2 % male. The sample was 79.5 % White, 12.9 % Black, and 7.6 % Other (Asian, Hispanic, American Indian). Of the sample, 17.1 % of the students received free or reduced lunch.

Measures

Student data were gathered using the *New Standards Reference Examination* (NSRE, for discussion of the exam see Briars and Resnick 2000; Wiley and Resnick 1997), published by Harcourt Educational Measurement (1996, 1997, 1998, 1999),[2] and the *Elementary Mathematics Attitude Survey* (EMAS; Wilkins, 2004a). Each of the variables used in the study is described below. Descriptive statistics for the variables for the whole sample are presented in Table 1. This study uses secondary data analysis as the data were collected for other purposes. However, although the measures for the beliefs component had to be modified because there was not a complete set of belief measures, the data included measures consistent with the earlier models of quantitative literacy (Wilkins, in press, 2010).

Table 1 Descriptive statistics for observed variables for full sample

	N	*M*	SD
Cognition			
Problem	2459	5.66	3.76
Concept	2459	32.83	8.48
Skills	2459	13.28	2.78
Disposition			
Interest	2211	3.92	1.01
Self-concept	2211	3.82	0.85
Utility	2211	4.05	0.67
Beliefs			
B1	2173	3.27	1.25
B2	2198	1.83	1.14
B3	2186	2.68	1.20
B4	2190	2.64	1.17
B5	2189	3.70	1.13
B6	2193	2.69	1.11
Background			
Gender	2490	0.49	0.50
White	2490	0.80	0.40
Black	2490	0.13	0.33
Other	2490	0.07	0.26
Free/reduced lunch	2485	0.18	0.39
Reading	2297	645.37	43.26

Mathematical cognition

Student mathematical cognition was assessed using the NSRE (Form E). The NSRE assesses students' mathematical knowledge in the different content strands of mathematics advocated by the NCTM (see Wiley and Resnick 1997; Briars and Resnick 2000). In addition, this knowledge is assessed at three process levels: problem-solving, concepts, and skills. The items on the test use multiple formats including multiple-choice and open-ended. Given that the test assesses children's content knowledge across the strands of the NCTM and also assesses children's problem-solving and reasoning, conceptual understanding, and skills, it provides a good measure of the mathematical cognition component of quantitative literacy. The raw scores from each of the three process levels were used as the three measures of mathematical cognition: *problem*, *concept*, and *skills*. The same test form was used for all three cohorts; thus, the raw scores were comparable across the three cohorts.

Mathematical disposition

Student mathematical disposition was assessed using items from the EMAS. This survey was designed using items from other sources (e.g., Third International Mathematics and Science Study [TIMSS], Gonzalez and Smith 1998; Second International Mathematics Study, Westbury and Thalathoti 1989; Fennema and Sherman 1976). Items were chosen to be appropriate for Grade 4 students. This survey consisted of 48 items rated on a 5-point Likert scale from *Strongly Agree* to *Strongly Disagree*. Consistent with Wilkins (in press, 2010), measures of student mathematics self-concept, interest, and utility value were created from the survey and included as part of the mathematics disposition factor. The self-concept scale contained six items (e.g., "I usually do well in math", "Math is harder for me than most people") with strong internal consistency ($\alpha_1 = 0.81$, $\alpha_2 = 0.83$, $\alpha_3 = 0.84$, $\alpha_{FULL} = 0.83$). The interest scale contained five items (e.g., "Math is interesting to me," "I like math") with strong internal consistency ($\alpha_1 = 0.91$, $\alpha_2 = 0.92$, $\alpha_3 = 0.90$, $\alpha_{FULL} = 0.91$). The utility value scale contained eight items (e.g., "I will use math in many ways as an adult", "Math is useful in everyone's life") with good internal consistency ($\alpha_1 = 0.77$, $\alpha_2 = 0.74$, $\alpha_3 = 0.76$, $\alpha_{FULL} = 0.76$).

Mathematical beliefs

The four components associated with epistemological beliefs related to mathematics (see Wilkins, in press; Hofer 2000) were not explicitly assessed within the EMAS. However, six items on the survey did have face validity in terms of the simplicity of knowledge component. These six individual items were used to measure the beliefs component: (B1) Learning math is mostly memorizing; (B2) Math problems should be solved the same way by everyone; (B3) In math, memorizing facts is more important than being a good problem solver; (B4) Math is a set of rules; (B5) There is always a rule to follow in solving a math problem; (B6) Math helps one to think according to strict rules. These six items did not overlap with the items used in the disposition factors. Given the age of the students, it was felt that these items were accessible to the children and provided a good representation for the beliefs component. The internal consistency of these six items is relatively low ($\alpha_1 = 0.51$, $\alpha_2 = 0.58$, $\alpha_3 = 0.56$, $\alpha_{FULL} = 0.56$), but along with the face validity of the items, provides some evidence that the scale will be useful as a measure of the simplicity of mathematical knowledge.

Curriculum

Because of the implementation schedule of the *Investigations* curriculum, the three cohorts of students had differing amounts of exposure to the curriculum. For Cohort 1, the district was not using *Investigations* for students in the grades being surveyed. For Cohorts 2 and 3, the district was using *Investigations*. More specifically, for Cohort 2 the curriculum had been implemented for 2 years (in grades 3 and 4), and for Cohort 3, the curriculum had been implemented for 4 years (in grades 1–4). By comparing the three cohorts of students, it is possible to investigate the relationship between curriculum exposure and level of quantitative literacy. In order to compare the level of quantitative literacy across the three cohorts, students were dummy coded by cohort to create three new variables: Cohort 1, Cohort 2, and Cohort 3 (e.g., 1 = member of Cohort 1, 0 = not a member of Cohort 1). By using this coding scheme, it is possible to test whether students in the school district using *Investigations* had higher quantitative literacy scores than students in the district not using *Investigations*. Moreover, because the three cohorts are coded separately, Cohorts 2 and Cohorts 3 can also be compared to test whether increased exposure leads to increased quantitative literacy. For the students in Cohort 1, it is not assumed that they did not have opportunities to learn mathematics and develop their quantitative literacy; it is only assumed that they were not using the *Investigations* curriculum.

Background measures

Student background measures included gender, race/ethnicity, free/reduced lunch status, and prior knowledge (reading). The three cohorts of students were collected from the same school district in three consecutive school years and thus likely provide three very similar samples of students for comparison. However, background variables were used to statistically control for differences that may exist across cohorts. Gender was coded 0 = male, 1 = female. Students' race/ethnicity was dummy coded into three categories: White, Black, and Other (Asian, Hispanic, American Indian). Free/reduced lunch status was used as a proxy for socioeconomic status (0 = regular lunch, 1 = free/reduced). Stanford 9 reading total scaled scores were included as a control for prior knowledge.

Analysis

In order to test for differences in quantitative literacy across the three different cohorts, it was necessary to build and test a baseline measurement model of quantitative literacy (QLT model) for these elementary-aged students. The building of the QLT model in this study followed a model generation scenario (Joreskog 1993). Quantitative literacy was posited as a second-order three-factor model (Wilkins, in press, 2010) and then tested for its fit to the data from the first cohort of students using a confirmatory factor analysis (CFA). Based on model fit, a series of post hoc respecifications were made to the model and retested to create a model that better fit the data. This new model was then cross-validated with data from the second and third cohorts of students. Model respecifications were guided by fit statistics, but changes were made only if they reflected meaningful relationships or were consistent with theory. The goal of these initial analyses was to create a baseline measurement model that was acceptable across all three cohorts.

Following model generation, a multiple-groups analysis was conducted to test for model structure invariance across the three cohorts of students. In order to validly compare quantitative literacy scores, it is necessary to test for model invariance to determine whether the same construct has been measured for all three groups. Model invariance provides evidence that any differences found between groups are not merely artifacts of measurement differences in the models.

Finally, using the QLT model, a test for differences in latent quantitative literacy scores by cohort was conducted. In this study, a quasi-experimental design was used. Student latent quantitative literacy scores were regressed on dummy coded variables representing cohort membership (i.e., opportunity to learn using *Investigations*) while controlling for student background characteristics.

Model creation and testing were conducted using AMOS 22.0.0 (IBM Corporation 2013). Judgment of model fit was guided by four fit indexes (Kline 2011; Byrne 2010): (a) the model chi-square statistic, (b) the comparative fit index (CFI), (c) the root mean square error of approximation (RMSEA) with it 90 % confidence interval, and (d) the standardized root mean square residual (SRMR). The chi-square statistic has been found to be sensitive to sample size and model complexity, and thus, other indexes are also considered that take into account sample size and model complexity. The CFI takes on values between 0 and 1 with values closer to 1 showing better fit; values greater than 0.90 usually show adequate model fit (Kline 1998; Hoyle 1995) with values close to 0.95 showing good model fit (Hu and Bentler 1999); although Marsh et al. (2004) have cautioned against applying 0.95 as a stringent cutoff. The RMSEA and SRMR take on values between 0 and 1 with values closer to 0 showing better model fit. Values for the SRMR less than 0.05 represent good model fit (Byrne 2010), although Hu and Bentler (1999) suggest that values as high as 0.08 show good model fit. Values of the RMSEA less than 0.05 show good model fit, and values between 0.05 and 0.08 represent reasonable model fit (Browne and Cudeck 1993). The 90 % confidence interval (CI) of the RMSEA with its associated p value is used to test hypotheses of close fit ($p > 0.05$) and poor fit (upper bound of CI < 0.10).

These statistics were also used to test for model invariance across the cohorts. Tests of model invariance compare fit statistics of a baseline model with subsequent models with additional constraints. For example, if the difference in the chi-square statistic from two models is not found to be statistically significant then the model is assumed to be invariant with respect to the given constraint. However, recent research has shown that the difference in chi-square is also sensitive to sample size and non-normality (Cheung and Rensvold 2002). Therefore, in this study, the difference in chi-square is reported, but final decisions of model invariance are based primarily on two criteria: (a) the fit of the constrained model to the data and (b) whether the difference in the CFI from one model to the next is less than 0.01 (Byrne and Stewart 2006).

Missing data existed for all variables in the sample (see Table 1). The amount of missing data differed by variable as different sets of variables were collected at different times. For the most part, student background variables were complete with the exception of the reading scores (7.8 %) and free/reduced lunch status for five students (0.2 %). Missing data were handled using pairwise deletion methods. Pairwise deletion removes missing data only for variables that are being used in a particular statistical computation. In this study, pairwise deletions were carried out by calculating the correlation matrix among all variables in the study; thus, correlations were calculated for available data for each pair of variables. This matrix was then used in AMOS to conduct the analyses described above.

If data are not missing completely at random, results from statistical analyses can be biased depending on the amount of data missing by different groups. For each of the cognitive measures, *problem*, *concept*, and *skills*, 1.2 % of the data was missing representing a relatively insignificant amount of missing data. For each of the disposition measures, Self-Concept, Interest, and Utility, 11.2 % of the data was missing. For the six items used to measure Beliefs, the percent of missing data ranged from 11.7 to 12.7 %. The amount of missing data for Beliefs and Dispositions, while not negligible, represents a reasonably small amount of missing data. The amount of missing data for these variables was examined by demographic groups (gender, race/ethnicity, and free/reduced lunch status); and missingness was further examined across variables created from the NSRE and EMAS as these surveys were administered at different times. A chi-square test of association found no relationship between amount of missing data and demographic group (i.e., gender, race/ethnicity, free/reduced lunch status). A test of association found no relationship between missingness for variables created from the NSRE and the EMAS (e.g., comparing missingness for the PROBLEM and Self-Concept variable). A t - test found no statistical difference in reading scores by missing data status for each of the Beliefs and Disposition variables. However, there was a statistically significant difference for the Cognition variables suggesting that, on average, the 31 students with missing data for the cognition variables tended to have lower reading scores (however, the small amount of missing data for the cognition variables seems to mitigate this finding). Taken all together, the evidence suggests that missing data cannot be systematically attributed to student demographics or completion of one or both of the NSRE or the EMAS, thus lessening the chance that statistical results will be biased due to missing data. However, it is important that results be interpreted in light of the potential biases that could be due to missing data.

Results and discussion

Establishing a baseline measurement model of quantitative literacy

In this study, quantitative literacy is modeled as a second-order factor (Wilkins, in press, 2010). That is, each of the three first-order factors (*Beliefs*, *Disposition*, and *Cognition*) is explained by a person's quantitative literacy (the second-order factor). Further, *Self-concept, Utility, and Interest* were used as measures of the three components related to student disposition (Wilkins, in press, 2010). The three sub-scores from the NSRE (*problem*, *concept*, and *skills*) were used as measures associated with students' mathematical cognition. Finally, the six items (B1–B6) identified to be associated with the simplicity component of epistemological beliefs associated with mathematics were used to form a latent measure, *Beliefs*.

It was first necessary to establish a baseline model that could be used to make comparisons across the three cohorts. Using the first cohort of students ($N = 815$), estimation of the QLT model described above resulted in an overall χ^2 value of 317.90, $p < 0.001$, with 51 degrees of freedom. Based on the χ^2 value, the exact-fit hypothesis was rejected. Together, the CFI = 0.89, SRMR = 0.069, and RMSEA = 0.08 also suggested inadequate model fit; however, the magnitude of the indexes suggested promise for the model and warranted inspection for potential model respecification. Furthermore, the pattern coefficients were all found to be statistically significant and consistent with the theorized model (cf. Wilkins, in press, 2010). An inspection of the standardized residual covariance matrix (SRCM) identified several large residuals associated with the covariances among the items within the *Beliefs* factor; the modification indices (MI) associated with these items also confirmed the possible underestimation of the covariances among these items and suggested that a model that estimated some of these covariances would better represent the data. An examination of the wording of the individual items with large residual covariances revealed three smaller clusters of items (items B1 and B3; items B4, B5, and B6; items B1, B4, and B5). Items B1 and B3 share a common theme related to equating mathematics to memorization; items B4, B5, and B6 share the common theme of mathematics as a set of rules; and items B1, B4, and B5 share a common theme of memorizing rules. Each of these sub-clusters reflects the larger notion of the simplicity of mathematics but also reflect a meaningful sub-theme within the larger *Beliefs* factor. Thus, it is reasonable that the items share residual covariance and it makes sense for this covariance to be estimated in the model. Other large residual covariances found between factors could not be substantively justified, and so covariances for these relationships were not specified in the model.

Thus, a series of model respecifications based on the SRCM and MI were made for the *Beliefs* factor and subsequent tests were conducted. Estimation of the final respecified model resulted in a χ^2 value of 211.94, $p < 0.001$, with 45 degrees of freedom. The reduction in the chi-square ($\Delta\chi^2 = 105.96$, $p < 0.001$, with 6 degrees of freedom) was statistically significant indicating a better fit to the data. Furthermore, the CFI = 0.934 and SRMR = 0.056 suggest adequate fit to the data. The RMSEA = 0.068, with 90 % CI = (0.059, 0.077), and pclose = 0.001, also suggests reasonable fit, although the close-fit hypothesis was rejected (i.e., pclose < 0.05), but the poor-fit hypothesis was also rejected (i.e., upper bound of the 90 % CI < 0.10). Again, all pattern coefficients were statistically significant and consistent with theory. This general QLT model is presented in Fig. 1 (note that the coefficients in the model are estimated for all three groups combined into one sample and will be discussed later).

This respecified model was cross-validated using the data from the second cohort ($N = 837$). Estimation of the QLT model using these data resulted in an overall χ^2 value of 161.65, $p < 0.001$, with 45 degrees of freedom. Based on the χ^2 value, the exact-fit hypothesis was rejected. However, based on the RMSEA = 0.056, with 90 % CI = (0.047, 0.065), and pclose = 0.148, the close-fit hypothesis was not rejected (i.e., pclose > 0.05), and the poor-fit hypothesis was rejected (i.e., upper bound <0.10). The CFI = 0.952 and SRMR = 0.048 suggest good fit to the data. An examination of the SRCM found no significant residual covariances among the items in the *Beliefs* factor. All pattern coefficients were statistically significant and consistent with theory. Furthermore, findings provide validation for the model respecifications made to the first model suggesting that the changes do not merely represent artifacts of the sample data.

The QLT model was then estimated using the data from the third cohort ($N = 838$). Estimation of the model using these data resulted in an overall χ^2 value of 203.53, $p < 0.001$, with 45 degrees of freedom. Based on the χ^2 value, the exact-fit hypothesis was rejected. However, the RMSEA = 0.065, with 90 % CI = (0.056, 0.074), and pclose = 0.003, suggests reasonable fit; the close-fit hypothesis was rejected (i.e., pclose < 0.05), but the poor-fit hypothesis was rejected (i.e., upper bound <0.10). The CFI = 0.942 and SRMR = 0.056 suggest reasonably good fit to the data. An examination of the SRCM found no significant residual covariances among the items in the *Beliefs* factor. All pattern coefficients were statistically significant and consistent with theory. Again, estimation of this model with the third sample of data provides additional validation for the model.

Testing model invariance across the three cohorts

A multiple-groups analysis was conducted to compare the measurement and structural invariance of the QLT model across the three cohorts. Based on the earlier model testing, a baseline multigroup model of quantitative literacy consistent with theory (Wilkins, in press, 2010) has now been created and found to fit the data from each cohort reasonably well. At this point, it is important to establish structural invariance for the model across the three cohorts. This provides evidence that the model operates similarly for each cohort, and thus, differences in the cohorts can be tested with confidence that the differences are more likely due to interventions and not an artifact of measurement differences. Testing for invariance of first- and second-order factor loadings and factor variances is usually sufficient to declare model invariance (Byrne 2010). First, a test for configural invariance was conducted to create a baseline for

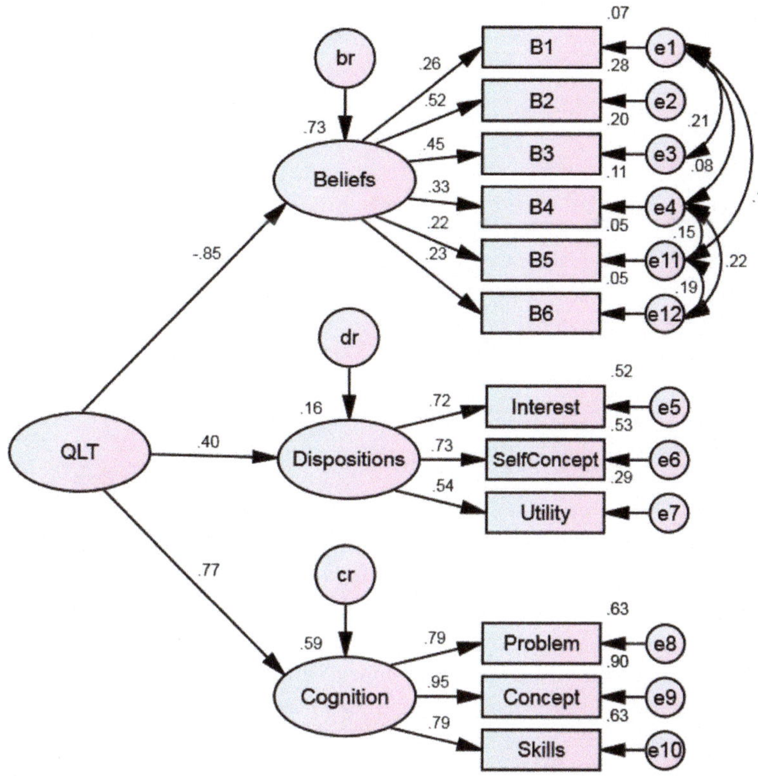

Fig. 1 Measurement model of quantitative literacy

subsequent comparisons. Next, tests for invariance of first-order factor loadings, second-order factor loadings, and structural variances were conducted. Beyond this, tests for invariance of structural residuals and measurement residuals were also conducted.

A test of configural invariance was conducted by estimating the QLT model for all three cohorts simultaneously. In this test, no constraints are imposed on the model. The goal of this test is to determine if the baseline model structure is the same for all three cohorts; further, this model provides baseline statistics for subsequent model comparisons with more strict constraints (see Table 2). Estimation of this unconstrained model (Model 1) resulted in the following fit indexes (see Table 2): $\chi^2 = 577.12$, $p < 0.001$, with 135 degrees of freedom; CFI = 0.942; and RMSEA = 0.036, with 90 % CI = (0.033, 0.039), and pclose = 1.00. Overall these indexes provide evidence of good fit to the data and evidence of configural invariance.

Given configural invariance, a series of tests was conducted (see Table 2). For each test, increased constraints were added to the model, first constraining the first-order factor loadings to be equal across the cohorts (Model 2). This was followed by constraining the second-order factor loadings to be equal across the three cohorts (Model 3). In Model 4, factor variances were constrained. Finally, structural residuals and measurement residuals were constrained in Model 5 and Model 6, respectively. In each case, the subsequent model was compared to the preceding model based on model fit and change in the CFI. Although, the change in chi-square value was significant for Model 2 and 6, in both cases, the Model was found to have good fit and the change in the CFI was less than 0.01. In all other comparisons, the models were found to have good fit, non-significant differences in chi-square and negligible differences in the CFIs. Based on these tests, the QLT model was determined to have structural and measurement invariance across the three cohorts.

A final model of quantitative literacy

Given model invariance across the three cohorts, the three samples of students were combined to estimate model fit for the entire sample. Using this sample of students, estimation of the QLT model resulted in an overall χ^2 value of 430.19, $p < 0.001$, with 45 degrees of freedom. Based on the χ^2 value, the exact-fit hypothesis was rejected. The RMSEA = 0.059, with 90 % CI = (0.054, 0.064), and pclose = 0.002, suggests reasonably good model fit, and the poor-fit hypothesis was rejected (upper bound of 90 % CI < 0.10). Furthermore, the CFI = 0.950 and the SRMR = 0.048 suggest good fit to the data. Overall these statistics provide evidence of good model fit and construct validity of the model. This final model is presented in Fig. 1. All pattern coefficients[3] were statistically significant (see Fig. 1 and Table 3) and

Table 2 Fit statistics for testing invariance of second-order factor model of QLT across cohorts

Model	χ^2	*df*	CFI	SRMR	RMSEA (90 % CI) (pclose)	Model comparison	ΔCFI	$\Delta\chi^2$	Δ*df*
Model 1 configural invariance	577.12***	135	0.942	0.056	0.036 (0.033–0.039) (1.00)	–			
Model 2 first-order factor loadings invariant	618.31***	153	0.939	0.061	0.035 (0.032–0.038) (1.00)	2 vs. 1	0.003	41.19***	18
Model 3 first- and second-order factor loadings invariant	621.67***	157	0.940	0.061	0.034 (0.032–0.037) (1.00)	3 vs. 2	0.001	3.36	4
Model 4 first- and second-order factor loadings and structural variances invariant	623.68***	159	0.940	0.062	0.034 (0.031-0.037) (1.00)	4 vs. 3	0.000	2.02	2
Model 5 first- and second-order factor loadings, structural variances, and structural residuals invariant	628.66***	165	0.940	0.062	0.034 (0.031–0.036) (1.00)	5 vs. 4	0.000	4.98	6
Model 6 first- and second-order factor loadings, structural variances, structural residuals, and measurement residuals invariant	713.26***	201	0.933	0.062	0.032 (0.029–0.035) (1.00)	6 vs. 5	0.007	84.98***	36

***$p < 0.001$

consistent with the theorized model (Wilkins, in press, 2010). That is, students' quantitative literacy was characterized by an interrelationship among mathematical cognition, disposition, and beliefs in the simplicity of mathematical knowledge, e.g., increased mathematical cognition is related to positive disposition and decreased beliefs in the simplicity of mathematics and inversely.

Predicting student quantitative literacy

The relationship between students' quantitative literacy and the opportunity to learn mathematics using a *Standards*-based mathematics curriculum was investigated at the district level using a series of regression models. Quantitative literacy was measured as a latent construct as described by the measurement model above (see Fig. 1, Table 2).

Table 3 Standardized regression weights for measurement model of quantitative literacy

	QLT	BELF	COG	DISP
Beliefs	-0.853			
Cognition	0.769			
Disposition	0.400			
B1		0.257		
B2		0.525		
B3		0.448		
B4		0.334		
B5		0.219		
B6		0.230		
Problem			0.794	
Concept			0.949	
Skills			0.792	
Interest				0.720
Self-Concept				0.728
Utility				0.543

All regression weights were statistically significant ($a < 0.001$). *QLT* = quantitative literacy, *BELF* = beliefs, *COG* = cognition, *DISP* = disposition. χ^2 (45) = 440.19, $p < 0.001$; CFI = 0.950; SRMR = 0.048; RMSEA = 0.059, 90 % CI = (0.054, 0.064) pclose = 0.002

First, a Baseline Model, regressing student quantitative literacy on student background variables was estimated (see Table 4). Because the design of the study was quasi-experimental, this baseline model served to statistically control for differences in these variables that might exist across cohorts. Prior knowledge was found to be a statistically significant predictor of student QLT scores ($\beta = 0.664$; $b = 0.003$, $SE < 0.001$, $p < 0.001$). That is, on average, students with higher reading scores were found to have increased quantitative literacy and inversely. Reading scores were found to be the strongest predictor of QLT. Students receiving free or reduced lunch, on average, were found to have lower QLT scores ($\beta = -0.161$; $b = -0.092$, $SE = 0.012$, $p < 0.001$). Gender was found to be a statistically significant predictor of QLT ($\beta = -0.033$; $b = 0.015$, $SE = 0.006$, $p < 0.05$), indicating that, on average, females have lower QLT scores. Furthermore, compared to students categorized as White, on average, students categorized as Black were found to have lower QLT scores, and this difference was statistically significant ($\beta = -0.135$; $b = -0.089$, $SE = 0.013$, $p < 0.001$). Students categorized as Other were not found to be statistically different from students categorized as White ($\beta = 0.023$; $b = -0.020$, $SE = 0.013$). Overall, these background variables explained 62.5 % of the variance in the latent QLT scores.

In order to investigate the relationship between QLT scores and exposure to *Investigations*, a second model, the Curriculum Model, was estimated (see Table 4). This model included dummy coded variables that made it possible to compare students in Cohorts 2 and 3 to students in Cohort 1. By not including the Cohort 1 variable in the model, coefficients for the Cohort 2 and Cohort 3 variables represented differences in QLT scores compared to Cohort 1. After controlling for student background

Table 4 Regression of student quantitative literacy on background variables and opportunity to use a *Standards*-based curriculum

	Baseline model			Curriculum model		
	β	b	SE	β	b	SE
Gender	−0.033	0.015*	0.006	−0.033	−0.014*	0.006
Black (compared to White)	−0.135	−0.089***	0.013	−0.136	−0.090***	0.012
Other (compared to White)	0.023	0.020	0.013	0.020	0.017	0.013
Free/reduced Lunch	−0.161	−0.092***	0.012	−0.159	−0.090***	0.012
Prior achievement	0.664	0.003***	0.000	0.668	0.003***	0.000
Cohort 2 (compared to Cohort 1)				0.041	0.019*	0.008
Cohort 3 (compared to Cohort 1)				0.102	0.048***	0.009
R^2	0.625			0.640		

*$p < 0.05$, ***$p < 0.001$

variables, the difference in QLT scores between Cohort 1 and Cohort 2 was found to be statistically significant ($\beta = 0.041$; $b = 0.019$, $SE = 0.008$, $p < 0.05$) in favor of Cohort 2. The difference in QLT scores between Cohort 1 and Cohort 3 was also found to be statistically significant ($\beta = 0.102$; $b = 0.048$, $SE = 0.009$, $p < 0.001$) in favor of Cohort 3. That is, on average, students in the school district who were surveyed after implementation of *Investigations* were found to have increased quantitative literacy when compared to students surveyed prior to the implementation of *Investigations*. The Curriculum Model explained 64.0 % of the variance in latent QLT scores. After controlling for background variables, the curriculum variables explained an additional 2.4 % of the variance in latent QLT scores relative to the variance explained by the Background Model. Furthermore, an additional test comparing QLT scores for Cohort 2 and Cohort 3 found the difference to be statistically significant ($\beta = 0.062$; $b = 0.029$, $SE = 0.008$, $p < 0.001$) indicating an overall increase for Cohort 3 above and beyond the increased change made by Cohort 2.

Conclusions

The purposes of this study were to create and validate a QLT model for elementary-aged students and to use this model to examine the relationship between student quantitative literacy and exposure to a *Standards*-based mathematics curriculum. The results of the study provide evidence for the validity of the QLT model for the sample of elementary-aged children. In this model, the quantitative literacy construct is represented as a second-order factor comprising three first-order factors: mathematical beliefs, mathematical disposition, and mathematical cognition (see Fig. 1). Furthermore, the model highlights the interrelationship among these factors that is consistent with the theoretical notion of quantitative literacy proposed by Wilkins (in press, 2010). By using a sample of elementary-aged students, the results of this study provide further evidence for the validity of a generalized model of quantitative literacy as previous research has validated the model for secondary and undergraduate students (Wilkins, in press, 2010).

Using the measurement model of quantitative literacy, QLT scores for students in the school district using *Investigations* were compared to scores for students in the same school district before the implementation of *Investigations*. Overall, Grade 4 students in the school district after implementation had increased QLT scores when compared to Grade 4 students in the district prior to the implementation of *Investigations*. Moreover, a comparison of students with 4 years of exposure to the curriculum to students with only 2 years of exposure, found, on average, a statistically significant increase in QLT scores for those students with 4 years of exposure. Compared with the amount of variance in QLT scores explained by the Background Model, the amount of additional variance explained by the Curriculum Model was relatively low, and its practical significance should be considered with caution. However, the evidence does suggest a positive relationship between the use of a *Standards*-based curriculum and the development of quantitative literacy. Compared with prior research that has only shown increased mathematics achievement (cf., Mokros 2003), findings from this study provide evidence that the use of a *Standards*-based curriculum may lead to increased overall quantitative literacy. By using a measurement model that portrays the holistic notion of quantitative literacy, instead of measuring different components and aggregating findings, we are better able to assess whether *Standards*-based curricula promote the whole of quantitative literacy.

In addition to the measurement of quantitative literacy, the findings from this study have implications for assessment and curriculum development. From an assessment perspective, this study provides an example of how quantitative literacy can be assessed in a holistic manner. Most often, quantitative literacy is assessed with a focus solely on mathematical and statistical content knowledge using tasks that contextualize the mathematics in real-world or problem-based situations (e.g., TIMSS [see Orpwood and Garden 1998; Mullis et al. 1998], and Programme for International Student Assessment [PISA, Organisation for Economic Cooperation and Development OECD 2000]). While this form of assessment does test an important aspect of being quantitatively literate, at best, the affective components of quantitative literacy are measured as a secondary consideration and discussed merely as they relate to achievement but not as they interrelate (e.g., TIMSS, PISA). In addition, many colleges and universities have developed quantitative literacy courses and standards (Gillman 2006a; Steen 2004), but again these standards are often assessed based on achievement tests of contextualized mathematics (e.g., Comaz and Martin 2006; Gillman 2006b). Findings from this study suggest that quantitative literacy can be assessed holistically as a single construct that considers the interrelationship among the different aspects of quantitative literacy.

From a curriculum perspective, *Investigations* seems to have the potential to promote quantitative literacy in elementary-aged students. Without further analysis, it cannot be generalized that *Investigations* is a "quantitative literacy curriculum," but it is possible that *Investigations* could serve as a model that could be further studied to understand the components of a curriculum that could potentially promote quantitative literacy. In order to promote the notion of quantitative literacy outlined in this study, it would be important to understand how best to motivate children in a way that builds quantitative literacy as a habit of mind. That is, to help students create beliefs about mathematics as accessible, constructible, and justifiable by all, coupled with a value for mathematics and a confidence and willingness to engage in quantitative situations.

Limitations and future research

While the conclusions of the current study seem promising, it is important to situate the findings within a larger research trajectory to test mathematics education interventions (cf., Sloane 2008). In other words, it is important to highlight what the current study does not tell us but how the findings add to the research literature. First, this study is limited by its unit of analysis. The unit of analysis is the student, and the "treatment" happens at the level of the school district. From the findings of this study, it is not clear how students within different schools compared across the three cohorts[4] nor is it clear how students within different classrooms or with different teachers compared across the three cohorts.[5] It is quite possible for the findings to be different or even opposite at different levels of analysis (see e.g., Wilkins, 2004b). For example, some schools could have shown an increase across the cohorts, while others could have shown a decrease, but on average, the school district could still show an increase. Similarly, this could have happened at the classroom level. Documenting the patterns of differences across schools and classrooms would enhance the current findings. In addition, by documenting these patterns of differences, they could potentially be modeled using other school- or teacher-level variables further adding to the understanding of how the intervention contributed to students' overall quantitative literacy.

In this study, implementation (i.e., treatment) means that the curriculum was adopted by the school district, and thus, it can only be said that students are in a district that adopted the curriculum. In this study, there was no statistical or design-based control for the fidelity of curriculum implementation. Thus, it cannot be assumed that all teachers used the curriculum in the same way nor that all students received the same opportunities to use the curriculum, except to say, that at least they are in a school district and school that has adopted *Investigations.* Teachers were involved in professional development experiences to help them implement the curriculum appropriately, but beyond this, except for documentation by the mathematics supervisors that teachers in the schools were using the curriculum, there was no systematic documentation of implementation.

Sloane (2008) points out that prior to effectiveness studies of interventions in mathematics education, it is important, if not necessary, to conduct smaller scale studies to determine the feasibility of such larger scale studies. For example, these smaller scale studies may contribute to the larger research trajectory by developing measures of constructs and by providing preliminary tests of interventions through student-level quasi-experimental studies. Despite its limitations, the current study did just that. In this study, a measurement model of quantitative literacy was tested, and preliminary evidence from the study that students in a school district using *Investigations* had higher levels of quantitative literacy was documented. Future studies would enhance these findings by expanding the scope to include a multilevel design that considers the effects of classroom and school as interacting units of analysis. Beyond the research design, having teachers randomly assigned to treatment groups representing controlled professional development and curriculum implementation would make it possible to test the efficacy of the intervention. The findings of the current study provide the groundwork for additional research with this broader scope and research design.

Endnotes

[1]In the first year that data was collected there were only 15 elementary schools in the district.

[2]Harcourt Brace, Inc. merged with Pearson in 2008.

[3]Structure coefficients were also examined. Structure coefficients are measures of association between variables. It is important that the correlations between variables not assigned to higher-order factors be less than those assigned to a factor. For example, the correlations between the three lower-order factors of cognition and the *Cognition* factor should be greater than the correlations between these three variables and the other higher-order factors, *Beliefs* and *Dispositions*. This was found to be the case for the factors and observed variables in the model.

[4]The small number of schools in the study makes a school-level analysis limited in statistical power. However, based on the use of a slopes-as-outcomes model (Burstein, 1980), the regression analysis was conducted separately for each school and regression coefficients compared across schools. One school's coefficients seemed to suggest that it was an outlier which was consistent with an earlier personal communication with the district mathematics supervisor. Once this school was removed from this analysis, the average school-level differences were relatively consistent with the district-level findings.

[5]Recall that it was not possible to link students and teachers across the different cohorts.

Abbreviations

CCSSO: Council of Chief State School Officers; CFA: Confirmatory Factor Analysis; CFI: Comparative Fit Index; CI: confidence interval; EMAS: Elementary Mathematics Attitude Survey; MI: modification index; NCTM: National Council of Teachers of Mathematics; NGA: National Governor's Association; NSRE: New Standards Reference Exam; OECD: Organisation for Economic Cooperation and Development; PISA: Programme for International Student Assessment; QLT: quantitative literacy; RMSEA: root mean square error of approximation; SIMS: Second International Mathematics Study; SRCM: standardized residual covariance matrix; SRMR: standardized root mean square residual; TIMSS: Third International Mathematics and Science Study.

Competing interests

The author declares that he has no competing interests.

Authors' contributions

JLMW is the sole author of the paper.

Acknowledgements

This study was supported in part by the National Science Foundation Grant #9911558. Any conclusions stated here are those of the author and do not necessarily reflect the position of the National Science Foundation. Virginia Tech's Open Access Subvention Fund supported the publication of this article.

References

American Association for the Advancement of Science. (1990). *Science for all Americans*. New York: Oxford University Press.

Atkins, M., & Helms, J. (1993). Getting serious about priorities in science education. *Studies in Science Education, 21*, 1–20.

Briars, D. J., & Resnick, L. B. (2000). *Standards, assessments—and what else? The essential elements of standards-based school improvement (CSE Technical Report 528)*. Los Angeles: National Center for Research on Evaluation, Standards, and Student Testing (CRESST). Available online: https://www.cse.ucla.edu/products/reports/TECH528.pdf.

Browne, M. W., & Cudeck, R. (1993). Alternative ways of assessing model fit. In K. A. Bollen & J. S. Long (Eds.), *Testing structural equation models* (pp. 445–455). Newbury Park: Sage.

Burstein, L. (1980). The analysis of multi-level data in educational research and evaluation. *Review of Research in Education, 8*, 158–233.

Byrne, B. M. (2010). *Structural equation modeling with AMOS: basics concepts, applications, and programming* (2nd ed.). New York: Routledge.

Byrne, B. M., & Stewart, S. M. (2006). The MACS approach to testing for multigroup invariance of a second-order structure: a walk through the process. *Structural Equation Modeling, 13*(2), 287–321.

Carroll, W. (1997). Results of third-grade students in a reform curriculum on the Illinois state mathematics test. *Journal for Research in Mathematics Education, 28*(2), 237–242.

Cheung, G. W., & Rensvold, R. B. (2002). Evaluating goodness-of-fit indexes for testing measurement invariance. *Structural Equation Modeling: A Multidisciplinary Journal, 9*(2), 233–255.

Cockcroft, W. H. (1982). *Mathematics counts*. London: Her Majesty's Stationary office.

Comaz, D., & Martin, W. O. (2006). Quantitative literacy as an integral component of mathematics curriculum, case at North Dakota State University. In R. Gillman (Ed.), *Current practices in quantitative literacy* (pp. 155–163). Washington, DC: Mathematical Association of America.

Dossey, J. A. (1997). Defining and measuring quantitative literacy. In L. A. Steen (Ed.), *Why numbers count: quantitative literacy for tomorrow's America* (pp. 173–186). New York: College Entrance Examination Board.

Eccles, J. S., & Wigfield, A. (1995). In the mind of an actor: the structure of adolescents' achievement task values and expectancy-related beliefs. *Personality and Social Psychology Bulletin, 21*, 215–225.

Eccles, J., Adler, T. F., Futterman, R., Goff, S. B., Kaczala, C. M., Meece, J. L., et al. (1983). Expectancies, values, and academic behaviors. In J. T. Spence (Ed.), *Achievement and Achievement Motives* (pp. 75–146). San Fransisco, CA: W. H. Freeman and Company.

Fennema, E., & Sherman, J. A. (1976). Fennema-Sherman mathematics attitude scales: instruments designed to measure attitudes toward the learning of mathematics by females and males. *Journal for Research in Mathematics Education, 7*, 324–326.

Gal, I. (1997). Numeracy: imperatives of a forgotten goal. In L. A. Steen (Ed.), *Why numbers count: quantitative literacy of tomorrow's America* (pp. 36–44). New York: College Entrance Examination Board.

Gillman, R. (Ed.) (2006a). *Current practices in quantitative literacy*. Washington: Mathematical Association of America

Gillman, R. (2006b). A case study of assessment practices in quantitative literacy. In R. Gillman (Ed.), *Current Practices in Quantitative Literacy* (pp. 165–169). Washington: Mathematical Association of America

Gonzalez, E. J., & Smith, T. A. (Eds.). (1998). *User guide for the TIMSS international database: primary and middle school years, 1995 assessment*. Chestnut Hill, MA: TIMSS International Study Center.

Harcourt Educational Measurement. (1996). *New standards reference exam—mathematics*. San Antonio: Harcourt, Inc.

Harcourt Educational Measurement. (1997). *New standards reference exam—mathematics*. San Antonio: Harcourt, Inc.

Harcourt Educational Measurement. (1998). *New standards reference exam—mathematics*. San Antonio: Harcourt, Inc.

Harcourt Educational Measurement. (1999). *New standards reference exam—mathematics*. San Antonio: Harcourt, Inc.

Harris, K., Marcus, R., McLaren, K., & Fey, J. (2001). Curriculum materials supporting problem-based teaching. *School Science and Mathematics, 101*(6), 310–318.

Hofer, B. K. (2000). Dimensionality and disciplinary differences in personal epistemology. *Contemporary Educational Psychology, 25*, 378–405.

Hofer, B. K., & Pintrich, P. R. (1997). The development of epistemological theories: beliefs about knowledge and knowing and their relation to learning. *Review of Educational Research, 67*(1), 88–140.

Hoyle, R. H. (1995). The structural equation modeling approach: basic concepts and fundamental issues. In R. H. Hoyle (Ed.), *Structural equation modeling: concepts, issues, and applications* (pp. 1–15). Thousand Oaks: Sage.

Hu, L., & Bentler, P. M. (1999). Cutoff criteria for fit indexes in covariance structure analysis: conventional criteria versus new alternatives. *Structural Equation Modeling: A Multidisciplinary Journal, 6*(1), 1–55.

IBM Corporation. (2013). *IBM SPSS AMOS, Version 22.0*. Armonk, NY: IBM Corporation.

Joreskog, K. G. (1993). Testing structural equation models. In K. A. Bollen & J. S. Long (Eds.), *Testing structural equation models* (pp. 294–316). Newbury Park: Sage.

Kline, R. B. (1998). *Principles and practice of structural equation modeling*. New York: The Guilford Press.

Kline, R. B. (2011). *Principles and practice of structural equation modeling* (3rd ed.). New York: The Guilford Press.

Madison, B. L., & Steen, L. A. (2003). *Quantitative literacy: why numeracy matters for schools and colleges*. Princeton: National Council on Education and the Disciplines. Retrieved from: http://www.maa.org/external_archive/QL/qltoc.html.

Marsh, H. W., Hau, K., & Wen, Z. (2004). In search of golden rules: comment on hypothesis-testing approaches to setting cutoff values for fit indexes and dangers in overgeneralizing Hu and Bentler's (1999) findings. *Structural Equation Modeling: A Multidisciplinary Journal, 11*(3), 320–341.

McCaffrey, D. F., Hamilton, L. S., Stecher, B. M., Klein, S. P., Buglari, D., & Robyn, A. (2001). Interactions among instructional practices, curriculum, and student achievement: the case of standards-based high school mathematics. *Journal for Research in Mathematics Education, 32*(5), 493–517.

Mokros, J. (2003). Learning to reason numerically: the impact of *Investigations*. In S. L. Senk & D. R. Thompson (Eds.), *Standards-based school mathematics curricula: what are they? What do students learn?* (pp. 109–131). Mahwah: Lawrence Erlbaum Associates.

Mullis, I. V. S., Martin, M. O., Beaton, A. E., Gonzalez, E. J., Kelly, D. L., & Smith, T. A. (1998). *Mathematics and science achievement in the final year of secondary school: IEA's Third International Mathematics and Science Study (TIMSS)*. Chestnut Hill, MA: Boston College.

National Commission on Excellence in Education. (1983). *A nation at risk: the imperative for education reform*. Washington: US Department of Education.

National Council of Teacher of Mathematics. (1989). *Curriculum and evaluation standards for school mathematics*. Reston: NCTM.

National Council of Teachers of Mathematics. (2000). *Principles and standards for school mathematics*. Reston: NCTM.

National Council of Teachers of Mathematics. (2006). *Curriculum focal points for prekindergarten through grade 8 mathematics: a quest for coherence*. Reston: NCTM.

National Governors Association Center for Best Practices, Council of Chief State School Officers. (2010). *Common core state standards (mathematics)*. Washington: NGA Center, CCSSO.

National Research Council. (1989). *Everybody counts: a report to the nation on the future of mathematics education*. Washington: National Academy Press.

Organisation for Economic Cooperation and Development (OECD). (2000). *Measuring student knowledge and skills. The PISA 2000 measurement of reading, mathematical and scientific literacy*. Paris: OECD.

Orpwood, G., & Garden, R. A. (1998). *Assessing mathematics and science literacy*. Vancouver: Pacific Educational Press.

Post, T. R., Harwell, M. R., Davis, J. D., Maeda, Y., Cutler, A., Andersen, E., et al. (2008). *Standards*-based mathematics curricula and middle-grades students' performance on standardized achievement tests. *Journal for Research in Mathematics Education, 39*(2), 184–212.

Reys, R., Reys, B., Lapan, R., Holliday, G., & Wasman, D. (2003). Assessing the impact of standards-based middle grades mathematics curriculum materials on student achievement. *Journal for Research in Mathematics Education., 34*(1), 74–95.

Riordan, J. E., & Noyce, P. E. (2001). The impact of two *Standards*-based mathematics curricula on student achievement in Massachusetts. *Journal for Research in Mathematics Education, 32*(4), 368–398.

Russell, S. J., Tierney, C., Mokros, J., & Economopoulos, K. (2004). *Investigations in number, data, and space*. Glenview: Scott Foresman.

Senk, S. L., & Thompson, D. R. (Eds.). (2003). *Standards-based school mathematics curricula: what are they? What do students learn?* Mahwah: Lawrence Erlbaum Associates.

Sloane, F. C. (2008). Randomized trials in mathematics education: recalibrating the proposed high watermark. *Educational Researcher, 37*(9), 624–630.

Steen, L. A. (Ed.). (1990). *On the shoulders of giants: new approaches to numeracy*. Washington: National Academy Press.

Steen, L. A. (1997). Preface: the new literacy. In L. A. Steen (Ed.), *Why numbers count: quantitative literacy for tomorrow's America (pp. xv-xxviii)*. New York: College Entrance Examination Board.

Steen, L. A. (1999). Numeracy: the new literacy for a data-drenched society. *Educational Leadership, 57*(2), 8–13.

Steen, L. A. (Ed.). (2001). *Mathematics and democracy: the case for quantitative literacy*. United States: The Woodrow Wilson National Fellowship Foundation.

Steen, L. A. (2004). *Achieving quantitative literacy: an urgent challenge for higher education*. Washington: Mathematical Association of America.

Thompson, D. R., & Senk, S. L. (2001). The effects of curriculum on achievement in second-year algebra: the example of the University of Chicago school mathematic project. *Journal for Research in Mathematics Education, 32*(1), 58–84.

Westbury, I., & Thalathoti, V. V. (1989). *United States—population B*. Urbana: The Board of Trustees of the University of Illinois.

Wiley, D. E., & Resnick, L. (1997). *The new standards reference examination standards-referenced scoring system (CSE Technical Report 470)*. Los Angeles: National Center for Research on Evaluation, Standards, and Student Testing (CRESST). Available online: http://www.cse.ucla.edu/products/Reports/TECH470.pdf.

Wilkins, J. L. M. (in press). An assessment of the quantitative literacy of undergraduate students. *Journal of Experimental Education*.

Wilkins, J. L. M. (2010). Modeling quantitative literacy. *Educational and Psychological Measurement, 70*(2), 267–290.

Wilkins, J. L. M. (2004a). *Elementary Mathematics Attitude Survey (EMAS)*. Blacksburg, VA: Virginia Tech.

Wilkins, J. L. M. (2004b). Mathematics and science self-concept: An international investigation. *Journal of Experimental Education, 72*(4), 331–346.

Wilkins, J. L. M. (2000). Preparing for the 21st century: The status of quantitative literacy in the United States. *School Science and Mathematics, 100*(8), 405–418.

11

Mathematical practices and mathematical modes of enquiry: same or different?

Hamsa Venkat[1,2]

Abstract

Background: In this paper, I share a case study of a teacher's work on mathematics tasks in the context of a 'mathematics for teaching' course aiming to develop mathematical content understandings and mathematical practices among primary teachers in one South African province. The course was developed in a national context of concerns about the nature and levels of primary teachers' mathematical knowledge. Theories viewing mathematical practices as fundamental, contrasted with those that view mathematical practices and mathematical content in more separate and 'to be integrated' ways, are used to frame the analysis and critically reflect on the findings.

Results: Data from this teacher's pre-test and selected course assessments and interactions suggest that while he was able to develop some aspects of the mathematical practices described in the literature, his overall orientation remained attuned to memorization and recall. Findings also pointed to an ongoing reliance on external validation of the 'correctness' of his answers.

Conclusions: The data suggest that the presence of elements of mathematical practices cannot be viewed as equivalent to the presence of mathematical modes of enquiry. The analysis presented in this paper suggests that while elements of mathematical practices can be developed, moving towards an encompassing orientation to mathematical modes of enquiry may require more central focus on problem-solving approaches to achieve a change in orientation.

Keywords: Mathematical practices; Mathematical modes of enquiry; South Africa; CCSM; Primary mathematics

Background

A significant body of writing in mathematics education points to the importance of mathematical processes/practices within mathematical working. Writing focused on the nature of mathematics has noted its 'autopoeitic' form, in that mathematics produces the objects it discusses, rather than describing objects or phenomena that exist externally in the physical world (Sfard 2008; Maturana and Varela 1980). A consequence of this view of the nature of mathematics is that the production of mathematical objects in non-mathematical ways produces a discourse that fundamentally disrupts the nature of mathematics as a discipline.

So what are considered to be mathematical practices? These practices have been described in a number of ways at more general and specific levels. The National Council of Teachers of Mathematics (NCTM), for example, described general mathematical processes in terms of representing, problem-solving, reasoning, connecting, communicating - with all of these acting as means of mathematizing (NCTM 2000). More specific descriptions of mathematical practices include attention to, e.g., ordering, structuring, reversing, abstracting, and generalizing (Mason et al. 1982).

In recent years, there has been an overt emphasis on incorporating attention to mathematical practices alongside content in many curricula, (e.g., NCTM 2000 in the United States). The ongoing emphases on coverage and accountability, though, continue to be reflected in concerns that mathematics is presented as its content-based 'products' rather than in terms of its processes leading to products.

In the South African context of this paper, post-apartheid curricula that placed greater emphases on mathematical practices have given way to a reversal back

Correspondence: hamsa.venkatakrishnan@wits.ac.za
[1]Wits School of Education, University of the Witwatersrand, Johannesburg, South Africa
[2]Wits School of Education, University of the Witwatersrand, Johannesburg, South Africa and Jönköping University, Jönköping, Sweden

to more traditional content specifications. A key driver for this reversal was extensive evidence of gaps in teachers' content knowledge which, in the terrain of the less explicitly specified and process-orientated versions of curricula, contributed to pedagogies that were criticized as mathematically hollow. This evidence on teachers' mathematical content knowledge, much of it focused on primary level mathematics, suggests gaps at or close to the level at which they are teaching (Carnoy et al. 2008; Taylor 2011). There is evidence too, though, of pedagogic shortcomings at the level of mathematical practices rather than at the level of content (Venkat 2013). These concerns are set within broad national and international acknowledgement that teachers are reproducing trained ways of working, with the added awareness in South Africa of a history of inequitable and disrupted access to education for the majority of teachers currently in the system.

In exploring mathematics teacher learning for teaching, Watson and Barton (2011) suggest a 'fundamental' view of mathematical practices in which 'mathematical modes of enquiry' are central:

> 'Knowing mathematics means being able to use mathematical concepts mathematically: the two cannot be separated'. (p. 66)

This fundamental view is contrasted in this paper with views that identify content and practices in what I describe as more 'separate but to be integrated' ways.

Within our work in the Johannesburg-based Wits Maths Connect-Primary (WMC-P) research and development project, we developed a 'primary mathematics knowledge for teaching' course that incorporated attention to mathematical practices within a structure that was delineated on the basis of broad content areas. The course consisted of 16 contact days spaced across the school year in 2-day blocks, with each block focused on a content area - e.g., numbers and number system, additive relations, multiplicative relations, etc. Our attention to mathematical practices was embedded within an overt framework based on developing teachers' awareness and explanations in relation to mathematical content areas, reflecting more the 'separate but integrated' position.

Work with teachers across three cohorts (2012-14) has indicated broad successes at the level of content knowledge gains (based on pre- and post-test results with each cohort) and in relation to some of the mathematical practices referred to above (based on course task assessments that placed emphasis on problem-solving through connecting, representing, communicating, and explaining). The successes were not universal though and led to the question driving this paper: the extent to which separate but integrated views of mathematical practices and content can be considered as consistent with or equivalent to the notion of mathematical modes of enquiry. This issue is explored through a focus on a teacher (Christopher, pseudonym) whose interactions and test performance indicated moves towards aspects of some mathematical practices but set within an overarching orientation that remained at some distance from mathematical modes of enquiry. Through looking at some of Christopher's task responses and interactions, I analyze instances of both his use and disruption of mathematical practices. I suggest that underlying the somewhat contradictory nature of his working is a failure, on our part, in shifting Christopher's overarching orientation to mathematics towards one that could work mathematically with mathematical objects. Rather, he maintained an orientation to mathematics that was about remembering and retrieving facts and processes, even while showing some evidence of being able to engage in reasoning and problem-solving activities.

Christopher's story takes current understandings of the development of mathematical practices in pedagogy forward in two ways. Firstly, it adds to the relatively limited body of knowledge that has explored shortcomings relating to mathematical practices within pedagogy providing exemplifications of how these limitations play out. Secondly, it allows for a critical consideration of different theorizations of mathematical practices in relation to mathematical content. Christopher's story suggests that our more 'separate and integrative' presentation of mathematical content and practices was not sufficient for eliciting broad-ranging moves towards mathematical modes of enquiry within the time frames that we had available.

Christopher's story is shared through the following structure: the paper begins with a literature review outlining the nature of mathematical practices and reasons for their advocacy. South African data that suggest some distance from mathematical practices, as vehicles for carrying and producing mathematical objects, are then shared. The data sources and case study methodology drawn on for sharing Christopher's story are detailed and followed by a section where his responses on key tasks and accompanying interactions are presented and analyzed. I conclude the paper by considering what this analysis suggests for ways of thinking about developing mathematical practices.

Mathematical practices - a literature review

Attention to mathematical practices continues to get wide attention in the international mathematics education literature. Writing emanating from the United States has been particularly influential in this regard. The current 'common core standards for mathematics' (CCSM) (Common Core State Standards Initiative 2010) include a set of 'Standards for Mathematical Practices'. This set, drawing from the NCTM list stated earlier and Kilpatrick et al. (2001) 'strands of mathematical proficiency', contains the following features:

- Make sense of problems and persevere in solving them
- Reason abstractly and quantitatively
- Construct viable arguments and critique the reasoning of others
- Model with mathematics
- Use appropriate tools strategically
- Attend to precision
- Look for and make use of structure
- Look for and express regularity in repeated reasoning (pp. 6 to 8)

Each of these practices has an extensive associated literature base. In this overview, I provide some detail on aspects of the practices that are relevant to issues that have been raised in the South African teaching landscape (and thus to our work within the course) and to the empirical data that follows.

Problem-solving

Polya's (1962) early but seminal work on problem-solving continues to be widely cited in the literature. Polya emphasized the importance of starting with situations that provide an authentic problem - a problem for which solution procedures are not known at the outset and have to be developed. The CCSM document reflects this notion, describing sense-making/problem-solving proficiency in terms of understanding problem situations in terms of 'givens, constraints, relationships, and goals' (p. 6), with this understanding, feeding in to the formulation of possible solution pathways.

Abstract/quantitative reasoning

Mason has written extensively about the nature of abstract reasoning and abstraction within mathematical working (e.g., Mason 1989). Working with abstract reasoning as a follow-up to generalizing activity, Mason describes these two practices as collectively representing a move from 'manipulating objects (physical, pictorial, symbolic, mental) to expressing properties or features of those objects in ways that can form the basis for further manipulations' (p. 3). Sfard's (2008) notion of mathematics developing through the production of 'discursive layers' provides a more condensed version of these processes. Schifter (2011) explains her emphasis on teaching driven towards helping children to reason quantitatively through considering the effects of operations on numbers, rather than practicing operational procedures through lists of calculations. Across this writing is a view of mathematical learning guided by the need to move beyond getting the answer to the immediate problem, to being able to abstract structural similarities between situations that allow for the generation of increasingly powerful, generalized problem-solving techniques.

Constructing viable arguments

The need to construct viable arguments draws from Kilpatrick et al. (2001) 'adaptive reasoning' strand. It involves developing the capacity to build networks of logical statements - argumentation chains with awareness of the warrants that underlie them. Over time, and through experience of the breadth and boundaries of associated example spaces, this standard also calls for awareness of the 'domains to which an argument applies'. Yackel (2001) notes that within teaching for the development of justification and argumentation practices:

> 'initially children had to learn that their explanations and justifications needed a mathematical, rather than a social, basis'. (p. 14)

Kazemi and Stipek (2001) contrast teachers' orchestration of 'mathematical arguments' with 'procedural descriptions', associating the former with classrooms characterized by a 'high conceptual press' and the latter with 'low conceptual press'.

Mathematical modeling

A key antecedent for emphasis on mathematical modeling is the Dutch work on 'Realistic Mathematics Education' (RME). A central assumption within RME is that mathematics emerges, or comes to be reinvented, through mathematization activity that seeks to understand and organize phenomena (Freudenthal 1983). Interpreting results in relation to the situation also features within this standard.

Mathematical structure and regularity

Attunement to noticing patterns and structure is a key part of the 'looking for structure' strand. Attention to juxtaposing examples in ways that draw attention to variations, invariances, and connections between examples has been argued as one way to develop this attunement (Watson and Mason 2006). Careful sequencing can draw attention to ideas like 'doing and undoing' and the regularities within sets of related examples in ways that draw attention to underlying mathematical structure.

Is attention to mathematical practices necessary?

At one level, the thrust of much of the work on mathematical practices appears to state the obvious, like Watson and Barton's (2011) emphasis on using 'mathematical concepts mathematically'. This view fails however to explain the ongoing attention to mathematical practices in the literature. In order to understand this emphasis, we need to seek out the phenomena within mathematics teaching and learning that have motivated these foci. To do this, I return to the writings mentioned above to note the shortcomings that their attention to mathematical practices seeks to address. This is followed by an outline of South African evidence on mathematics teaching and learning related to mathematical practices that led to the choice to orient our primary mathematics knowledge for teaching course in particular ways.

Polya's interest in problem-solving heuristics was driven by observations of the absence in much of mathematics teaching of genuine problems - problems set, not with the intention of repeatedly practicing a previously taught procedure, but instead, problems for which a solution path is not known:

> 'to have a problem means: to search consciously for some action appropriate to attain a clearly conceived, but not immediately attainable aim. To solve the problem means to find such action'. (p. 117)

Mason (1989) highlights the difficulties that students often have with abstracting and generalizing in mathematics. He speculates that these difficulties may relate to the frequent presentation in mathematics lessons of abstract forms, divorced from the generalizing and abstracting activities that have produced them: 'there is a huge difference between expressing your own generality and doing someone else's algebra' (p. 3). Freudenthal (1973) takes this issue as the central pedagogic problem of 'anti-didactical inversion' wherein 'ready made' models that have emerged from the 'crystallized' products of prior mathematical activity are presented to children without giving them any access to the problems that produced them, nor to the contours of the models and the purposes that they are useful for. The need for a mathematical working guided by mathematizing activity is thus foregrounded in this literature.

Moving beyond generalizations and models more broadly into mathematical learning, Vinner (1997), p. 101 contrasts 'conceptual' and 'analytical' behaviors with 'pseudo-conceptual' and 'pseudo-analytical' behaviors:

> 'In mental processes that produce conceptual behaviors, words are associated with ideas, whereas in mental processes that produce pseudo-conceptual behaviors, words are associated with words; ideas are not involved'.

Vinner is careful to distinguish between pseudo-conceptual modes of thinking and misconceptions, noting that the latter have definite cognitive involvement while the former are characterized by the lack of cognitive involvement. He argues that pseudo-analytical ways of working primarily involve reactions to stimuli or cues, rather than cognitive engagement (Vinner 1997, p. 121). Of interest in relation to the analysis that I present later is Vinner's acknowledgement that pseudo-conceptual behavior still involves attention to similarities between situation and model and between different task situations and their associated procedures. The problem is that these practices play out in ways that ignore logical reasoning chains or violate definitions. Superficial similarities, rather than similarities that are critical features of the topic or concept being handled, are instead noticed and followed up.

This brief overview highlights that the notion of working mathematically with mathematics, far from being an underpinning fundamental of school mathematical activity, is considered rather rare. A key outcome of Vinner's pseudo-conceptual orientations to mathematics is a heavy reliance on memorizing associations between perceptual features of situations and use of specific and localized procedural responses.

South African evidence on primary mathematics teaching

The South African landscape reflects the concerns identified above, sometimes in quite extreme forms. The terrain is marked by low performance in mathematics at all levels of schooling. In primary mathematics, substantial gaps between the advocated curriculum and attainment of large numbers of children are apparent by the end of grade 3 (DBE 2013). As noted already, larger scale studies have pointed to serious gaps at the level of teachers' mathematical content knowledge, with some of these studies showing gaps at or very close to the levels at which these teachers are teaching (Taylor 2011; Carnoy et al. 2008). Highly procedural orientations to teaching with lack of incorporation of problem-solving tasks have also been noted in teaching in the intermediate grades (grades 4 to 6) (Ally and Christiansen 2013; Sorto and Sapire 2011).

Smaller scale qualitative studies have investigated the nature of pedagogy. Hoadley (2007), using sociological lenses, drew attention to classrooms in which no criteria for the appropriateness of answers were provided. Adler and Venkat's studies have focused attention on the teachers' explanations, set within what they have termed teachers' 'Mathematical discourse in instruction' (MDI). While some of their episodes indicate breakdowns between tasks and representations (Venkat and Adler 2012), Adler and Venkat (2014) also draw attention to narratives that reflect 'ritualized' activity (drawing on Sfard 2008) in which:

> 'Talk is about actions on discrete symbol parts, and these processes are asserted, with substantiation that relies on perceptual features'. (p. 144)

Across Hoadley's work and Adler and Venkat's papers, we see patterns of working in which mathematics is often produced and proceeds in the absence of mathematical argumentation. This teaching embodies many of Vinner's (1997) characterizations of pseudo-conceptual behavior, and Adler and Venkat (2014) note that such behaviors within learning reflect what is enacted in teaching:

> 'what is made available to learn through the teacher's MDI, and the substantiating narratives at work, relies on memory and visual cues'. (p. 144)

Venkat (2013) identifies instances where correct answers are produced in classroom teaching but in ways that disrupt notions of mathematical practices leading to the production of mathematical outcomes and objects. Her illustrative examples indicate a lack of attunement to how givens and unknowns are configured within problem-solving practices. Verificational processes occur in the absence of a preceding derivational process. Possibilities for students to independently produce correct answers to similar questions are severely disrupted here, with trial-and-error guessing representing the only option for pupils who do not know the answer at the outset.

Theorizing integrative views of mathematical practices

In the opening section, I contrasted a 'fundamental' view of mathematical practices with a 'separate but to be integrated' view of mathematical content and practices. The CCSM, in their separate listing of content and practice standards, tend to fall into the latter category. Further supporting this position is that while the CCSM document stresses the need to connect practice and content standards within teaching (p. 8), it suggests also that content standards containing the word 'understand' provide particularly fertile ground for such integration. This points to a more selective integration than the position proposed by Watson and Barton (2011), who offer a more fundamentally integrative view, with particular interests in mathematics teacher knowledge and education. They emphasize that mathematics teaching activity should center around enacting mathematics and that 'mathematical modes of enquiry' are central to this enactment. A consequence of this orientation for them is that discussions about what teachers of mathematics know cannot be divorced from the ways in which they know mathematics:

> 'It is not just a question of what teachers know, but how they know it, how they are aware of it, how they use it and how they exemplify it'. (p. 67)

Differences in the descriptions of mathematical practices in the 'separate but integrated' view and the 'mathematical modes of enquiry' view point to subtle differences in how mathematical working is conceptualized. In the CCSM view, mathematical practices are viewed as an outcome of well-connected understanding of content (p. 8). Mathematical modes of enquiry, in contrast, tend to point to mathematical practices as fundamental to developing mathematical understanding.

It could be argued that there is not really a distinction here between the more separate integrative (CCSM) and more fundamental (Watson and Barton) views; rather, the issues and gaps seen in mathematics teaching and learning lead to the need to make visible the mathematical practices that seem to 'fall out' of enactments of mathematics in classrooms. Listing practices separately from content, as in the CCSM formulation, provides one way of highlighting mathematical practices and drawing attention to their nature and range. Watson and Barton (ibid), however, tend to disagree with this view, arguing that curriculum lists are: 'hypothetical until mathematical modes of seeking, using, and exemplifying understanding are understood' (p. 66). Schoenfeld's (1987) attention to mathematical problem-solving echoes the fundamental view, with mathematical enactment, in his view, connected to developing capacities that link discourses, activities, and identities within a mathematical culture wherein mathematics functions as 'the medium of exchange' (p. 213).

In the next section, the teacher development course model is outlined and critically considered in terms of its orientation towards mathematical practices.

The course model and orientation

The South African evidence on content knowledge gaps and the nature of primary mathematics classroom teaching led to our development of a 'primary mathematics knowledge for teaching' course. As noted already, each 2-day block across the 16 contact days was focused on a content domain, with mathematics homework and classroom teaching tasks completed between contact sessions. While course pre- and post-test assessments featured items drawn from prior studies focused on conceptual understanding of key mathematical ideas, in-course assessments incorporated attention to constructing and communicating mathematical arguments within problem-solving and using emergent representations to model situations in ways that would allow for purposive selections of operations, rather than guessing or recalling the operations required. These latter tasks reflected multiple elements of the mathematical practices highlighted in the literature section above.

I noted in the introductory sections that gains at the level of content knowledge and mathematical practices were seen in our assessments across three cycles of the course (2012-14). Teacher evaluations of the course suggested awareness of better understandings of content and growing awareness of the need for at least some of the mathematical practices noted in the literature review above. Learning related to explaining 'why' steps work was one of the most common comments on teacher feedback, alongside comments on learning related to specific content/representations/procedures. This feedback suggested some successes in making mathematical practices 'visible' in the course alongside mathematical content, while reflecting also the 'separate and integrative' position seen in the CCSM, rather than Watson and Barton's fundamental position on mathematical modes of enquiry.

Methods

A case study design is used in this paper. The case in focus relates to excerpts of mathematical working and accompanying talk on tasks completed by a teacher, Christopher, who was a course participant in 2013. The case is framed thus because the ways in which mathematical practices and/or mathematical modes of enquiry played out within this dataset was the 'phenomenon ... in a bounded context' (Miles and Huberman 1994, p. 25) that I was interested in. Christopher was not teaching mathematics in school in 2013 but was interested in doing so. Selected excerpts of his work from across the year and my fieldnote records of his commentaries and our interactions around this work are drawn on within the analysis. Christopher was an enthusiastic and vocal participant in our course sessions and was quickly willing to admit that while he often knew what to do, he frequently did not have any reasons for why he was performing the selected sequence of steps - redolent of Skemp's (1976) 'instrumental' understanding. Christopher's enthusiastic participation means that we have more evidence from him in terms of verbal commentary and interaction around his work than for most of the other teachers on the course, leading to my selection of him as a particularly illustrative or 'telling' case (Mitchell 1984). However, comments from other teachers suggest that the phenomena that he provided a case of - the ability to produce and expand a repertoire related to some mathematical practices without an overall shift in orientation towards mathematical modes of enquiry - were more widespread.

Christopher was teaching social science, natural science, and technology in grades 6 and 7 in a suburban primary school in Johannesburg. Christopher told us that he came on to the course because he was interested in teaching mathematics but had not done so previously. His academic background (a BA Honours degree in Education) represented a higher level of education than many of his peers, and his pre- and post-test scores were above the cohort's mean scores in both tests.

The data I draw on to analyze Christopher's mathematical working are drawn from three points in the year. The first excerpt of his working is on an item in the pre-test. The second excerpt, drawing on his workings and his commentary and interactions on this working, occurred halfway through the course in the context of an assessment focused on multiplying decimals. The third excerpt is also located in his working and related commentary (recreated from my fieldnotes in this case) and is drawn from an additional voluntary revision session that we offered at the end of the year before the final post-test where participants were asked to bring problems that they had tried and were having difficulty with. Broader background data on Christopher's performance are drawn from the datasets that we keep for all the teachers detailing their performance across all course tasks. These data are selected because they are usefully illustrative of 'recurring regularities' (Guba 1978, p. 53) in Christopher's responses at points when he was not completely certain of the procedure being worked with. As noted already, sporadic responses from other teachers across all three years indicate that presences of aspects of mathematical practices allied with absences in relation to an overarching orientation to mathematical modes of enquiry were more broadly prevalent.

My analysis of this data links to interpreting presences and absences in relation to the literature-based identification of markers of mathematical practices overviewed earlier. Ethical clearances for data collection, analysis and anonymized reporting in the course were granted by the university and the provincial education department, with informed consents for use of course-related data for research purposes granted by participating teachers.

Results and discussion

Excerpt 1

While Christopher's performance on the pre-test indicated that he was well above the group mean in terms of his mathematical content knowledge, his ways of working indicated an orientation that swung towards operational techniques more often than towards structure or generality. For example, three items on the pre-test, shown in Table 1, were focused on using rounding to estimate answers to decimal multiplication and division calculations:

Christopher had circled the correct answer in all three cases. His work on these three problems (scribbled on a rough piece of paper inside his test script) is shown in Figure 1.

Table 1 Pre-test items

Circle the number that is nearest in size to the answer (do not work out the answer)							
2.9 × 7	0.002	0.02	0.2	2	20	200	2000
0.29 × 7.1	0.002	0.02	0.2	2	20	200	2000
59 ÷ 190	0.003	0.03	0.3	3	30	300	3000

This work shows that for questions 1 and 2, in contradiction to the instruction, Christopher calculated actual answers using traditional column multiplication methods (with an error in the second calculation) and then rounded. The work seen on the third problem is interesting because Christopher tried two related problems (190 ÷ 59 and 590 ÷ 190) and used repeated addition to get 3 as the rough answer for both of these problems. The correct approximate answer (0.3) is written below but whether this was arrived at through an awareness of reciprocal or scaling down relationships, or simply by guessing, is not known.

Part of the complexity of Christopher's orientation is that his work indicates that he has at least some of the quantitative reasoning skills needed to work out the answers to the first two problems by rounding (e.g., he is able to round his answer of 20.3 correctly to 20). The issue here is not that he does not know how to round off to the nearest whole number. Instead, it would appear that the presence of a problem in mathematics is viewed as a trigger for a calculation, regardless of an instruction that calls for a solution through quantitative reasoning. The instruction is returned to after the exact answer has been calculated. This routine is followed in the second example as well, where, in spite of a calculation error, his answer still takes him to 2 as the nearest answer. Thus, while relevant reasoning practices are sporadically evident here relating to rounding and possibly scaling up and reversing downwards, these are not set holistically within either the quantitative reasoning (Schifter 2011) or the strategic working (Kilpatrick et al. 2001) that are described as part of the mathematical practices canon or mathematical modes of enquiry frame.

In Christopher's response to the third question, his selection of two associated, simpler calculations suggests some awareness of quantitative relations. I cannot tell from the marks on the paper whether Christopher used scaling down to get from 3 to 0.3, mirroring the relationship between 590 and 59. What we can see is that this technique was not brought into play in question 2, where it could also have been applied. In combination, a highly localized approach to techniques is seen and further, thinking about quantitative relations appears to come into play only when a procedure is not immediately at hand, pointing to a prioritization of content and techniques over a more fundamental integration of mathematical modes of enquiry. Thus, the evidence taken together indicates a lack of consistent attunement to reasoning quantitatively, rather than an inability to do so.

Excerpt 2a

The second excerpt relates to Christopher's responses and interactions on a decimal multiplication task halfway through the course. The course was structured such that the topic in focus in each 2-day block had a short assessment associated with it in the following 2-day block. Days 5 and 6 had been focused on multiplication and division. Various models for representing multiplication and division situations had been discussed during the 2 days, with 'area' models of multiplication developed out of more basic array models in the context of early multiplication. The assessment on day 8 included the question shown in Figure 2.

Christopher's solutions to this particular set of problems are shown in Figure 3. This work followed a word problem asking for the area of a rectangular field

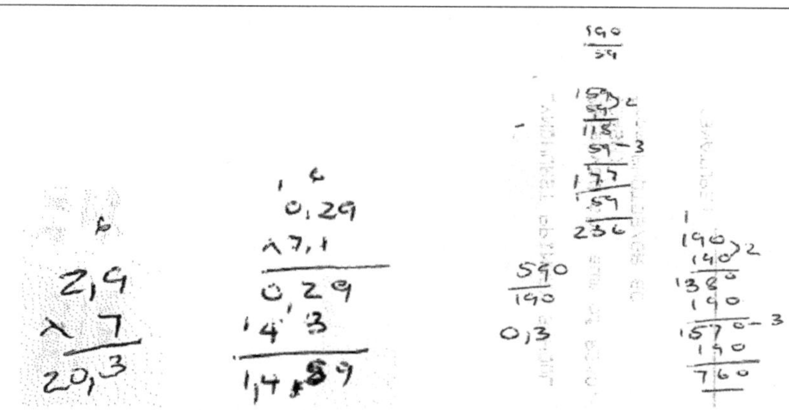

Figure 1 Christopher's working on Table1 pre-test items.

involving two integer value dimensions. Christopher had calculated the answer to this first problem correctly using a traditional column algorithm method.

Discussion 2a

We see here and following from the work seen above in the pre-test that Christopher appears to have difficulty with multi-digit long multiplication involving decimal numbers. The consistency in his problem setup indicates fragments of remembered rules - 'the decimal point has to line up', 'move a column across each time you deal with a new partial product', and 'the number of digits after the decimal point is the sum of the number of digits after the decimal point in the numbers being multiplied'. However, 'carrying' within the partial products appears haphazard - sometimes applied and other times missed. As in his pre-test working, his exact answer (incorrect) is rounded for the estimate, in spite of the repeated addition of 13 three times alongside the calculation.

Beneath the request for an area method, there is an attempt at some elements of the 'form' that accompanies area models - a grid that looks like a table. However, the partitioning of number that can be used within area-based models is absent, and instead, his own long multiplication column model is placed within the grid. Alongside this diagram, the calculation above is repeated with the same incorrect answer. Here, the association of the area model with the visual grid format is evident and points to the pseudo-conceptual behaviors described by Vinner (1997).

Excerpt 2b

In the course, we follow interim assessments with a subsequent feedback session where common errors, misconceptions, or shortcomings are discussed. A follow-up repeat opportunity to do a similar task is offered. In Christopher's case, the repeat assessment was on day 9 of the course (about a month after the earlier task). The repeat assessment task involved calculating the area of a strip of field 42.5 m long and 2.15 m wide. While completing this task, Christopher called me over. He asked me to look at his written script - which, at this point, contained the working shown in Figure 4.

In his working, two models had been juxtaposed alongside each other - the area model on the left and a column algorithm model placed within a place value frame. The answer for his area model working was written in the middle of the page (91.375 m^2). His answer for the column model working was 9,137.50. Christopher had noticed that the two answers were different and was perturbed enough to call me over. Our conversation proceeded thus:

> Hamsa: Yes?
> Christopher: There's a problem here.
> Hamsa: Oh, what?
> Christopher: See this, there are two different answers.
> Hamsa: Yes, I see. Is that a problem?
> Christopher: Yes, they should be the same.
> Hamsa: Ok. And they are not. So is one of them right and not the other?
> Christopher: Yes, but I don't know which.
> Hamsa: So how could you decide?
> Christopher: I don't know. I've checked all the numbers on both sides. They are right.
> Hamsa: So if we look at the question, roughly how big do you think that field should be? Do you think you could use that to help you decide?

I left Christopher at that point to carry on. In the version we took in, Christopher had added the line shown in Figure 5 to his working:

Discussion 2b

Several aspects of Christopher's work are of interest here. The first point is that he has expanded his representational repertoire to include the area model for the first time voluntarily in an assessment and used this model to calculate the correct answer. His writing above the models indicates also that he is strategically aware of the extent of scaling up required to move from 42.5 to

2	Ntombi works out the answer to 13,2 × 3,16 as follows: 132 316 × 792 132 396 1320 Ntombi says that the answer is 1,320	
	What should Ntombi's answer be roughly? Use rounding to estimate this answer.	Use the area method to find the exact answer.

Figure 2 Day 8 assessment question.

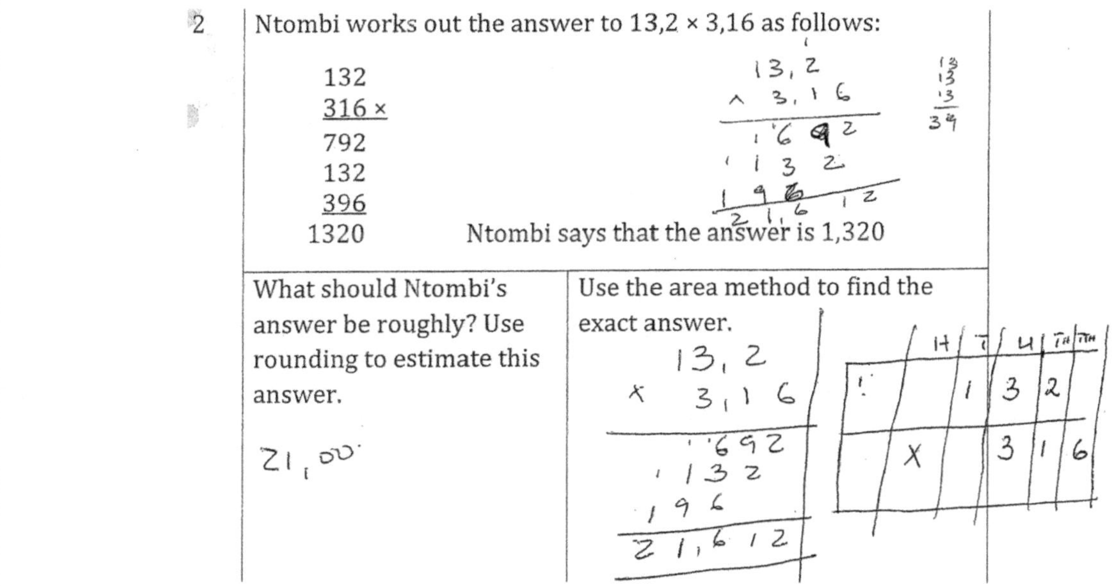

Figure 3 Christopher's written response to day 8 assessment question.

425 and from 2.15 to 215, i.e., to produce a related integer value, with the reverse scaling down applied appropriately to the answer at the end. Strategic selections within problem-solving and awareness of how to reverse operational effects - highlighted as important aspects of mathematical thinking (Mason et al. 1982) - both feature prominently within descriptions of mathematical practices.

However, Christopher appears to remain uncertain about this new method and repeats the calculation in column form. In placing the problem in a place value grid, he adds a '0' onto 42.5 to make 42.50 in the calculation. The carrying is error free here within all the partial products, but the decimal point is re-inserted in the wrong position in the bottom line. On completion, Christopher's appeal to me for resolution coupled with the seeming absence of mathematical resources for dealing with two inconsistent answers indicates a lack of development of the sociomathematical norms (Yackel 2001) described as critical to mathematical enquiry. When a 'path' is suggested though, he is able to enact the calculation required with the rounded numbers and, on the basis of this, decides that his area model answer is the correct one. There is no mathematical curiosity though, to understand why or where the second method went wrong. Schoenfeld (1987) has noted that students holding beliefs about mathematics as devoid of meaning-making frequently write contradictory statements in sequence. Christopher interprets the difference between the two answers as a problem. However, his resolution

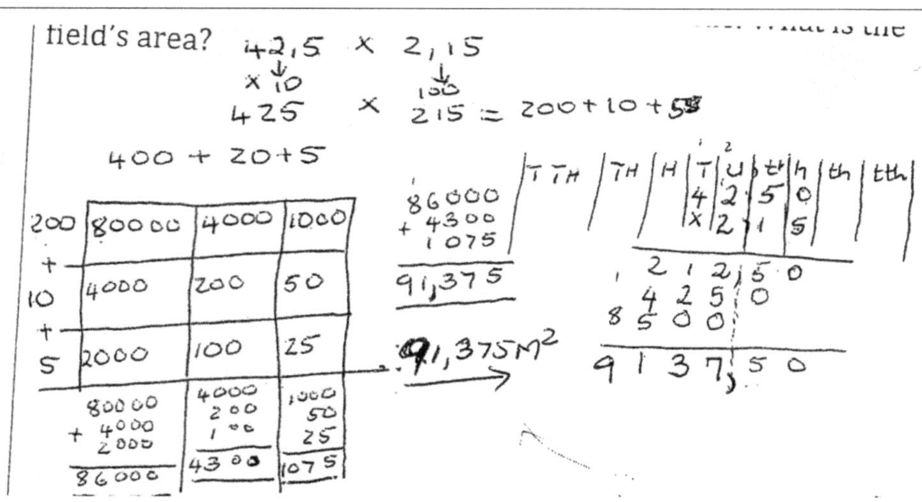

Figure 4 Day 9 repeat assessment working.

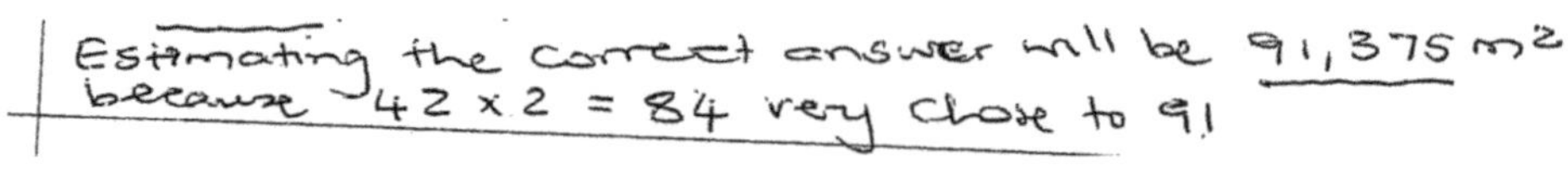

Figure 5 Added working.

remained reliant on external direction and ended with a decision on which answer was correct, without wanting to find out what was wrong with the rejected answer. Given the importance accorded to dealing with learner errors within the mathematics teacher knowledge literature (Ball et al. 2005), Christopher's lack of interest in probing his own mathematical error is particularly problematic. The disposition to view mathematics as reasonable is notably absent here, pointing to lack of shift in some aspects of mathematical practices in the midst of evidence of other elements.

Excerpt 3

The next excerpt is drawn from an optional additional revision session held towards the end of the year in early October, where teachers were invited to bring tasks that they had tried but were having difficulty with. One problem that some teachers asked for help with was the 'Hi-fives' task (Beckmann 2011) asking for the number of hi-fives needed between a group of 20 people if each one hi-fived everyone else. Our support consisted of prompts based on many of the problem-solving heuristics that Mason et al. (1982) and Schoenfeld (1985) have suggested:

> Hamsa: 20 is quite a large number of people to work. Can we think about the situation with a smaller number of people to make it more manageable?

'Four people' was suggested. Four participants came up and acted the problem out, the first person hi-fiving the other three, the next hi-fiving the two that she has not hi-fived, and so on. We then 're-played' the actions with a mathematical representation for the number of hi-fives. The group told me that the total would be:

$$3 + 2 + 1 + 0 = \text{total number of hi-fives}$$

They calculated this total by adding. I asked them to think about the situation for five people. In groups, with some acting out and some moving straight into the symbolic expression, all reached the expression 4 + 3 + 2 + 1 + 0 and calculated the answer. Returning to the original problem, most (including Christopher) were able to directly write down the expression representing the total number of hi-fives for 20 people as: 19 + 18 + ... + 1 + 0. Some started complaining that this was a very long sum to work out. Noting that part of working mathematically involves trying to find shortcuts for long-winded calculations, we ended up, after some discussion, with the annotated expression shown in Figure 6.

Some said that the ten groups of 19 in this list made 190 the total. Most seemed satisfied with this, but one teacher asked if the same method could be used for 15 people. I suggested they try this problem to decide if they could use the same method. Christopher was working with a group on this problem. After a spell working with his group, he asked me to look at his working - recreated from my notes (Figure 7).

Below, Christopher had written the following sequence of additions:

$$14 + 0 = 14$$
$$13 + 1 = 14$$
$$12 + 2 = 14$$
$$11 + 3 = 14$$
$$10 + 4 = 14$$
$$9 + 5 = 14$$
$$8 + 6 = 14$$
$$7 + 7 = 14$$

Adding up the eight groups of 14, Christopher had arrived at 112 as his answer. His calling me was prompted by the fact that others in his group had a different answer: 105. Once again, there is evidence here of Christopher's ceding authority for 'correctness' to me as the teacher (after discussion with his colleagues here) - retaining Yackel's (2001) social, rather than mathematical, bases for judgment. Together, we traced through his connecting arrows over the total expression and linked them to the list of sums below - e.g., the 14 and 0 pair links to the 14 + 0 sum. Reaching the 7 in the middle, I noted that there was only one 7 in his total expression but there was a 7 + 7 (i.e., two 7 s in his list of sums). Christopher responded thus:

> 'Oh, so I must not have 7 + 7. But you put an arrow over all the numbers in the list'.

Pointing to his working on the 20-person example, I responded that there had been two numbers in the middle in that case that I could connect.

Christopher nodded slowly and said: 'So if there is a number in the middle on its own, I don't put an arrow in the middle over it, I just add it on its own'. A colleague on his table interjected that odd numbers of people would leave a number on its own in the total expression. Christopher listened and responded: 'So I must remember

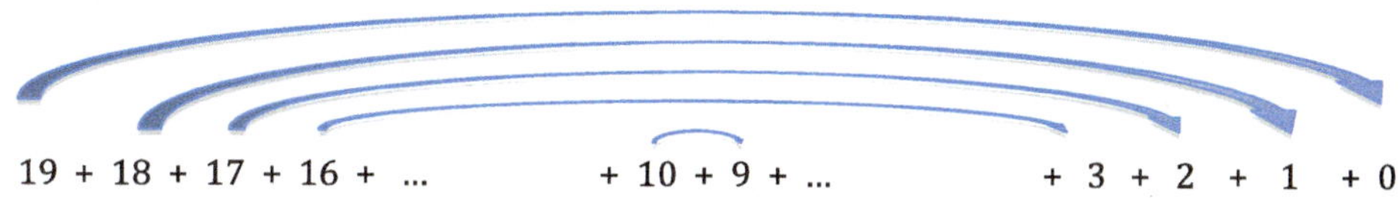

Figure 6 Annotated expression.

that odd numbers will leave a number on its own in the middle without an arrow and even numbers won't have a number on its own'. He annotated his working with the words 'Odd number' and underlined them. I ventured that as he had just figured the expression out, he probably did not need to commit this fact to memory. I noted later that he had annotated his earlier copying down of the answer for 20 people with the words 'Even number' underlined.

Discussion 3

Vinner's (1997) identification of attention to 'superficial similarity' within pseudo-analytical working is apposite here. Christopher's initial response, setting up the addition string for calculating the total number of hi-fives, shows evidence of some facility in construction of problem solutions through the initial setting up of an appropriate model. In making this construction, there is attention to the pattern seen in earlier examples and to generalizing what he has noticed to a new case. However, the need to make sense of this emergent representation and to attend to its structure in order to transform it appropriately are lost in his next steps, pointing to sporadic and partial presence of some mathematical practices. Christopher's attention is directed instead to incidental perceptual features - connecting arrows between terms in the numerical string, rather than the values they are connecting. His response to the discrepancy between his addition list and this numerical string illustrates his belief that he needs to remember what to do in the context of different cues. A dominant reliance on memory is therefore apparent in Christopher's comments and responses, again in the midst of indications that sense-making is within his grasp.

Conclusions

The analysis suggests that the presence of, even multiple elements of, mathematical practices cannot necessarily be considered equivalent to take up of mathematical modes of enquiry. Christopher retains a view of mathematics as dependent on memory and external validation through instances of strategic adaptation and abstraction. Framing his recruitment of mathematical practices is a recurring incidence of working and interaction driven by the need to 'pin down' the procedure that will produce the answer, rather than attend to structure and sense-making. As Schoenfeld (1987) has noted, these ways of working with mathematics run concurrently, in many instances, with the underlying content knowledge needed to reason in the problem contexts described.

Empirically, this analysis suggests that presenting mathematical practices in terms of separate strands alongside content strands can create situations in which specific practices are produced but set within a broader orientation that remains procedure and answer driven. In this 'separate and integrative' frame, where mathematical practices are selectively, rather than fundamentally, drawn upon, it would appear that a possible outcome of sporadic absence of explicit attention to mathematical practices is the disruption of mathematical modes of enquiry. Watson and Barton (2011) might consider this outcome to be the consequence of failing to view mathematical modes of enquiry as fundamental to all mathematical working.

In the course teaching, while mathematical enquiry modes were never disrupted, they were not always centrally the focus of discussion and reflection. It could be the case that it is the limited timeframe of the course rather than the mode of engagement with mathematical practices that is critical. In any case, the evidence presented in this paper points at the very least to the need for greater attention to mathematical practices within our work with teachers. A concluding post-script supporting this conclusion came from another teacher who attended the course in 2014. Her performance on the

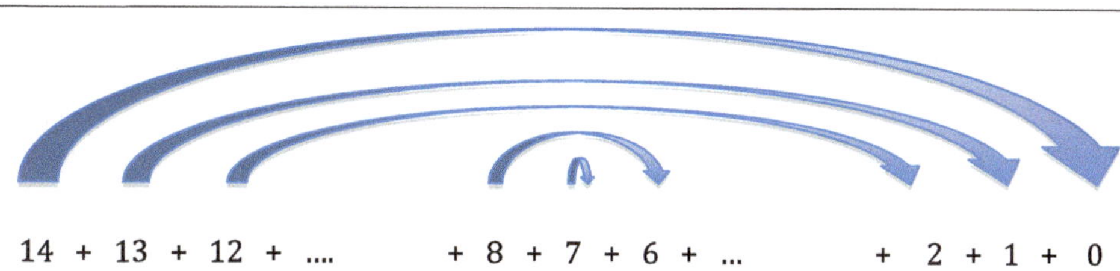

Figure 7 Christopher's working.

pre-test was similar to Christopher's and her post-test score was higher than his. Like him, she was positive and enthusiastic about the course. In the 2014 late-year revision session, she offered an entirely coherent explanation of how to produce the 'rule' for a linear sequence, with the mathematical arguments that Kazemi and Stipek (2001) describe as important for a high conceptual press communicated across all her steps. Several of the mathematical practices detailed in this paper were marshaled within her problem-solving and associated explanation. She paused at the end, looking doubtful, and asked: 'Was that right?' While assuring her that it was, her response provided further support for the view that accretions of mathematical practices, even when enacted without the disruptions seen in Christopher's working and commentary, may yet not amount to a practice driven fundamentally by trust in mathematical modes of enquiry. The analysis suggests that while elements of mathematical practices can be developed, moving towards mathematical modes of enquiry may require more explicit, consistent, and longitudinal attention to problem-solving approaches to support orientational change.

Competing interests
The author declares that she has no competing interests.

Authors' information
HV holds the SA Numeracy Chair and leads the WMC-P project within which the data reported on in this study was collected. HV was also the coordinator and tutor, with doctoral students Lawan Abdulhamid and Samantha Morrison, on the 'mathematics for teaching' course that provides the context of this paper.

Authors' contributions
HV is the sole author of this research article.

Acknowledgements
This paper forms part of the work in progress within the Wits SA Numeracy Chair project, entitled the Wits Maths Connect - Primary project. It is generously funded by the FirstRand Foundation, Anglo American, Rand Merchant Bank, and the Department of Science and Technology and is administered by the National Research Foundation.

References
Adler, J, & Venkat, H. (2014). Teachers' mathematical discourse in instruction: focus on examples and explanations. In H Venkat, M Rollnick, J Loughran, & M Askew (Eds.), *Exploring mathematics and science teachers' knowledge: windows into teacher thinking* (pp. 132–146). Abingdon, Oxon: Routledge.

Ally, N, & Christiansen, I. (2013). Opportunities to develop mathematical proficiency in grade 6 mathematics classrooms in KwaZulu-Natal. *Perspectives in Education, 31*(3), 106–121.

Ball, DL, Hill, H, & Bass, H. (2005). Knowing mathematics for teaching: who knows mathematics well enough to teach third grade, and how can we decide? *American Educator, 29*, 14–22.

Beckmann, S. (2011). *Mathematics for Elementary Teachers with Activity Manual, 3rd edition: Pearson*

Carnoy, M, Chisholm, L, Arends, F, Baloyi, H, Hoadley, U, wa Kiwilu, M, et al. (2008). *Towards understanding student academic performance in South Africa: a pilot study of grade 6 mathematics lessons in South Africa.* Pretoria: HSRC.

Common Core State Standards Initiative. (2010). *Common core state standards for mathematics.*

DBE. (2013). *Report on the Annual National Assessment of 2013: Grades 1 to 6 and 9.* Pretoria: Department of Basic Education.

Freudenthal, H. (1973). *Mathematics as an educational task.* Dordrecht: Reidel.

Freudenthal, H. (1983). *Didactical phenomenology of mathematical structures.* Dordrecht: Reidel.

Guba, EG. (1978). *Toward a methodology of naturalistic inquiry in educational evaluation. Monograph 8.* Los Angeles: UCLA Center for the Study of Evaluation.

Hoadley, U. (2007). The reproduction of social class inequalities through mathematics pedagogies in South African primary schools. *Journal of Curriculum Studies, 39*(6), 679–706.

Kazemi, E, & Stipek, D. (2001). Promoting conceptual thinking in four upper-elementary mathematics classrooms. *Elementary School Journal, 102*, 59–80.

Kilpatrick, J, Swafford, J, & Findell, B. (2001). *Adding it up: helping children learn mathematics.* Washington, D.C.: National Academy Press.

Mason, J. (1989). Mathematical abstraction as the result of a delicate shift of attention. *For the Learning of Mathematics, 9*(2), 2–8.

Mason, J, Burton, L, & Stacey, K. (1982). *Thinking mathematically.* London: Addison-Wesley.

Maturana, H, & Varela, FJ. (1980). *Autopoiesis and cognition: the organization of the living.* Boston: Reidel.

Miles, MB, & Huberman, AM. (1994). *Qualitative data analysis: an expanded source, book* (2nd ed.). Thousand Oaks, CA: Sage.

Mitchell, J. (1984). Typicality and the case study. In RF Ellen (Ed.), *Ethnographic Research: A guide to conduct* (pp. 238–241). New York: Academic.

National Council of Teachers of Mathematics. (2000). *Principles and standards for school mathematics.* Reston, VA: NCTM.

Polya, G. (1962). *Mathematical discovery: on understanding, learning and teaching problem-solving.* New York: Wiley.

Schifter, D. (2011). Examining the behavior of operations: noticing early algebraic ideas. In M Gamoran Sherin, VR Jacobs, & RA Philipp (Eds.), *Mathematics teacher noticing: seeing through teachers' eyes* (pp. 204–220). New York and London: Routledge.

Schoenfeld, AH. (1985). *Mathematical problem solving.* New York: Academic.

Schoenfeld, AH. (1987). What's all the fuss about metacognition? In AH Schoenfeld (Ed.), *Cognitive science and mathematics education* (pp. 189–215). Hillsdale, NJ: Lawrence Erlbaum Associates.

Sfard, A. (2008). *Thinking as communicating.* Cambridge: Cambridge University Press.

Skemp, R. (1976). Relational understanding and instrumental understanding. *Mathematics Teaching, 77*, 20–26.

Sorto, A, & Sapire, I. (2011). The teaching quality of mathematics lessons in South African schools. *Journal of Education, 51*, 1–22.

Taylor, N. (2011). *The National School Effectiveness Study (NSES): Summary for the synthesis report.* Johannesburg: JET Education Services.

Venkat, H. (2013). Curriculum development minus teacher development ≠ mathematics education. In Z Davis & S Jaffer (Eds.), *Proceedings of the 19th Annual National Congress of the Association for Mathematics Education of South Africa, 24-28th June.* Bellville, Cape Town: University of the Western Cape.

Venkat, H, & Adler, J. (2012). Coherence and connections in teachers' mathematical discourses in instruction. *Pythagoras, 33*(3), 25–32.

Vinner, S. (1997). The pseudo-conceptual and the pseudo-analytical thought processes in mathematics learning. *Educational Studies in Mathematics, 34*(2), 97–129.

Watson, A, & Barton, B. (2011). Teaching mathematics as the contextual application of mathematical modes of enquiry. In T Rowland & K Ruthven (Eds.), *Mathematical knowledge in teaching* (pp. 65–82). Dordrecht: Springer.

Watson, A, & Mason, J. (2006). Seeing an exercise as a single mathematical object: using variation to structure sense-making. *Mathematical Thinking and Learning, 8*(2), 91–111.

Yackel, E (2001) Explanation, justification and argumentation in mathematics classrooms. In *25th Conference of the International Group for the Psychology of Mathematics Education.* Utrecht, The Netherlands, July 12-17 (Vol. 1, pp. 9-24).

12

Developing preservice elementary teachers' specialized content knowledge: the case of associative property

Meixia Ding

Abstract

Background: Specialized content knowledge (SCK) is a type of mathematical content knowledge specifically needed for teaching. This type of knowledge, although serving as a critical component for preservice teacher education, is often challenging to develop with preservice elementary teachers (PTs). The purpose of this study is to investigate PTs' development of SCK for teaching fundamental mathematical ideas in a university methods course. Focusing on the case of the associative property (AP) of multiplication, the author as the course instructor identified three instructional opportunities (a formal introduction and two delayed revisits) to stress two SCK components, representations, and explanations. PTs' learning progresses were assessed through three diagnostic tests (a pretest, a mid-term exam, and a final exam) and two prompts, which informed the upcoming lesson design. Meanwhile, the course instructor conducted ongoing reflections on PTs' learning, which also informed the corresponding lessons.

Results: It was found that PTs initially generated abstract number sentences without reasoning about the contexts of word problems. This representational sequence indicates a symbol precedence view. When prompted for explanations, PTs focused on individual numbers rather than quantitative relationships, and they could not consistently apply the basic meaning of multiplication for reasoning. The methods course, when designed to address these issues, promoted PTs' SCK development. At the end of the course, the majority of PTs were able to generate number sentences based on the word problem structures and provided reasonable explanations; however, the methods course also faced dilemmas due to PTs' robust symbol precedence view and the tension between PTs' learning and children's learning.

Conclusions: Very few studies have explored ways to support PTs' knowledge growth in SCK, especially for teaching fundamental mathematical ideas. This study, by carefully documenting the successes and challenges in developing PTs' SCK, contributes to the existing literature. Based on our findings, this study highlights the importance of stressing basic meanings so as to develop PTs' explanation skills. Meanwhile, to develop PTs' representation skills, university instructors should be aware of the tension between PTs' and children's learning as manifested by PTs' symbol precedence view. Finally, to support PTs' SCK growth, it is also important to emphasize the role of elementary textbooks.

Keywords: Preservice elementary teachers, Specialized content knowledge, Fundamental mathematical ideas, Associative property of multiplication, Methods course

Correspondence: meixia.ding@temple.edu
Temple University, 436 Ritter Hall, 1301 Cecil B. Moore Avenue, Philadelphia, PA 19122-6091, USA

Background

Mathematics education programs should support preservice elementary teachers' (PTs) learning of specialized content knowledge (SCK), which is a type of mathematical content knowledge specifically needed for teaching (Ball et al. 2008). Such knowledge addresses both mathematics substance and pedagogical appropriateness. For example, in order to help elementary students make sense of abstract mathematical ideas such as the associative property (AP), a teacher may need to know how to illustrate AP through concrete word problem contexts. According to Morris et al. (2009), SCK is critical for teaching but often challenging to develop. This is because this type of knowledge focuses on unpacking a mathematical concept into its subcomponents to make it comprehensible for children. Thus, SCK does not rely on particular teaching contexts or particular students and therefore can be developed through university education programs. However, the acquisition of SCK demands PTs' well-connected mathematical knowledge and the awareness of children's learning, which is often found to be lacking in PT's existing conception (Borko et al. 1992; Ding et al. 2013; Morris and Hiebert 2009; Simon and Blume 1994). Such deficiency may be more problematic when developing PTs' SCK for teaching fundamental mathematical ideas (e.g., basic properties of operations) that are the core principles of mathematics but too abstract for children. As such, in order to better teach elementary children fundamental mathematical ideas, there is a need to investigate ways to support PTs development of SCK. The purpose of this study is to explore, through the case of the AP of multiplication, PTs' development of SCK and ways to support PTs' SCK development in a mathematics methods course. By documenting PTs' knowledge growth and the successes and challenges in learning to teach AP of multiplication, this study aims to contribute a small but vital piece to the knowledge base of teacher education (Morris et al. 2009), particularly in the area of teaching fundamental mathematical ideas.

Literature review

Teaching fundamental mathematical ideas: the case of AP

The associative property (AP) is a representative among fundamental mathematical ideas. This property, together with the commutative property (CP), and distributive property (DP) are the basic laws of arithmetic, which can be learned in early grades and will lay a foundation for future learning of algebra such as solving equations. As such, researchers view these fundamental mathematical ideas as early algebra topics (Carpenter et al. 2003; Kaput et al. 2008). Due to the limited scope, this study will focus only on the AP of multiplication $(ab)c = a(bc)$, which is harder than AP of addition (Carpenter et al. 2003). The significance of the AP of multiplication warrants this focus. For instance, the Common Core State Standards (Common Core State Standards Initiative 2010) has clearly stressed that elementary students should learn and understand the AP of multiplication starting from the third grade. Ding et al. (2013) also reviewed several important aspects of this property. First, along with the other properties, the AP provides tremendous flexibility for computation (Bruner 1960). For instance, to compute $(3 \times 4) \times 25$, one may use the AP to first multiply the latter two numbers, $3 \times (4 \times 25)$, and obtain the answer quickly. Second, the AP of multiplication may serve as a powerful tool for justification, reasoning, and proof (Carpenter et al. 2003). The example given by Carpenter et al. was to prove the following mathematical statement, "when you multiply an even number times any whole number, you get an even number." One may use "$2n$" and "m" to represent any even number and whole number, respectively, and then use the AP to obtain $(2n)m = 2(nm)$. Third, students' understanding of the AP may be transferred to later learning to solve algebraic equations and to learn more advanced concepts such as elementary group theory (Larsen 2010). Due to the significance of AP of multiplication, it is reasonable to expect PTs to obtain the necessary SCK for teaching this property through methods courses. Due to the fact that AP of multiplication is only one of the many fundamental mathematical ideas (e.g., CP, DP, inverse relations), findings from this study are also expected to serve as a window for developing PTs' SCK to teach other fundamental mathematical ideas.

Although fundamental mathematical ideas like the AP of multiplication are powerful, they are abstract in nature (Goldstone and Son 2005). Very often, students obtain only inert knowledge of these ideas (e.g., memorization of formulas) but lack the ability to flexibly retrieve them. For instance, when facing $(3 \times 4) \times 25$, a student may compute from the left to the right, $(3 \times 4) \times 25 = 12 \times 25$, without noticing the possibility of applying the AP. Such an inability to activate the AP is likely due to a lack of deep and meaningful initial learning (Chi and VanLehn 2012). In order to help students obtain meaningful initial learning, it is important for teachers (including PTs) to develop specialized content knowledge that will enable them to unpack an abstract concept in meaningful ways.

Specialized content knowledge

SCK is a key component of *mathematical knowledge for teaching,* a notion developed by Ball and colleagues (Ball et al. 2008) including common content knowledge (CCK), specialized content knowledge (SCK), knowledge of content and students (KCS), and knowledge of content and teaching (KCT). According to these researchers, SCK is a type of mathematical knowledge that is needed only for teaching rather than any other work. "This work involves an uncanny kind of unpacking of mathematics that is not needed—or even desirable—in settings other than teaching." (Ball et al. 2008, p. 400). SCK is different from CCK in that it is possessed by every educated adult; it is also different from KCS and KCT, which demand knowledge of specific students and teaching context. Therefore, SCK serves as a good candidate for topics to be covered in preservice teacher education (Morris et al. 2009). Note that although these knowledge components are distinguished in theory, they are not disjoint in actual teaching. For instance, SCK demands but also promotes CCK.

Even though Ball et al. (2008) provided a list of SCK tasks that are unique for teaching mathematics (e.g., "explaining mathematical goals and purposes to parents," "inspecting equivalencies," p. 400), this study focused mostly on teachers' representations and explanations, which are the core to unpacking a concept to make it visible and meaningful for students. Venkat (2015) argued that a focus on representations and explanations can simultaneously support teachers' mathematical learning and their learning about mathematics teaching. In fact, representations and explanations are not disjoint (e.g., one may explain the connections between representations). This study mainly stresses PTs' ability in (a) making connections between representations through a specific sequence, from concrete to abstract, and (b) explaining the meaning of an abstract number sentence by referring it to concrete contexts. As to be reviewed below, these two SCK components are largely emphasized by the existing literature, serving as a theoretical framework for this study.

Representations Ball et al. (2008) stressed teachers' ability in "selecting representations for particular purposes," "recognizing what is involved in using a particular representation," and "linking representations to underlying ideas and to other representations" (p. 400). Representations can be concrete (manipulatives, visual images, real-world contexts) or abstract (symbols). Both types of representations have strengths and limitations. For instance, concrete representations can activate students' personal experiences to aid sensemaking; however, these representations can contain irrelevant information that may hinder students from seeing the underlying mathematical ideas (Kaminski et al. 2008). Abstract representations support students' learning of powerful mathematical ideas; yet, these representations are often distant from students' personal experiences and thus may be learned in the form of inert knowledge. As such, it was suggested that teachers should help students make connections between concrete and abstract representations (National Mathematics Advisory Panel 2008; Pashler et al. 2007). Recent research particularly stresses a sequence of fading from concrete into abstract (also called "concreteness fading," Goldstone and Son 2005). This representational sequence is well aligned with how students learn and has been found to be effective in supporting both learning and transfer (Goldstone and Son 2005; McNeil and Fyfe 2012).

In this study, we expect PTs to illustrate fundamental ideas through word problem contexts. Thus, the representational sequence begins from concrete word problem situations. We consider word problems as concrete because the real-world situations provided by such problems "have the potential to offer memorable imagery that can act as a touchstone for teachers and learners in building and discussing abstract concepts" (Gerofsky 2009, p. 36). However, in order to make the underlying fundamental mathematical ideas explicit, we also expect that PTs will solve word problems symbolically, which can be generalized to reveal the underlying mathematical principle. The above sequence is consistent with a *verbal precedence view* (Nathan and Koedinger 2000) that emphasizes reasoning from verbal to symbol. This sequence is found well aligned with students' mathematical development (Koedinger and Nathan 2004; Nathan et al. 2002).

Explanations The second SCK component target in this study is explanation of mathematical ideas. Ball et al. (2008) highlighted tasks of "presenting mathematical ideas," "finding an example to make a specific mathematical point," and "giving or evaluating mathematical explanations" (p. 400). Prior studies have pointed out that students' self-explanations of mathematical ideas promote learning (Chi et al. 1994; Cobb 1994; Hiebert et al. 1997; Lewis 1988). However, in order to facilitate student explanations, teachers themselves should be able to explain. At times, teachers who are able to ask good question may not necessarily know the deep explanations to their own questions (Ding and Carlson 2013). Therefore, it is important to develop teachers' deep and meaningful explanations of a mathematical concept. According to Chi and VanLehn (2012), deep explanations refer to structural relationships rather than surface features or interactions among quantities rather than only individual numbers. Teachers whose explanations focus on structural relationships or quantitative interactions will likely have a better chance to develop students' self-explanations of the target concepts and thus decreases the risk of rote memorization.

SCK for teaching AP of multiplication Based on the above SCK framework, we expect PTs to situate the teaching of AP of multiplication in word problem contexts, which can be unpacked through representation uses and explanations. Ding et al. (2012) reported that a widely used US textbook (Greenes et al. 2005) introduced AP through the following word problem

"Mr. Levin's students are tasting foods grown in rainforests. He put 5 pieces of mango on each plate and put 2 plates on each table. There are 3 tables. How many pieces of mango are there?" (see Fig. 1). One may notice that the number choices in this problem do not effectively show the power of the AP as in the instance of (3 × 4) × 25 = 3 × (4 × 25); yet, for initial learning where the goal was to help student make sense of the AP, this mango problem context has a potential to serve the purpose. According to Ding et al., a teacher with SCK may first draw a diagram to represent the problem structure: 3 tables of 2 plates of 5 mangos (see Fig. 2). Such a diagram may serve as a mediating tool for classroom discussion and facilitate students' schema acquisition (Larkin and Simon 1987). Next, a teacher may guide students to reason by using the diagram to generate two mathematical solutions: (3 × 2) × 5 and 3 × (2 × 5). Finally, a teacher may guide students to compare two solutions to generate an instance of the AP, (3 × 2) × 5 = 3 × (2 × 5), which may lead to further generalization of the algebraic formula, $(ab)c = a(bc)$. The above representational sequence—word problem, diagram, arithmetic solutions, and algebraic formula—indicates an inductive reasoning sequence, moving from concrete to abstract and from specific to general (see Fig. 2).

To ensure students' understanding of the numerical solutions, explanations should be incorporated so students could understand the meaning of these number sentences. For example, a teacher should help students understand why one multiplies certain numbers together (e.g., 3 × 2, 6 × 5, 2 × 5, 3 × 10) and what each step actually meant. According to the problem structure, one may first find out how many plates are in total (3 tables of 2 plates thus 3 × 2 = 6 [1]) and then how many mangoes are in total (6 plates of 5 mangos thus 6 × 5 = 30), resulting in the first solution (3 × 2) × 5. Alternatively, one may first find out how many mangos are on one table (2 plates of 5 mangos thus 2 × 5 = 10) and then how many mangos are in total (3 tables of 10 mangos thus 3 × 10 = 30), resulting in the second solution, 3 × (2 × 5). The above explanations of the meaning of each step demands one's understanding of the quantitative definition of multiplication $a \times b$, which refers to "a groups of b." This definition or the basic meaning of multiplication is the core in the multiplicative conceptual field serving as a foundation for mathematical reasoning (Beckmann and Izsák 2015; Beckmann et al. 2015). More importantly, this definition should be used consistently to enable the reasoning process (Beckmann et al. 2015). Consider, for example, if a teacher sometimes uses 3 × 2 to refer to 3 groups of 2 and then other times to refer to 2 groups of 3, students will have difficulties constructing an understanding of multiplication and mathematics will become spurious and meaningless (Schwartz 2008). With a consistent use of the basic meaning, students will be

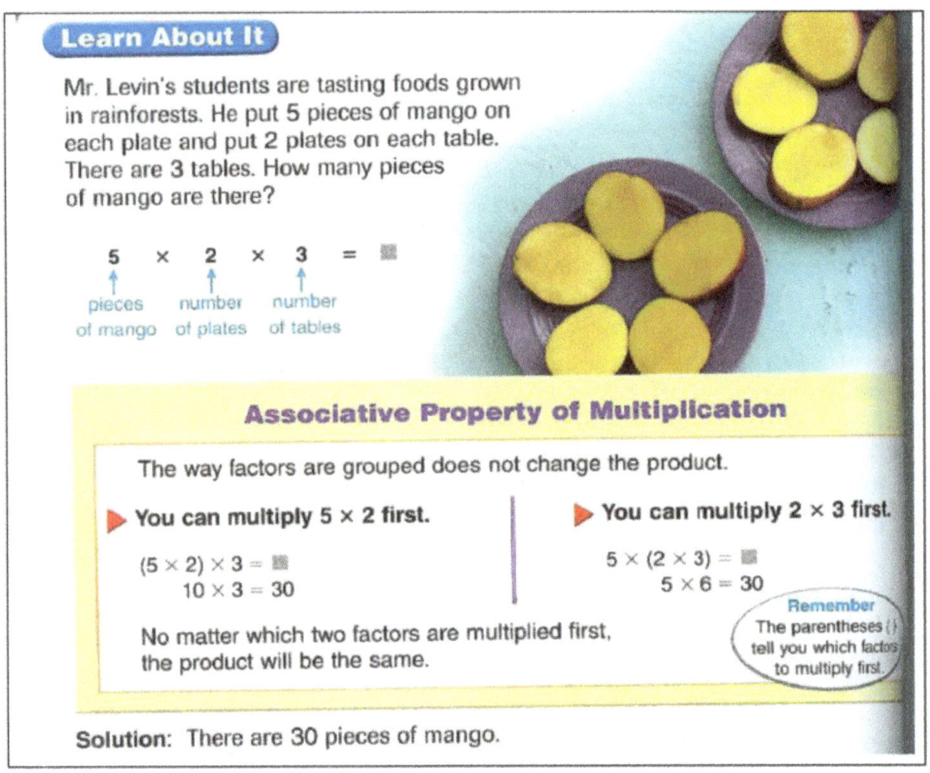

Fig. 1 The third grade elementary textbook page that presents the mango problem in *Houghton Mifflin* (Greenes et al. 2005)

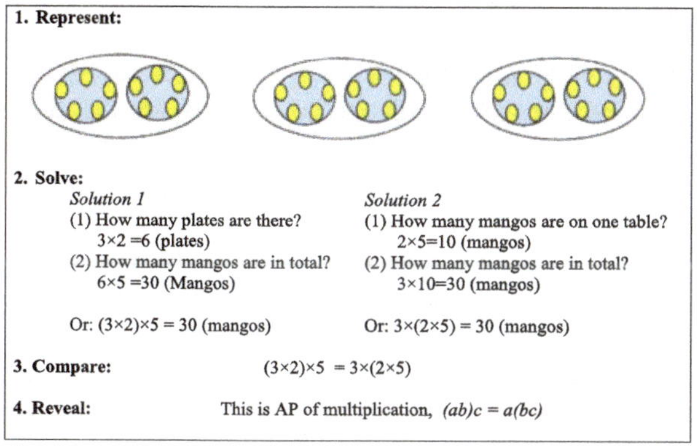

Fig. 2 The suggested teaching approach in Ding et al. (2012)

able to make inferences and link a number sentence back to the story problem situation to provide meaningful explanations.

Developing PTs' SCK: the challenges

PTs, as well as many other educated adults, possess compressed and abstract knowledge when they enter education programs. This type of knowledge, although demonstrating procedural fluency, is not sufficient for teaching children who need to construct knowledge based on their prior understanding. In particular with the AP of multiplication, Ding et al. (2013) reported that, when PTs first entered education programs, many of them did not remember the AP (CCK). For those who did remember, they had difficulties in illustrating the AP through concrete contexts (SCK). For instance, for a word problem with a structure of 3 groups of 2 groups of 4, many PTs generated number sentences such as $(3 \times 4) \times 2$, or $(4 \times 3) \times 2$, or $2 \times (3 \times 4)$. Although all these number sentences can produce a correct answer, they were not aligned with the word problem structure and each step cannot be explained in terms of the word problem situation. When prompted to explain these number sentences, PTs attended to the individual quantities (e.g., 3 boxes, 2 sets, 4 pencils) but not the interactions between them or the meaning of each step (e.g., 3 boxes of 2 sets thus $3 \times 2 = 6$ sets). These findings indicate PTs' procedural knowledge and their attention to number manipulation rather than quantitative relationships. In addition, many PTs directly presented the number sentences without reasoning upon the word problem situations (e.g., no pictures were drawn before presenting a number sentence). This finding echoes prior reports that US teachers (and textbooks) commonly possessed a *symbol precedence view* (as opposed to a *verbal precedence view*, Nathan and Koedinger 2000; Nathan et al. 2002). With this view, teachers and textbooks tended to treat manipulation with symbols as easier than word problems. Therefore, they often presented computations earlier than word problems because they thought word problems were too complex for students to learn. However, these researchers' experimental studies show that students indeed performed much better on word problems than the parallel algebraic equations, likely due to the fact that word problem contexts have elicited students personal knowledge to aid students' problem solving. Nathan and others' findings show that the commonly held symbol precedence view contradicts how students learn (Koedinger and Nathan 2004).

Prior findings on PTs' SCK for the AP of multiplication were consistent with a broader literature on PTs' learning to teach. Simon and Blume (1994) found that many PTs know the area formula "length × width," yet they could not explain why this formula worked through illustrations. Recently, Morris et al. (2009) found that PTs had incredible difficulty in unpacking decimal addition into sub-concepts that involve decimal units and the corresponding relations. These findings indicate the challenge to help PTs unpack their compressed knowledge. When getting frustrated, some PTs complained about these tasks as "the needlessly complicating things that should be straightforward" (Suzuka et al. 2010, p. 17). In fact, PTs who have taken methods courses may still not be able to unpack a task in ways that are comprehensible for children. As reported by Borko et al. (1992), when a student asked for the reasons of the inverse and multiply procedure for computing fraction division, a PT attempted to draw pictures to explain the process but failed to do so. This PT ended up telling students to just follow the procedure she provided. These findings call for a greater endeavor in developing PTs' SCK and a closer investigation of the role that university methods courses may play in supporting PTs' SCK development.

Prior research has shed light on this study; however, most of the SCK-related studies (e.g., Borko et al. 1992; Simon and Blume 1994; Morris and Hiebert 2009) have not explored the area of teaching fundamental mathematical ideas that undergird the mathematical system. Ding et al. (2013) did focus on SCK for teaching fundamental mathematical ideas and reported the levels of SCK PTs brought to teacher education; yet, this study did not investigate how PTs may be supported to grow this type of knowledge. Indeed, very few studies have tracked PTs' growth with SCK in university classrooms. The current study therefore aims to extend and continue this line of research. In particular, this research explores two questions: (1) How do PTs develop SCK for teaching the AP of multiplication through word problem contexts? and (2) How does the methods course instruction play a role in developing PTs' SCK?

Methods

This study employs a case study model (Stake 1995). The case in focus is PTs' learning to teach the AP of multiplication, which serves as a window that foreshadows the process of PTs' SCK development and the ways in which a methods course may support PTs' SCK development for teaching fundamental mathematical ideas.

Participants

This study was part of a methods course in a 4-year university in the USA. As the course instructor, the author conducted systemic reflections and improvements over a semester. Among the six course goals, one of them was to develop PTs' SCK for teaching fundamental mathematical ideas, which was discussed mainly through the case of teaching the AP of multiplication. It was expected that the intended SCK for teaching the AP of multiplication would help develop PTs' teaching schema and would enable them to teach other fundamental mathematical ideas such as CP, DP, and beyond. The current study documents the part of investigation with the AP of multiplication.

There were 25 PTs who took the methods course. This is the first but also the last course for PTs to learn to teach mathematics before they leave for elementary school jobs. Among these PTs, 24 PTs were female (96 %) and one was a male (4.0 %). All of the PTs were Caucasian. At the beginning of this course, the PTs were presented with an approved consent form and encouraged to participate in this study by providing permission for the instructor to use their coursework. It was also made clear that PTs' choices of participation would make no impact on their course grades. Supportively, all the PTs provided permission.

Course design and procedures

The course design contained at least three features. First, the instructor spaced the relevant learning over time (Pashler et al. 2007). As the mathematics methods course involves many topics, it is infeasible to spend too much time on the teaching of AP. However, since the targeted SCK is challenging to develop, it is also inappropriate to spend too little time on it. As such, the instructor spaced the learning across three existing curriculum opportunities. This included an initial math method lesson focused on the intended approach and two follow-up lessons arranged during the discussion of other topics. The second feature was to build the methods course instruction on the PTs' own learning. To understand PTs' learning processes, three diagnostics tests along with two prompts were administered, which informed the corresponding course instruction. In addition, the instructor conducted self-reflections on classroom instruction after each lesson. Finally, this methods course incorporated elementary textbook tasks into classroom discussions. This is because the method textbook (Reys et al. 2009) only briefly presented the definition, arithmetic examples, and the algebraic formula for the AP of multiplication, which targeted only the CCK but not SCK. To address this limitation, the instructor supplemented class discussion with the aforementioned mango problem (see Fig. 1). This mango task was selected from the third grade mathematics textbook of *Houghton Mifflin* (Greenes et al. 2005), a textbook series used by the participating PTs in their teaching practicum. Incorporating elementary textbook tasks into the methods course was recommended as an effective way to support PTs' learning and growth (Lloyd and Behm 2005). Indeed, incorporating elementary textbook tasks also made the methods course instruction more relevant to PTs' teaching practices. Figure 3 shows the procedures of data collection over the semester, which included three diagnostic tests, two prompts, and three methods course lessons.

As indicated by Fig. 3, a pretest using the mango problem (February 21) was conducted before lesson 1 (February 23). After lesson 1, PTs' SCK was reassessed through the mid-term exam (posttest 1, March 7). PTs' performance on both tests was suggested for comparison in prompt 1 (March 18), which informed lesson 2 (April 6) and lesson 3 (April 27). A second posttest was conducted through the final exam (posttest II, May 2), which contained prompt 2

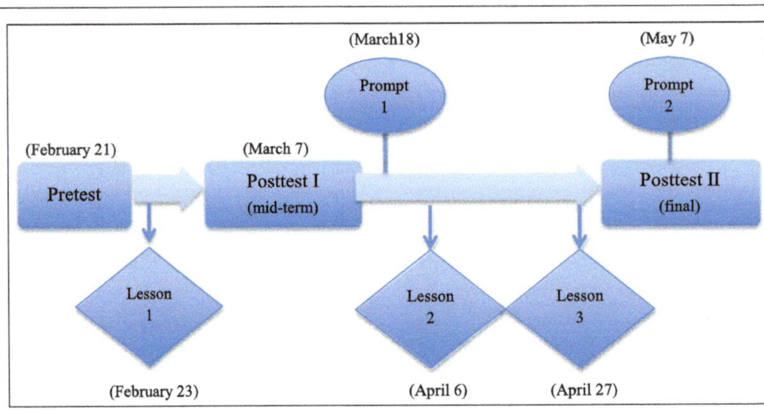

Fig. 3 Procedures of data collection over the semester

requesting the PTs to reflect upon their overall learning progress.

Data collection and data analysis

The data presented in Fig. 3 were collected and analyzed to answer the two research questions. For question 1, the three diagnostic tests along with the two prompts were analyzed to identify PTs' knowledge changes. For the second research question, the three lessons were analyzed and compared with PTs' performance in the diagnostic tests and prompts so as to identify the role that the methods course instruction played in PTs' learning. Elaboration follows.

Three diagnostic tests

In all the diagnostic tests, the PTs were asked "How will you use the following word problem to teach the Associative Property of multiplication?" The word problems used in the tests were the mango, string, and cup tasks, respectively (see Table 1).

All these tasks demand PTs' SCK in that the PTs were expected to analyze the actual problem structures and solve them in ways that could help children make sense of the AP. These word problems shared the same problem structures (e.g., 3 tables of 2 plates of 5 mangos, 3 boxes of 2 sets of 4 strings, and 4 boxes of 3 cups of $5, see Table 1). The mango and string problems also shared surface similarities, because the literal order of numbers in the problem situation (e.g., 4 strings-2 sets-3 boxes) was exactly opposite to the order in the problem structure (e.g., 3 boxes of 2 sets of 4 strings). The cup problem did not share the same problem structure, and its context also contained "money," which was a continuous quantity. The intention of using this cup problem was to measure students' transferability with a new context with a slightly different problem structure. Regardless of the differences in the surface features, all of these word problems should be unpacked in the same way as with the previously discussed mango problem (see Fig. 2).

It should be noted that the actual textbook presentation of the mango problem has shortcomings related to explanations and representations, respectively (see Fig. 1). In terms of explanations, the textbook directly presented a two-step numerical solution, $5 \times 2 \times 3$, which could not be explained based on the problem structure, 3 tables of 2 plates of 5 mangos. For instance, the meaning of each step could not be explained by referring to the word problem situation (e.g., for "5×2," one could not find 5 groups of 2 but 2 groups of 5). Moreover, the textbook only explained the literal meaning of each number (5 mangos, 2 plates, 3 tables). The second shortcoming is related to representations. The textbook directly introduced the AP and then applied it for computation whereas the mango problem was not used for sensemaking. This sequence indicated a *symbol* but not *verbal precedence view* (Nathan et al. 2002). Despite the shortcomings, this study deemed the mango problem a great learning opportunity to develop PTs' critical thinking skills and SCK for teaching fundamental mathematical ideas.

To analyze PT's knowledge change, PTs' responses to the mango, string, and cup problems were coded. We first coded whether a PT knew what the AP is (CCK). For example, if a PT provided a pair of solutions that switched numbers around [e.g., $(3 \times 2) \times 5$ and $(5 \times 3) \times 2$], we considered it as an indicator of lacking understanding of the AP of multiplication. We then coded the PTs' representations and explanations (SCK), which were detailed into the following aspects: (a) Does the PT draw a correct diagram to represent the problem structure? (b) Are the number sentences mathematically correct? (c) Are the explanations of each step meaningful? and (d) Does the solution sequence show a verbal precedence view? For each aspect, PTs' responses were coded using either "1" or "0" to indicate the presence of the knowledge component. All data were re-coded by the author 4 months later to check the reliability (96 %). A second coder was also trained to re-code 20 % of PTs' responses with a coding reliability of 98 %. The mean score of each aspect in each exam was computed. Given the small sample size and categorical nature of this data, nonparametric tests were used for analysis. This included the use of the Friedman test to identify any differences between groups and the Wilcoxon test to identify changes over time (Leech et al. 2008; Nussbaum 2014). These tests indicated PTs' deficiency

Table 1 The tasks used in three diagnostic tests

Exam	Name	Problem situation	Problem structure	Two solutions	Source
Pretest	Mango	Mr. Levin's students are tasting foods grown in rainforests. He put 5 pieces of mango on each plate and put 2 plates on each table. There are 3 tables. How many pieces of mango are there?	3 tables of 2 plates of 5 mangos	$(3 \times 2) \times 5 = 3 \times (2 \times 5)$	*Houghton Mifflin*—3rd grade
Posttest I (mid-term exam)	String	Upright bass strings come in sets of 4. Suppose one box holds 2 sets of strings. If a musician orders 3 boxes, how many strings will there be?	3 boxes of 2 sets of 4 strings	$(3 \times 2) \times 4 = 3 \times (2 \times 4)$	*Houghton Mifflin*—4th grade
Posttest II (final exam)	Cup	Each cup costs $5. Mom wants to purchase 4 boxes of cups with each box holds 3 cups. How much does mom need to pay?	3 cups of 4 boxes of $5	$(4 \times 3) \times 5 = 4 \times (3 \times 5)$	Chinese 3rd grade textbook (adapted)

in explanations and representational sequences. As such, PTs' responses to each of these aspects were further inspected and classified to identify the types of difficulties that the PTs had.

Two prompts

Along with the diagnostic tests, the PTs were asked to self-reflect on their performances. As previously mentioned, prompt 1 was conducted after the mid-term exam. The PTs were asked to compare their responses to the posttest 1 (string problem) and the pretest (mango problem), reporting the progress they made and the confusion that remained. Prompt 2 was part of the final exam. the PTs were asked to reflect, based on the cup problem, what they had learned about teaching fundamental mathematical ideas through word problems. Responses were coded to capture (a) PTs' insights on representations and explanations when unpacking a word problem to teach fundamental ideas and (b) PTs' remaining difficulties or their attitude changes.

Three lessons

To support PTs' learning to teach the AP, three lessons were spaced over the semester. By the time of lesson 1, the instructor had read PTs' responses to the pretest and was aware of the PTs' difficulties in representations and explanations. Lesson 1 (75 min) then formally discussed the mango problem using PTs' self-generated work. The purpose of using PTs' own work was to build on classroom instruction based on PTs' existing conceptions and engage them in course discussion. Lesson 2 reviewed AP in a chapter titled "Algebraic Thinking" (Reys et al. 2009) where the modeling perspective was involved. As one of the early algebra topics, it is appropriate to use AP, along with CP and DP, as an example to show how these fundamental ideas can be illustrated. As part of this lesson, the PTs were asked to create a word problem for a given instance of AP, $(4 \times 3) \times 2 = 4 \times (3 \times 2)$. These students then modeled and solved the problems. The relevant discussion on AP in lesson 2 took about 30 min. Lesson 3 was a final review of the course and thus was mostly open-ended. To revisit the course goals of teaching fundamental mathematical ideas, AP of multiplication was reviewed. PTs in small groups were asked to create a word problem that can be used to illustrate AP. The created problems were then exchanged among groups for peer solutions. This activity took approximately 20 min. In all three lessons, PTs' representations and explanations were the targets of class discussion.

To identify how the methods course may have played a role in PTs' learning, all relevant instruction in three lessons were audio-recorded, transcribed, and analyzed in a qualitative manner. Each lesson was first segmented into small chunks, which was analyzed from the aspects of representations and explanations. After this, relevant excerpts were compared in terms of PTs' representation uses and explanations, respectively. Meanwhile, these excerpts were linked back to three diagnostic tests and two prompts so as to confirm PTs' SCK changes and explain how classroom instruction may have supported or failed to support PTs' knowledge growth. For instance, if there was a shift of PTs' explanations or representations between two diagnostic tests, the author went back to the lesson that occurred between the two tests (see Fig. 3) to identify the typical instructional moves that might have made an impact on PTs' learning. If there was no change in PTs' SCK between the diagnostic tests, the author also examined the corresponding lesson to understand why it failed to promote SCK changes. The next section reports findings for each research question.

Results

How do PTs develop SCK for teaching AP through word problem contexts?

Overall performance

Findings about PTs' knowledge for teaching AP across the three exams are presented in Table 2.

Table 2 demonstrates PTs' knowledge growth over the semester. Given the pretest was conducted after the class had discussed what AP was, most PTs demonstrated sound CCK. In addition, most PTs in the pretest performed well on drawing a diagram to represent the problem. Indeed, the PTs performed well on these two skills across three tests ($M_{\text{CCK}} = 0.84$, 0.92, and 1 across three tests; $M_{\text{diagram}} = 0.92$, 0.92, and 1 across three tests). The Friedman test indicated no changes over the course of the semester for both CCK and drawing a diagram to represent the word problem.

However, the PTs in the pretest had difficulties generating correct number sentences and providing meaningful explanations (see Table 2). Results from the Friedman test for these two aspects indicated progress was made over the course of the semester, x^2_{sentence} $(2, n = 25) = 25.2$, $p < 0.001$; $x^2_{\text{explanation}}$ $(2, n = 25) = 19.18$, $p < 0.001$. In addition, the Wilcoxon test was used to compare two

Table 2 PTs' overall performance across three diagnostic tests

		Pretest		Posttest I (mid-term exam)		Posttest II (final exam)	
		M	SD	*M*	SD	*M*	SD
CCK	What is AP	0.84	0.37	0.92	0.28	1	0
SCK	Drawing a diagram	0.92	0.28	0.92	0.28	1	0
	Correct number sentences	0.24	0.44	0.48	0.51	0.96	0.2
	Meaningful explanations	0.04	0.2	0.16	0.37	0.6	0.5
	Verbal precedence view	0.04	0.2	0.16	0.37	0.28	0.46

orthogonal contrasts for each aspect (Leech et al. 2008). The posttest II (final) and posttest I (mid-term) contrast was found to be significant for both aspects: $r_{sentence} = 0.69$, $r_{explanations} = 0.61$; however, the posttest I (mid-term) and pretest contrast was not significant for either aspect. This suggests that the PTs' difficulties found in the pretests remained in the mid-term exam but changed significantly from the mid-term to the final exam.

With regard to the representational sequence, PTs were expected to possess a *verbal precedence view* that started with reasoning upon the diagrams. Only one PT demonstrated this view in the pretest. Over time, there was an increased number of PTs who obtained this view ($n = 1$, 4, and 7 across three tests; $M_{verbal} = 0.04$, 0.16, and 0.28, respectively). Yet, the Friedman test showed that this change was not significant.

Issues with explanations

Table 3 presents the results of PTs' explanations for the number sentences they generated in three diagnostic tests. In the pretest, the major difficulties were that PTs (72 %) generated number sentences based on the literal order of the numbers in the problem statement (e.g., 5, 2, and 3, see Table 4a, b for examples), and when explaining their number sentences, 76 % of the PTs explained only individual numbers (e.g., 5 mangos, 2 plates, and 3 tables) without considering the meaning of each step (see Table 4a). This confirms the findings of Ding et al. (2013). With instruction, the number sentence mistake decreased in posttest I (32 %) and disappeared completely in posttest II. Yet, the explanation mistake remained robust in posttest I (72 %) and then decreased in posttest II (24 %). In addition, there were minor issues that seemed to indicate a middle status of PTs' understanding. For instance, some PTs (4 % in pretest, 20 % in posttest I) provided a correct first step but incorrect second step for the number sentence (see Table 4c). With regard to explanations, some PTs provided partial- or pseudo-explanations (20, 12, and 16 %, respectively). These PTs appeared to acknowledge the importance of giving meaning to each step; however, because of the mismatch between their number sentences and the explanations, their explanations were inaccurate (see Table 4b, c).

Issues with representational sequence

Examination of PTs' representational sequence reveals PTs' lack of verbal precedence view. First, many PTs directly provided their numerical solution even before drawing a diagram (see Tables 4b and 5a, b), which indicates a symbol precedence view. Second, there seemed to be a "blending" view that mixed verbal and symbol precedence views. That is, some PTs first drew a diagram to represent the word problem. After that, they wrote a numerical solution, followed by explanations of the diagram (see Tables 4a and 5c, d). Given the diagram in this situation was not utilized to generate a number sentence, this blending view was in nature symbol precedence, which was termed as "semi-symbol precedence view" in this study. Across the three tests, only a few PTs demonstrated a verbal precedence view (see Tables 4c and 5e, f). Fig. 4 summarizes the number of PTs who heldeach view across the three tests. While the symbol precedence view decreased ($n = 10$, 4, and 2, respectively) and verbal precedence view increased ($n = 1$, 4, and 7, respectively), the semi-symbol precedence view was consistently the most prevalent ($n = 14$, 17, and 16, respectively), which may partially explain why many PTs drew sound diagrams yet did not provide solutions that bear contextual inferences.

PTs' voice in prompts

Consistent with the results in the diagnostic tests, PTs' voice in two prompts indicated their learning and changes. In prompt 1, PTs self-compared their performance on the string and mango problems and reflected upon their progresses in representations and explanations, which suggested different levels of understanding after the first formal instruction (see Table 6).

As indicated by Table 6, among the 24 PTs (one response missing), 11 of them (45.7 %) stated that they did not have any confusion, which was consistent with the results of the posttest I (mid-term). Four of them (16.7 %) suggested the need for further practice. Six PTs (25 %) admitted that they were uncertain about how to

Table 3 Issues about the number sentences and explanations

	Illustrating AP	Pretest		Posttest I (mid-term exam)		Posttest II (final exam)	
		Freq	%	Freq	%	Freq	%
Generating number sentences	Attending to the literal order	18	72	8	32	0	0
	Having no meaning in the 2nd step	1	4	5	20	1	4
	Correct number sentences	6	24	12	48	24	96
Providing explanations	Explaining numbers only	19	76	18	72	6	24
	Partial- or pseudo-explanations	5	20	3	12	4	16
	Complete explanations	1	4	4	16	15	60

Table 4 Issues of PTs' number sentences and explanations in the pretest

	Explaining numbers not operations	Partial/pseudo-explanation
Number sentence: Attending the literal order	a. 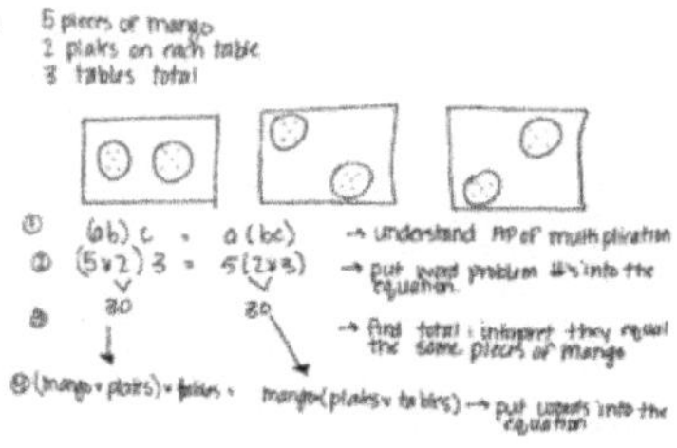	b. 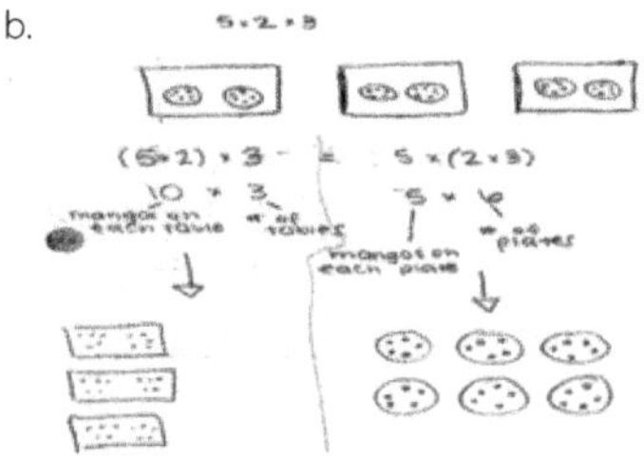
Number sentence: Having no meaning in the 2nd step		c. 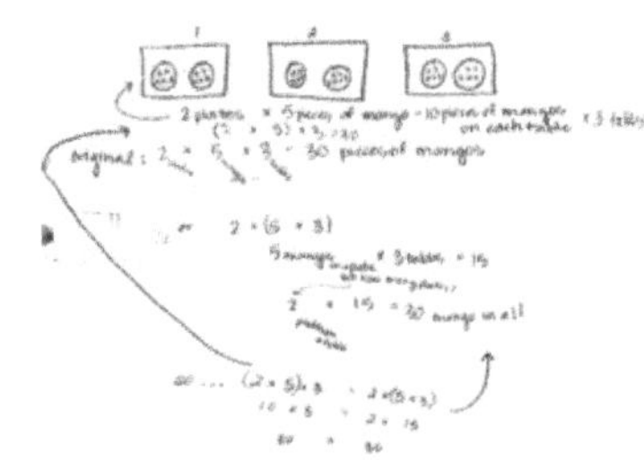

generate a number sentence that may refer back to the story situation, and three PTs (12.5 %) expressed frustration about the intended approach and refused to change their existing conceptions. For example, one PT stated, "I don't understand why you have to know exactly what object it refers to. I just think it would confuse kids if it confuses me and I would never teach this way" (see Table 6). After continuous instruction, PTs' responses in prompt 2 uniformly suggested their improved understanding and more positive views. In particular, those PTs who initially had refused to change clearly acknowledged the role of word problem contexts, especially the role of diagrams in developing children's understanding of fundamental mathematical ideas. For instance, one PT stated, "If you draw the word problem out it is much easier for students to understand the concept. The associative property is much easier to understand where you first draw out the picture." Another PT wrote, "I've learned to first draw a picture to help them see the groups because some word problems can be tricky.... I think a picture also let them see how the two problems are equivalent and see the associative property of multiplication as more concrete." In summary, PTs' responses to the three diagnostic tests, along with their voice in the two prompts revealed progress with their remaining difficulties. The next section reports how the methods course instruction played a role in PTs' learning.

How does the methods course instruction play a role in developing PTs' SCK?

To support PTs' learning, the instructor provided interventions that aimed to enhance PTs' representation uses and explanations. As mentioned in the "Methods" section, this process included an initial formal discussion (lesson 1) incorporating the mango problem to address issues with explanations and representations. After this, two follow-up lessons were provided to continuously address these issues (see Fig. 3). In lesson 2, PTs were asked to create a word problem to illustrate a given arithmetic example of the AP.[2] In lesson 3, PTs were asked to create a word problem for the AP and then exchange it with peers for solutions. Across these lessons, PTs demonstrated progress in some aspects but still had difficulties with others.

Addressing explanation issues

During lesson 1, the instructor handed back the pretest (mango problem) without grading marks and suggested PTs share their work within small groups. Each group then came up with a representative solution for class discussion (see Fig. 5). Among five groups, only one contained correct number sentences, three were incorrect, and one was incomplete. This overall result was consistent with the pretest (see Table 2). Using the work of group 1 that contained a mistake, the instructor led a whole-class discussion of the step-by-step meanings.

Focusing on step-by-step meaning

One PT in group 1 explained their solution $(5 \times 3) \times 2 = 5\times\ (3 \times 2)$, "You can put 5, or 2, or 3 in any order and you can always get the answer."

> Instructor (I): Assuming that I am a third grader and don't understand why you did 5×3, as a teacher, can you help me understand what it means by 5×3 using your picture?

Table 5 Examples of symbol, semi-symbol, and verbal precedence views

	Posttest I (mid-term) (the string problem)	Posttest II (final) (the cup problem)
Symbol precedence	a. *(PT4)* 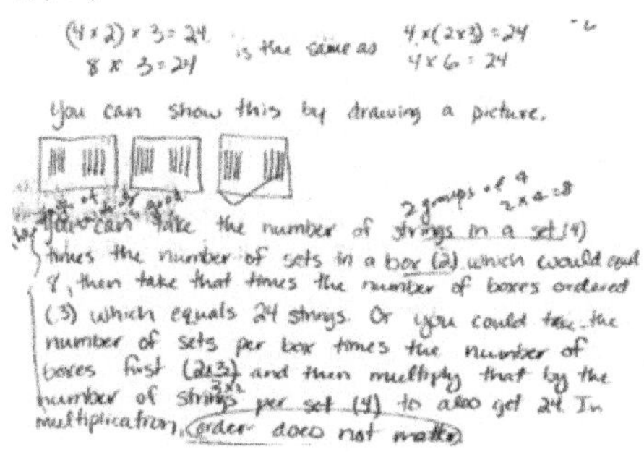	b. *(PT7)* 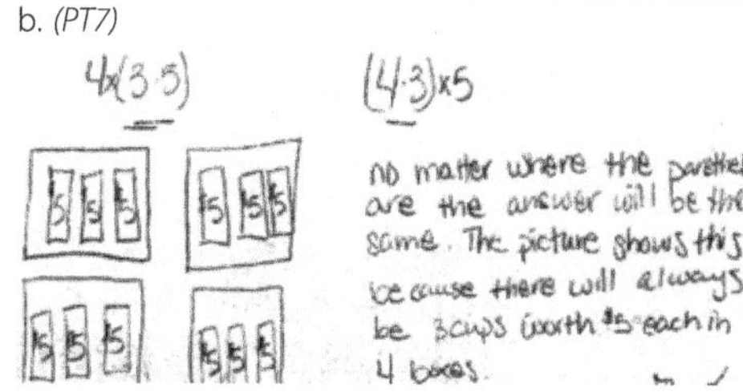
Semi-symbol precedence	c. *(PT12)* 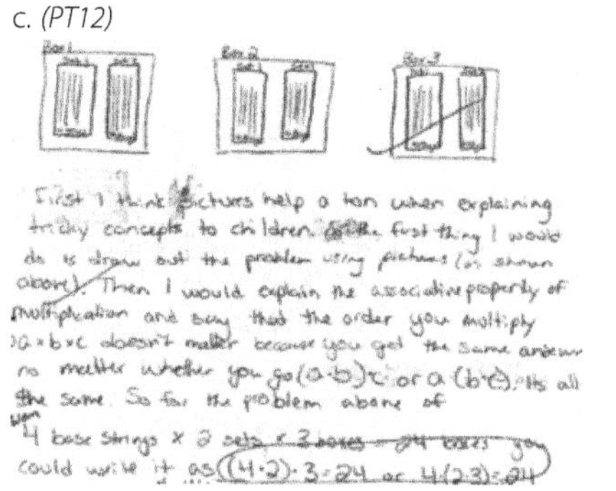	d. (PT6) 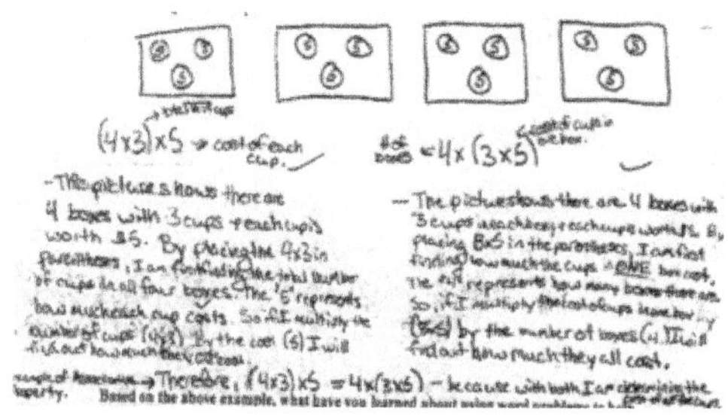
Verbal precedence	e. (PT19) 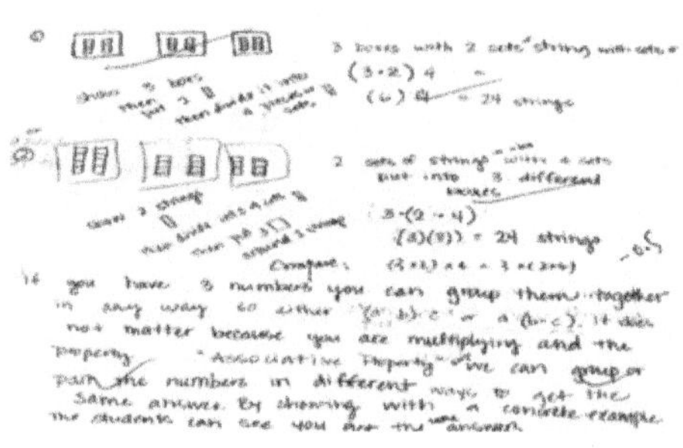	f. (PT25) 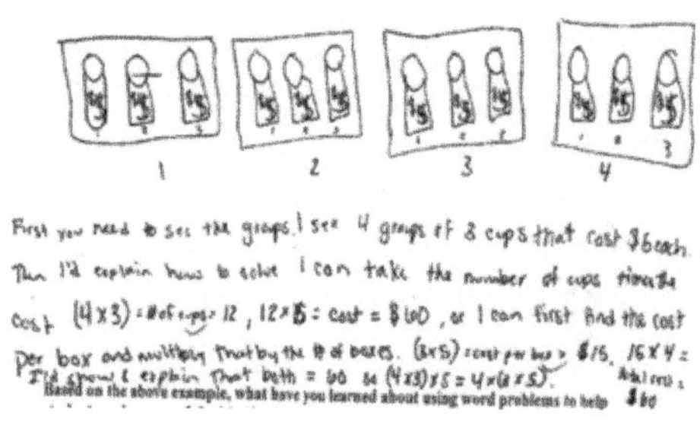

PT2: (from group 1): There are 5 pieces of mango, time 3 tables, equals 15. And we take that to time 2 plates on each table.

PT2's explanation indicates that she attended to the meaning of each number (5 and 3) but not the interaction between them (5 × 3). This is similar to the major issue observed in the pretest. The instructor asked if the other groups were convinced. One PT commented that there were no 5 groups of 3 in the picture, indicating the consideration of the meaning for each step. The instructor then asked whether 5 × 3 had a referent in this problem situation. This led to group 1's self-correction, "So, we actually should do 5 × 2 ... 5 groups of 2, oh, 2 groups of 5 so 2 × 5 ..." With the back-and-forth discussion of the meaning of the first step, the class reached an agreement that the first step should be 2 × 5, which represents 10 mangos on one table.

Surprisingly, PTs' understanding of the first step did not spontaneously transfer to the second step. A few PTs quickly suggested that the next step was to "find 3 tables," "time 3," or "10 × 3." These responses, accepted by the class, did not reflect the problem situation, 3 tables of 10 mangos. This observation confirmed the findings in the diagnostic tests that the PTs could not consistently apply the meaning of multiplication to the second step. To facilitate discussion, the instructor drew PTs' attention back to the diagram:

I: So, here is one table, how many mangoes on each table?

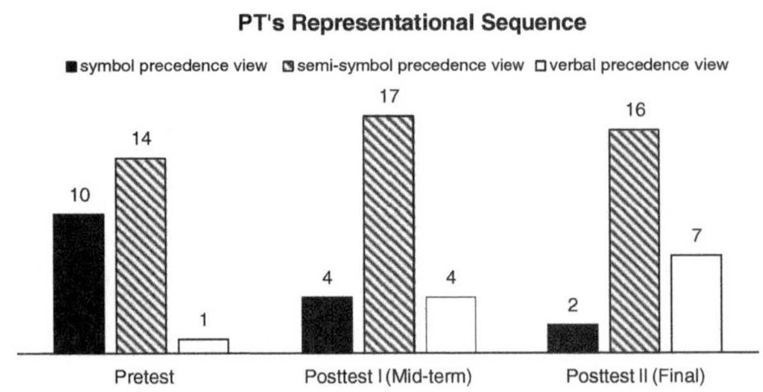

Fig. 4 Number of PTs who demonstrated different views across three diagnostic tests

PTs: 10

I: (labeled a "10" for each table in their picture, see the first picture in Fig. 5) Now, you have *how many groups of what*?

PTs: 3 groups of 10

I: So, what would be your number sentence?

PT: 3×10 ....It represents 30 mangos in total.

In the above discussion, PTs' attention was consistently oriented to the definition or the basic meaning of multiplication—how many groups of what. Note that even though these class discussions involved PTs who provided correct responses, these discussions seemed not to produce a success in PTs' understanding. One evidence was that at the end of lesson 1, the instructor handed out the actual textbook page of the mango problem (see Fig. 1) and asked the PTs to discuss it. Surprisingly, except for two PTs who commented on the textbook issue with explanations, no one showed any interest for further discussion. Further evidence revealed that only 48 % of the PTs could generate a meaningful number sentence in the mid-term exam (see Table 2). The instructor pondered whether the emphasis on step-by-step meaning in lesson 1 had overwhelmed PTs so that they saw only pieces of information but not the general problem structure.

Focusing on global meaning

The instructor made an effort to stress the issue with explanations by discussing the global meaning of the two-step problem ("groups of groups of something") so as to back up PTs' understanding with a schema. This took place in lesson 2 after the mid-term exam (April 6), through a chapter titled "Algebraic Thinking" (Reys et al. 2009). Using $(4 \times 3) \times 2 = 4 \times (3 \times 2)$, the instructor asked the PTs to create word problems to illustrate the AP. One group created a story problem showing "2 groups of (4×3)," which has no meaning in the second step. This scenario once again signified a need to build PTs' structural understanding. As such, the instructor provided a whole-group discussion:

I: If we discard the context and only look at this number sentence, what does it mean by $4 \times 3 \times 2$?

PT: You have 4 groups of 3 groups of 2.

I: In this equation that shows AP, we have $(4 \times 3) \times 2$ and $4 \times (3 \times 2)$. The first expression indicates 12 groups of 2, right? (Uniformly agree). For the second expression $4 \times (3 \times 2)$, you have how many groups of what?
PT: 4 groups of 6

I: We can sketch a picture to illustrate this problem structure, 4 groups of 3 groups of 2. You can imagine the picture from outside to the inside, that is, you first see 4 groups, then 3 subgroups in each, and eventually, 2 objects inside each subgroup (The instructor sketched a picture on the board). This picture indicates the structure of the word problem that you will *create.*

I: Later, when you try to *solve* your story problem, you may reason upon this picture in two ways, resulting in $(4 \times 3) \times 2$ and $4 \times (3 \times 2)$ that correspond to "12 groups of 2" and "4 groups of 6" respectively. Do you see 12 groups of 2?

PT: Yes! (Confidently)

I: Do you see 4 groups of 6?

PT: Yes!!! (Confidently)

In the above episode, the instructor consistently emphasized the definition or basic meaning of multiplication (how many groups of what) but at a global level that targets the hierarchical structure of multiplication. The instruction also contained "shortcuts," viewing a picture from outside to inside and viewing a picture two ways. These discussions seemed to generate a positive outcome by offering the PTs a schema that enabled all groups to create appropriate word problems (e.g., about 4 tables of 2 plates of 3 cookies, 4 flowerpots of 3 tulip of 2 ladybugs, and 4 boxes of 3 vases of 2 flowers). Each group explained their story problems and solutions that together illustrated AP, $(4 \times 3) \times 2 = 4 \times (3 \times 2)$. The class ended with widespread excitement, indicating the PTs enhanced motivation in learning. This success continued in lesson 3 when PTs created and solved each other's word problems in order to illustrate the AP.

Table 6 PTs' self-reflection on learning to teach AP in prompt 1

Levels of understanding	Frequency (%)	Example responses
No confusion	11 (45.7)	I have learned that when teaching the associative property I need to order the numbers so that they represent the number of groups and then how many are in each group. I did not know about this before taking this class. I have also learned how to write word problems to help explain this. I dont have any confusions about this.
Basically understand and practice needed	4 (16.7)	Knowledge that I have gained for future teaching of fundamental ideas includes the fact that concepts can be made clearer by the use of pictures. Drawing out the situation and clearly identifying the numbers involved and what they stand for may be extremely helpful when teaching students. With question #4 specifically, I still find it difficult to relate the property being taught directly to the story problem. However, I feel that I will develop a better understanding of this with more practice.
Still have confusion about the "order"	6 (25)	This problem is where I learned the most— I never realized how the associative problem works into these problems, but know it do ☺. I understand for future teaching I need to understand the idea clearly before I even approach my students about the problem. I am still confused by how to order the problem. So that certain groups [illegible]
Question this approach and refuse to change	3 (12.5)	Well when I learned the associative property we never used pictures to explain it. We were probably taught the properties in junior high and never used pictures to show them. I would say that as long as you are using the same three numbers I don't understand why you have to know exactly what object it refers to. I just think it would confuse kids if it confuses me and I would never teach it this way.

Interestingly, in lesson 3 while PTs were creating story problems, one PT shouted out her surprising findings about the previously discussed mango problem, "So even on this (pointing to the actual textbook page handed out during Lesson 1), it is not right? … Oh!!! …Yes, I agree now! We created a problem similar to this. But now I think the textbook, it is wrong!" This response was in sharp contrast to PTs' responses at the end of lesson 1 where most PTs could not recognize the textbook issue with explanations.

Indeed, PTs' improved understanding was confirmed by their performance on the final exam (see Table 2) where 96 % of the PTs generated correct number sentences (as opposed to 48 % on the mid-term exam) and 60 % provided meaningful explanations (as opposed to 16 % on the mid-term exam). It appears that the instruction of global meaning has provided strong support for PTs to generate meaningful number sentences and explicitly explain them.

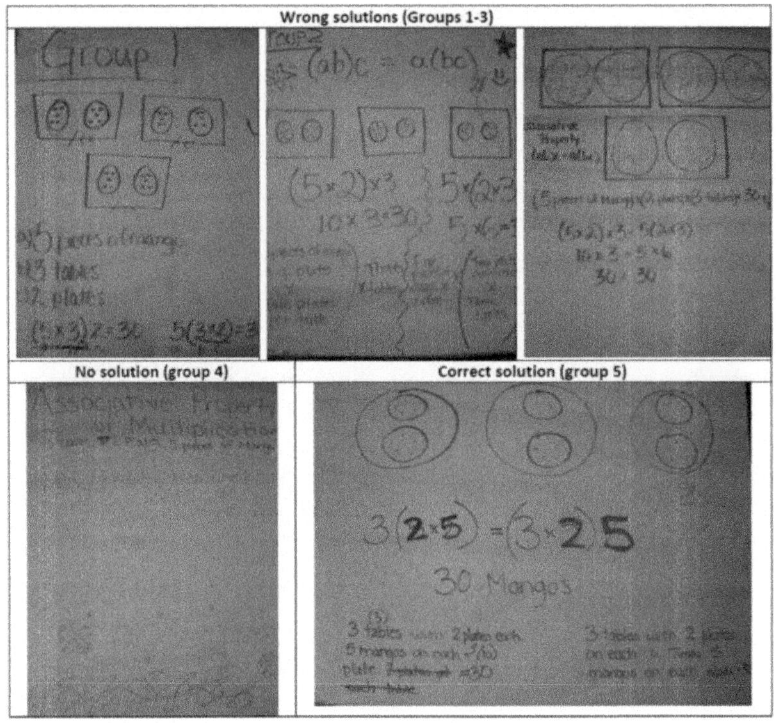

Fig. 5 PTs' group work during the first formal instruction

Addressing representation issues

In terms of representations, we expect PTs to start with concrete contexts to conduct verbal reasoning (e.g., drawing diagrams and reason upon the problem situation). From there, they should fade concreteness into abstract representations (generate number sentences to reveal AP). This representational sequence, however, did not occur smoothly, likely due to the PTs' symbol precedence review that was hard to overcome.

Challenging PTs' symbol precedence view partially

In lesson 1, after the discussion of the first solution based on verbal reasoning, the class was asked to figure out the second solution. A PT quickly suggested the second solution based on her knowledge of the AP formula, $(ab)c = a(bc)$: "Just like to show AP, like we have parentheses, like we can do in different order..." S4's suggestion indicated a symbol precedence view because she came up with the second solution based on her prior abstract knowledge rather than reasoning upon the mango problem. To challenge this unexpected view, the instructor commented:

> T: But children don't know AP of multiplication yet, right? That's why you need to teach them and reveal this property through this word problem context.
>
> S4: Ok, so in parenthesis, we have 3 × 2, five in the end. 3 tables and 2 plates on each table.
>
> T: If we teach elementary children, we need to slow down and they need to see what it means by 3 × 2. So, do we see 3 groups of 2?
>
> S. Yes... it represents the number of plates.

In this episode, the instructor's first suggestion, "reveal this property through this word problem context," demanded verbal reasoning. However, this was not understood by the PT as a challenge to her thinking. Rather, she continued with symbolic reasoning, which, however, was not criticized by the instructor who asked only for an explanation of those symbols. As such, the challenge to PT's symbol precedence view did not reach its potential. It should be noted that the instructor did purposely record the class conversation on the board in the sequence of represent-solve-compare-reveal (see Fig. 2) and guided the class to look back at this general teaching approach, which implicitly lined up with a verbal precedence view.

Reinforcing PTs' symbol precedence view unintentionally

Even though verbal precedence view was an expectation from the PTs, course instruction unintentionally reinforced the symbol precedence view. In the second lesson, the PTs were asked to create a story problem to illustrate $(4 \times 3) \times 2 = 4 \times (3 \times 2)$. Once an appropriate word problem is created, they should reason upon the word problem inductively to illustrate the AP. However, during the class discussion of the global meaning of $4 \times 3 \times 2$, the instructor introduced a shortcut of visualizing 4 groups of 3 groups of 2 from outside to inside, which was quickly taken by the PTs as a crutch for problem solving. This observation was most apparent in lesson 3 where the PTs were asked to solve peers' word problems to illustrate AP. Instead of reasoning upon the word problems, some PTs immediately generated a number sentence like $2 \times 6 \times 3$ by viewing the picture in a particular order (from outside to inside). From there, they added parentheses based on their knowledge of AP and explained the meaning of each step of these solutions. The above sequence reflected the semi-symbol precedence view, which was further seen on the final exam. For instance, a few PTs wrote, "from outside to inside" on the final exam and PT5's explanation was procedural, "First we have 4 boxes so boxes is our largest so it comes first; Second, we have 3 cups in each box, so that comes next; Finally, each cup cost $5 that is our smallest amount." Such explanations did not make meaningful reasoning based on the word problem situations, which may have explained why only 60 % of the PTs in the final exam could provide complete explanations (see Table 3) and why the verbal precedence view did not increase as expected on the final exam (see Table 2).

Discussion

Developing PTs' SCK is an important and much needed area of research, which has been regarded as challenging (Morris et al. 2009; Suzuka et al. 2010). How to support PTs' growth in such knowledge has been rarely studied. In particular with developing PTs' SCK for teaching fundamental mathematical ideas, there are very few studies that have reported such effort in mathematics courses. The present study, by carefully documenting the successes and challenges in developing PTs' SCK, contributes to the existing literature. For instance, while Ding et al. (2013) reported that PTs lack CCK and SCK when they first enter education program, our findings indicate that it is relatively easy to develop PTs' CCK but challenging to develop their SCK. This might be due to the fact that SCK is a new form of knowledge that requires a new mode of thinking. In particular, this study has focused on two SCK components, explanations and representations (Ball et al. 2008). We have obtained greater success in supporting PTs' meaningful explanations but less success in representational sequence, likely due to PTs' robust symbol precedence view. Even though we only have studied two SCK components, our findings shed light on the mathematics education field because the work of building a knowledge base calls for small tests for small changes (Morris and Hiebert 2009).

Developing PTs' explanation skills: the importance of stressing basic meanings

In this study, one SCK-related difficulty seen in the PTs involved explaining the meaning of number sentences when referring back to the concrete story situations. Some PTs tended to focus on the individual quantities rather than the interactions between them. Others cannot consistently apply the definition or the basic meaning of multiplication across two steps for quantitative reasoning. Such levels of understanding may lead to missing opportunities for deep initial learning with their future students (Chi and VanLehn 2012; Richland et al. 2012). In this sense, the current study adds to Ding et al. (2013) by highlighting the directions that teacher education courses may take when developing PT's SCK.

When the methods course is designed to deliberately address PTs' difficulties in explanations, PTs can grow their SCK as indicated by the diagnostic tests. We acknowledge the possibility that the consecutive testing on similar tasks might have contributed to PTs' performance; however, it should also be noted that the assessment task in the posttest II (final exam) was indeed more complex than the previous tasks. The success in developing PTs' explanations may be partially attributed to the instructor's consistent emphasis on the definition or the basic meaning of multiplication. For instance, the instructor kept asking for the meaning of each step, "how many groups of what?" and stressed the mapping process between number sentences and diagrams. This finding echoes Beckmann et al. (2015) where preservice middle school teachers succeed in proportional reasoning lessons due to the instructors' consistent emphasis of the definition of multiplication. As these researchers suggested, consistent and explicit use of the definition of multiplication can support the development of teachers' proficiency with quantitative reasoning, which may further provide a basis for PTs to unpack mathematical tasks in ways that prompt students' mathematical reasoning and explanations. This adds to the literature of SCK as it illuminates a detailed path to support PTs' explanations of mathematical ideas (Ball et al. 2008).

It should be noted that PTs' development of explanation skills was gradual. In this study, the development process involved different formats of instructional support ranging from stressing the step-by-step meaning to the global meaning. To stress the step-by-step meaning, the instructor asked PTs to reason upon the concrete story situation to write each step based on the basic meaning of multiplication ("a groups of b" is represented as $a \times b$). The two solutions were then compared to generate an instance of AP. This bottom-up approach indicates deductive reasoning. In contrast, to stress the global meaning, the instructor first helped students understand the meaning of a two-step multiplication $a \times b \times c$, which represents a groups of b groups of c. This was further mapped to two solutions $(a \times b)$ groups of c, and a groups of $(b \times c)$, and each step of the two solutions was further referred back to the story situation. This top-down approach indicates deductive reasoning. With this instructional effort, the major issues (attending to the literal order, explaining numbers only) decreased and the expected explanations increased. However, there still exists a middle status (e.g., having no meaning in the second step, pseudo- or partial explanations). This indicates that PTs' SCK development is not an all-or-nothing phenomenon. Given that PTs generally possessed weak knowledge when they enter education program (Borko et al. 1992; Simon and Blume 1994; Morris and Hiebert 2009), it takes time to shift their attention from surface to deep explanations. Future studies may explore this interesting middle status phenomenon and seek better ways to promote greater success.

Developing PTs' representation skills: tension between PTs' and children's learning

To support elementary students' learning, within classrooms, PTs should be able to move flexibly between concrete and abstract representations in responsive ways (National Mathematics Advisory Panel 2008; Pashler et al. 2007). In this study, given that the initial learning of a fundamental mathematical idea is situated in a word problem context, we expect PTs to develop a particular type of SCK skill, reasoning from concrete to abstract, which is well supported by the literature (Goldstone and Son 2005; McNeil and Fyfe 2012; Pashler et al. 2007). However, the PTs demonstrated difficulties in using this intended representational sequence. This may reflect PTs' challenge in linking representations to the underlying ideas or making connections between different representations. As indicated by Table 2, even though the classroom instruction has helped the PTs understand such connections, PTs who were good at drawing a diagram from the beginning did not see the connections among diagram, number sentences, and the corresponding explanations. Another interpretation of the representational difficulties may be attributed to PTs' robust symbol precedence view, which may have hindered PTs' representational uses. As observed from this study, some PTs tended to operate directly on the given numbers of a word problem without reasoning upon the word problem situation or without drawing a diagram. This finding echoes prior studies where US secondary school teachers were found to possess a symbol precedence view because they believed that symbol manipulation is easier than word problems and thus should come before verbal reasoning (Nathan et al. 2002; Nathan and Koedinger 2000). Our finding suggests that elementary preservice teachers hold the same view, which is likely related to PTs' existing compressed knowledge. This interpretation is supported by prior studies suggesting that PTs are often familiar with computation procedures but lack the ability to illustrate, explain, or unpack them (Borko et al. 1992; Morris et al. 2009; Simon and Blume 1994). More interestingly, our emerged findings on PTs' semi-symbolic review contribute to new insights in the literature. As reported, some PTs did draw diagrams to represent the word problem situation; yet, they did not actually use the diagrams to generate number sentences. Still, some PTs used the diagram to generate number sentences but in procedural ways, such as looking at a picture from outside to inside to determine the number orders. In both occasions, diagrams of the given word problem were not utilized to support mathematical reasoning and explanations, which distinguishes the semi-symbol precedence view from the verbal precedence view. The detour from verbal to symbol reasoning further indicates the robustness of PTs' symbol precedence view that may even occur in a single word problem context involving diagrams. Given that prior studies only reported the symbol precedence view with a full lesson or a textbook series (Nathan et al. 2002; Koedinger and Nathan 2004) but not a concrete context that has apparent verbal advantages, our study calls for greater attention to PTs' use of concrete representations. Instead of "whether" concrete representations (e.g., drawing diagrams) are involved in teaching, we should focus on "how" the concrete aids are actually used in ways to support symbolic reasoning.

PTs' robust symbol precedence view presents great challenges for methods courses that aim to develop SCK. University instruction usually starts with PTs' existing concepts that are stored in compressed formats, making the instructional sequence deductive (from abstract to concrete). This sequence is opposite to elementary students' learning process (inductive, from concrete to abstract). The tension between PTs' and children's learning demands a paradigm shift of PTs' existing views, which may cause frustration with some PTs who may question this approach (Suzuka et al. 2010) or give up easily (Borko et al. 1992). Other PTs may revert to their old habits. For instance, when the course instructor provided a shortcut to help PTs visualize the problem structure so as to *create* a story problem, PTs quickly took it as a crutch for *solving* the problem based on their compressed knowledge of AP. This, however, conflicts children's learning because children often do not have any prior knowledge of the AP. These findings join the literature on expert blindspots (Nathan and Koedinger 2000), suggesting PTs may simply assume children see what they see. These findings also suggest the complexity in developing PTs' SCK due to the tension between PTs' compressed knowledge and children's learning process.

In retrospect, the above tension between PTs' and children's learning may be reduced by improving the methods course instruction. First, the instructor could have acknowledged the tension between PTs' and elementary children's learning, but still *explicitly* emphasized the importance of reasoning upon a word problem situation from the perspective of children. Helping PTs explicitly see the value of the intended instructional approach may motivate them to struggle for success (Eccles et al. 1983). Second, the instructor could have helped PTs develop a stronger understanding of the definition or the basic meaning of multiplication before offering the shortcuts. With a stronger understanding, PTs may find it easier to conduct mathematical reasoning (Beckmann et al. 2015). In fact, the shortcut may not even be needed during the process of problem solving. This may minimize the risk of reinforcing PTs' procedural foci and symbol precedence view that contradict children's learning.

The role of elementary textbooks in developing PTs' SCK

Findings from this study suggest that incorporating discussions of elementary textbook tasks may serve as an effective path to developing PTs' SCK. This is aligned with research assertions that textbooks should serve as educative materials (Ball 1996; Davis and Krajcik 2005). In this study, the textbook presentation of the mango problem contained similar mistakes as those of the PTs. It is predicted that if PTs have never been exposed to critical discussions like the one in this study, they may teach future students in the same way as the textbook does. As Nathan et al. (2002) pointed out, questionable textbook presentations "can go unchecked and can be implemented throughout the educational system, to the potential detriment of students and teachers" (p. 18). As seen from this study, the in-depth discussion of the mango task as a source problem has served as a worked example of a general teaching approach, which has enabled PTs' various degrees of transfer of the learned SCK.

How and to what extent elementary textbooks support PTs' learning, however, is not straightforward. It seems that there is an interaction between textbook presentation and PTs' own knowledge. When PTs do not possess sophisticated understanding of the intended approach, the issues of textbook presentation are unlikely identified and thus not critically analyzed. This was evident by the PTs' silence at the end of the first lesson when they were invited to comment publically on the textbook presentation. Possibly, when PTs themselves were striving for understanding of the new approach, asking them to analyze a problematic textbook page would increase their work-load. This may explain why many PTs did not acknowledge the textbook issues in a cognitively comfortable manner. In contrast, when equipped with the necessary knowledge, some PTs could spontaneously capture the textbook issue and learn from it. This was evident in lesson 3.

Conclusions

There are a few limitations of this study. First of all, it involves a small group of PTs ($N = 25$). As such, findings should not be over-generalized. In addition, this study only explores PTs' course work without investigating the field experiences; therefore, it is not clear how PTs may actually transform learned knowledge into classroom settings. Furthermore, this study has a narrowed focus because it mainly involves representations and explanations, whereas the SCK skills may demand other skills such as having ready strategies to respond to common mistakes (Ball et al. 2008). Indeed, the teaching of fundamental mathematical ideas does not necessarily involve word problems (e.g., a volume model is an alternative candidate for teaching AP, National Research Council 2001). Nevertheless, our findings have several implications for teacher education.

First, PTs' SCK acquisition appears to be gradual and takes time, which aligns with the literature assertion of spaced learning (Pashler et al. 2007). This brings a challenge to teacher education. While the current study targets only one fundamental idea, a methods course usually covers many more mathematical topics and thus has limited opportunities to revisit them. A possible solution to this challenge is to set up course goals centering on the teaching of *fundamental mathematical ideas* that transcend across various contexts. Second, because PTs lacked the ability and habit to explain quantitative relationships based on concrete contexts, this study has identified PTs' robust symbol precedence view. Teacher education programs need to be aware that activities involving word problems and diagrams do not guarantee PTs' sound use of those verbal and visual contexts. Teacher education programs should explicitly challenge PTs' symbol precedence view and stress the importance of quantitative reasoning, which may enable PTs to understand why they should construct a verbal precedence view; however, simply conveying general instructional principles, such as grounding abstract ideas in concrete contexts, may still be ineffective. Methods course instructors should encourage PTs to experience "productive struggles" (Richland et al. 2012, p. 196) without giving out shortcuts too quickly. Finally, this study incorporated elementary textbook pages that contained mistakes as methods course materials. It is clear that these mistakes may not be recognized by PTs without discussion. As such, it is critical for textbook authors to enhance their textbook presentations to better support teacher learning. On the other hand, methods courses could use flawed textbook tasks as counter-examples for course discussion. Future studies may explore when, how, and under what circumstances the different types of elementary textbook examples (correct and flawed) may be utilized to support PTs' learning. With continuous research on the ways to overcome PTs' misconceptions and prior views, future elementary teachers can be better equipped with the necessary SCK to teach fundamental mathematical ideas, which in turn may enhance children's learning.

Endnotes

[1]There is no agreement on the meaning of multiplication. Some define 3×2 as 3 groups of 2 $(2 + 2 + 2)$ while the others define it as 2 groups of 3 $(3 + 3)$. This debate goes beyond the scope of this study. Regardless of the differences, we and other researchers (e.g., Beckmann and colleagues) argue that in order to facilitate students' mathematical reasoning, the definition of multiplication should be applied consistently. The textbooks involved in this study initially defines 3×2 as 3 groups of 2.

[2]The PTs in lesson 2 were asked to illustrate the AP, CP, and DP by creating story problems or drawing pictures or using manipulatives. It was found that they had an easy time illustrating both CP of addition $a + b = b + a$ and the AP of addition $(a + b) + c = a + (b + c)$. For the properties that involve multiplication, the PTs were able to illustrate the CP of multiplication $(a \times b = b \times a)$ when they were reminded about the basic meaning of multiplication and the array model. For the DP $(a + b) \times c = ac + bc$, when PTs were reminded about the basic meaning of multiplication, they were also able to create story problems along with pictures to illustrate this property. However, the AP of multiplication $(a \times b) \times c = a \times (b \times c)$ appeared to be most challenging for PTs, likely due to the fact that this property involves two steps of multiplication.

Competing interests

The author declares that she has no competing interests.

Acknowledgements

This study is partially supported by the National Science Foundation CAREER program under Grant No. DRL-1350068 at Temple University. Any opinions, findings, and conclusions in this study are those of the author and do not necessarily reflect the views of the National Science Foundation. The author is grateful to the editor and the three anonymous reviewers for their constructive feedback. Thanks also go to Ryan Hassler for editorial assistance.

References

Ball, DL (1996). Teacher learning and the mathematics reforms: what we think we know and what we need to learn. *Phi Delta Kappan, 77*, 500–508.

Ball, DL, Thames, MH, & Phelps, G (2008). Content knowledge for teaching: what makes it special? *Journal of Teacher Education, 59*, 389–407.

Beckmann, S, & Izsák, A (2015). Two perspectives on proportional relationships: extending complementary origins of multiplication in terms of quantities. *Journal for Research in Mathematics Education, 46*, 17–38.

Beckmann, S, Izsák, A, & Ölmert, i. B. (2015). From multiplication to proportional relationships. In X. Sun, B. Kaur, & J. Novotná (Eds.), *Conference proceedings of ICMI study 23: primary mathematics study on whole numbers* (pp. 518–525). Macau: University of Macau.

Borko, H, Eisenhart, M, Brown, CA, Underhill, RG, Jones, D, & Agard, PC (1992). Learning to teach hard mathematics: do novice teachers and their instructors give up too easily? *Journal for Research in Mathematics Education, 23*, 194–222.

Bruner, JS (1960). *The process of education*. Cambridge: Harvard University Press.

Carpenter, TP, Franke, ML, & Levi, L (2003). *Thinking mathematically: integrating arithmetic & algebra in elementary school*. Portsmouth: Heinemann.

Chi, MTH, & VanLehn, KA (2012). Seeing deep structure from the interactions of surface features. *Educational Psychologist, 47*(3), 177–188.

Chi, MTH, de Leeuw, N, Chiu, M, & LaVancher, C (1994). Eliciting self-explanations improves understanding. *Cognitive Science, 18*, 439–477.

Cobb, P (1994). Where is the mind? Constructivist and sociocultural perspectives on mathematical development. *Educational Researcher, 23*(7), 13–20.

Common Core State Standards Initiative (2010). Common core state standards for mathematics. Retrieved from http://www.corestandards.org/Math/. Accessed 1 May 2013.

Davis, EA, & Krajcik, J (2005). Designing educative curriculum materials to promote teacher learning. *Educational Researcher, 34*(3), 3–14.

Ding, M, & Carlson, MA (2013). Elementary teachers' learning to construct high quality mathematics lesson plans: a use of IES recommendations. *The Elementary School Journal, 113*, 359–385.

Ding, M, Li, X, Capraro, MM, & Capraro, RM (2012). Supporting meaningful initial learning of the associative property: cross-cultural differences in textbook presentations. *International Journal for Studies in Mathematics Education, 5*(1), 114–130.

Ding, M, Li, X, & Capraro, M (2013). Preservice elementary teachers' knowledge for teaching the associative property: a preliminary analysis. *Journal of Mathematical Behavior, 32*, 36–52.

Eccles, JS, Adler, TF, Futterman, R, Goff, SB, Kaczala, CM, Meece, JL, & Midgley, C (1983). Expectancies, values, and academic behaviors. In J. T. Spence (Ed.), *Achievement and achievement motivation* (pp. 75–146). San Francisco: W. H. Freeman.

Gerofsky, S (2009). Genre, simulacra, impossible exchange, and the real: How postmodern theory problematises word problems. In L. Verschaffel, B. Greer, & W. V. Dooren (Eds.), *Words and worlds: Modeling verbal descriptions of situations* (pp. 21–38). Rotterdam: The sense publisher.

Goldstone, RL, & Son, JY (2005). The transfer of scientific principles using concrete and idealized simulations. *The Journal of the Learning Sciences, 14*, 69–110.

Greenes, C, Larson, M, Leiva, MA, Shaw, JM, Stiff, L., Vogeli, BR, & Yeatts, K (2005). *Houghton Mifflin*. Boston: Houghton Mifflin Company.

Hiebert, J, Carpenter, TP, Fennema, E, Fuson, KC, Wearne, D, Murray, H, et al. (1997). *Making sense: teaching and learning mathematics with understanding*. Portsmouth: Heinemann.

Kaminski, JA, Sloutsky, VM, & Heckler, AF (2008). The advantage of abstract examples in learning math. *Science, 320*, 454–455.

Kaput, JJ, Carraher, DW, & Blanton, ML (Eds.). (2008). *Algebra in the early grades*. New York: Lawrence Erlbaum Associates.

Koedinger, KR, & Nathan, MJ (2004). The real story behind story problems: effects of representations on quantitative reasoning. *Journal of the Leaning Sciences, 13*, 129–164.

Larkin, JH, & Simon, HA (1987). Why is a diagram is (sometimes) worth ten thousand words. *Cognitive Science, 11*, 65–100.

Larsen, S (2010). Struggling to disentangle the associative and commutative properties. *For the Learning of Mathematics, 30*(1), 37–42.

Leech, NL, Barrett, KC, & Morgan, GA (2008). *SPSS for intermediate statistics: use and interpretation* (3rd ed.). New York: Erlbaum.

Lewis, C (1988). Why and how to learn why: analysis-based generalization of procedures. *Cognitive Science, 12*, 211–256.

Lloyd, GM, & Behm, SL (2005). Preservice elementary teachers' analysis of mathematics instructional materials. *Action in Teacher Education, 26*(4), 48–62.

McNeil, NM, & Fyfe, ER (2012). "Concreteness fading" promotes transfer of mathematical knowledge. *Learning and Instruction, 22*, 440–448.

Morris, A, & Hiebert, J (2009). Introduction: building knowledge bases and improving systems of practice. *Elementary School Journal, 109*, 429–441.

Morris, A, Heibert, J, & Spitzer, S (2009). Mathematical knowledge for teaching in planning and evaluating instruction: what can preservice teachers learn? *Journal for Research in Mathematics Education, 2009*(40), 491–529.

Nathan, MJ, & Koedinger, KR (2000). An investigation of teachers' beliefs of students' algebra development. *Cognition and Instruction, 18*, 209–237.
Nathan, MJ, Long, SD, & Alibali, MW (2002). The symbol precedence view of mathematical development: a corpus analysis of the rhetorical structure of textbook. *Discourse Processes, 33*, 1–12.
National Mathematics Advisory Panel. (2008). *Foundations for success: The final report of the National Mathematics Advisory Panel*. Washington: U.S. Department of Education.
National Research Council. (2001). *Adding it up: helping children learn mathematics*. Washington: National Academy Press.
Nussbaum, EM (2014). *Categorical and nonparametric data analysis: choosing the best statistical technique*. New York: Taylor & Francis.
Pashler, H, Bain, PM, Bottge, BA, Graesser, A, Koedinger, K, McGaniel, M, et al. (2007). *Organizing instruction and study to improve student learning (NCER 2007-2004)*. Washington: National Center for Education Research.
Reys, RE, Lindquist, MM, Lambdin, DV, & Smith, N (2009). *Helping children learn mathematics* (9th ed.). Hoboken: John Wiley & Sons.
Richland, LE, Stigler, JW, & Holyoak, KJ (2012). Teaching the conceptual structure of mathematics. *Educational Psychologist, 47*, 189–203.
Schwartz, JE (2008). *Elementary mathematics pedagogical content knowledge: powerful ideas for teachers*. Boston: Allyn & Bacon.
Simon, MA, & Blume, GW (1994). Building and understanding multiplicative relationships: a study of prospective elementary teachers. *Journal for Research in Mathematics Education, 25*, 472–494.
Stake, RE (1995). *The art of case study research*. Thousand Oaks: Sage.
Suzuka, K, Sleep, L, Ball, DL, Bass, H, Lewis, JM, & Thames, M (2010). Designing and using tasks to teach mathematical knowledge for teaching. *Association of Mathematics Teacher Educators, Monograph, 4*, 7–23.
Venkat, H (2015). Representational approaches to primary teacher development in South Africa. In X. Sun, B. Kaur, & J. Novotná (Eds.). *Conference proceedings of ICMI study 23: Primary mathematics study on whole numbers* (pp. 583-588). Macau, China: University of Macau.

13

Get a room: the role of classroom space in sustained implementation of studio style instruction

Alexis V. Knaub[1*], Kathleen T. Foote[2], Charles Henderson[1], Melissa Dancy[3] and Robert J. Beichner[4]

Abstract

Background: The characteristics of the classroom environment play an important role in shaping teaching practices and supporting research-based instructional strategies. One instructional strategy that has reimagined the classroom is the Student-Centered Active Learning Environment with Upside-Down Pedagogies (SCALE-UP). SCALE-UP uses studio-style instruction to facilitate student collaboration. Although there is significant interest in studio-style instruction, there is not much research-based guidance available for institutions interested in setting up a classroom, especially for secondary users interested in using this in different academic settings and contexts. We interviewed key informants involved in 21 successful secondary implementations of SCALE-UP about creating, using, and spreading studio-style classrooms. This paper summarizes respondent's perceptions of (1) how these classrooms are initiated; (2) which classroom features are helpful, non-essential, and unhelpful; (3) how professional development efforts support SCALE-UP instructors; and (4) how the classroom indirectly affects the department and/or institution.

Results: *Room initiation* Interviewees engaged in multiple activities to obtain a studio-style classroom. The majority of interviewees worked in teams created by faculty or administrators, with the participation from both groups. Interviewees typically sought institutional funding to develop the rooms.
Classroom features When developing the room, implementers used many key characteristics of the recommended classroom, such as collaborative workspace (e.g., special tables) for students, but they generally did not replicate all of the recommended features. Interviewees had mixed opinions about the importance of classroom technology.
Professional development and support Interviewees noted the importance of professional development for teaching staff (instructors and teaching assistants) new to the SCALE-UP teaching environment.
Indirect effects Beyond direct benefits to the teachers and learners, our interviewees reported that the classrooms had larger impacts including attracting visitors to the institution and encouraging the use of active learning in non-SCALE-UP classes.

Conclusions: There are many paths to successful development of a studio-style classroom. The process can be initiated by faculty or administrators. Classroom designs can vary to suit the local environment as long as they maintain the intent of the space: to support peer collaboration. Beyond improving student outcomes, these classrooms have additional benefits for institutions that include transforming instructor approaches to teaching and symbolizing the institution's commitment to quality teaching.

Keywords: SCALE-UP, Studio-style instruction, Classroom design, Modifying education innovation, Active learning spaces

* Correspondence: avknaub@gmail.com
[1]Department of Physics, Western Michigan University, 1903 West Michigan Ave, Michigan 49008, USA
Full list of author information is available at the end of the article

Background

Teaching practices are affected by the characteristics of both the individual instructor (i.e., beliefs, experience, desires, etc.) and the environment (i.e., physical space, local culture, and available resources) (Beggs 2000; Martin 2002; Cotner et al. 2013). Therefore, the design of the physical classroom space plays an important role in shaping the learning environment. From seating configuration to furniture to technology, the classroom and its features can encourage or discourage particular activities. For example, seating bolted to the floor facing forward toward a projection screen encourages instructor presentations, while round tables with no discernable front of the classroom facilitate group work. Developing non-traditional classroom space can support many active learning instructional strategies that have been shown to produce high student learning (Beichner et al. 2007; Dori et al. 2007; Walker et al. 2011; Narum 2013; Cotner et al. 2013).

Creating such classroom space is not a trivial undertaking, and there is little guidance available for those interested in building non-traditional classroom space. We conducted an interview study of 21 successful initiations of Student-Centered Active Learning Environment with Upside-Down Pedagogies (SCALE-UP), a well-tested instructional reform that radically re-envisions pedagogy and the instructional space (Beichner et al. 2007). SCALE-UP is a studio-style reform primarily used in higher education STEM settings, although instructors in other disciplines have implemented SCALE-UP (Foote et al. 2014).

The goal of this study is to better understand how secondary implementers, those who are not the initial developer but adopt the innovation, created successful and sustainable SCALE-UP classrooms. We provide practical advice for those seeking to create a SCALE-UP classroom as well as explore wider implications for other structural reforms. Specific research questions are discussed later in this paper.

What is SCALE-UP and how does it relate to this study?

Robert Beichner developed SCALE-UP in 1995 at North Carolina State University (NCSU) as an affordable way to bring the benefits of studio-style instruction to his large enrollment introductory physics classes (Narum 2013). SCALE-UP is an example of a broader class of studio-style reforms (Beichner et al. 2007). Studio-style teaching combines lecture and lab into one class, frequently incorporating collaborative active learning activities to engage students (Beichner 2014). While students are working on activities, the instructor moves around the classroom to interact with and encourage interaction among students. Other studio-style reforms include workshop physics and studio physics at Renneselaer Polytechnic Institute (Beichner 2014).

The SCALE-UP classroom features special tables, whiteboards, and technology to facilitate collaborative and hands-on learning. It represents a radical departure from a typical lecture hall. The SCALE-UP room design evolved through both experience and research (Beichner et al. 2007). NCSU's current SCALE-UP room is designed for 99 students and has 7-ft-diameter round tables that each can accommodate three groups of three students (Beichner et al. 2007; Narum 2013). The 7-ft-diameter tables allow students to have enough space for activities and also communicate across the table at a reasonable speaking volume (Beichner et al. 2007). While this table size and shape works well for large classes, other SCALE-UP implementations use other table shapes, for example, D-shaped tables in smaller classes. Instructional technology, such as laptops, and whiteboards are frequently incorporated into the room (Beichner 2014). Laptops are recommended, because they are smaller than desktops and can be stored when not needed (Beichner et al. 2007). Display screens or monitors around the room allow the instructor to show student work to the entire class. Students also use simulations and course software such as WebAssign, an electronic homework and assignment delivery system. Technology can help with course organization (e.g., storing the syllabus online) and promote flexible student-instructor interaction (e.g., groups submit work online so that instructors can identify and work with groups that need additional assistance).

Why study SCALE-UP?

We chose to study SCALE-UP for the following reasons:

- *Demonstrated student success.* The results of SCALE-UP style teaching are extremely positive. SCALE-UP has been shown to improve student retention, student problem solving, and success in subsequent courses (Beichner et al. 2007; Dori et al. 2007; Narum 2013). Particularly striking is that the drop, fail, and withdraw (DFW) rates dramatically decrease for women and underrepresented racial minorities and become comparable to non-underrepresented populations (Beichner 2008).
- Supports development of the twenty-first century skills. While the learning goals vary from instructor to instructor, Beichner (2014) points out that these goals frequently include "twenty-first century skills," which include using technology, working in teams, communicating effectively, and conducting experiments. SCALE-UP classrooms provide an environment where students can practice these skills. National organizations, including the American Institute of Physics (Czujko et al. 2014), the National Academies (Cooke and Hilton 2015), and the White House (President's Council of

Advisors on Science and Technology 2010) have identified these skills as being valuable for future STEM professionals to develop.

- Widespread usage. A Fall 2013 Survey found that SCALE-UP is used in 114 physics departments, 140 non-physics STEM departments, and 60 non-STEM (social sciences, arts, business, humanities departments worldwide (Foote et al. 2014). This number has increased as of mid-2015, when 259 colleges and universities have reported their SCALE-UP implementation to Beichner via the SCALE-UP website.
- Requires structural changes. One of the prominent features of SCALE-UP is the redesigned room. A previous study hypothesized that the room may facilitate the spread of SCALE-UP (Foote et al. 2014). Understanding the role of physical changes in education innovation is relevant not only to SCALE-UP but also other structural innovations.

As indicated by the widespread usage, SCALE-UP has numerous secondary implementers, faculty, and staff who have adopted the SCALE-UP innovation and created classrooms in their institutions.

Because there are many secondary implementers, fidelity to the original design varies. Although SCALE-UP has recommended room features as described by Beichner (see Table 3 for specific room features), secondary implementers do not always, and are not expected to, strictly adopt the SCALE-UP recommended layout from the NCSU development site. This may be obvious to some readers, but in our experiences, there sometimes are misconceptions that the room design must include all recommended features in order to do SCALE-UP. The SCALE-UP website includes recommendations for different designs (Beichner 2015) based on room size, shape, and class size. Practical constraints, such as current building architecture and costs, also limit what is possible. Beichner (2014) stresses maximizing student-student interactions, and fulfilling the learning goals of the instructor should be primary considerations when developing a SCALE-UP classroom.

Lack of SCALE-UP abandoners speaks to the significance of the room

This paper is a part of a larger study on SCALE-UP secondary implementation. Our initial intent was to study both successful and unsuccessful (i.e., abandoned) implementations of SCALE-UP, defining abandoned SCALE-UP users as those who had modified a classroom but then no longer used the room and were not likely to do so in the future. Those who had considered SCALE-UP but did not create a classroom were not included, as they did not implement the innovation.

In our initial survey which was used to identify the sample reported on in this paper, no clear abandoners were identified. We then set out to find them by posting on LISTSERVs such as PHYSLrnr and PHYS-L, asking for information on abandoned implementations either through direct involvement or through rumor. In the end, we received ten emails that identified ten possible abandoners. We were only able to identify one site that had once implemented SCALE-UP with a redesigned room that is no longer doing SCALE-UP and did not foresee doing it again in the near future, along with one site that abandoned SCALE-UP but would consider trying again. The site that considered revisiting SCALE-UP in the future had one semester where students were enthusiastic toward it and another semester where they were not, resulting in poor grades and low instructor evaluations. The one genuine abandoner has several possibilities why they abandoned it including the lack of departmental buy-in, the room located in a building that was infrequently used by other faculty in the department, and that SCALE-UP was not significantly different enough from current teaching practices to justify the logistical challenges entailing equipment.

This is indicative that if a SCALE-UP implementation can get as far as having an appropriately designed classroom space, there is an excellent chance it will be sustained. In contrast, Henderson et al. (2012) found in a survey of USA physics faculty that approximately one third of faculty who report tying a research-based instructional strategy in general abandon it. The significance of the room to SCALE-UP is why it is the focus of this paper. We want to explore not only the process of secondary SCALE-UP implementation but also what specifically about the room makes SCALE-UP implementation sustained.

Implementation of educational innovations

SCALE-UP reforms both the classroom space and pedagogy. In order for any innovation, SCALE-UP or otherwise, to be implemented successfully, the organizational climate should be supportive of the implementation (Klein and Sorra 1996; Zhu and Engels 2013). Collaborative efforts at implementation can lead to more successful adoption than those who attempt to implement an innovation individually (Zhu and Engels 2013). The literature in this section makes two important claims about secondary implementations.

Innovations are typically modified to match local characteristics

When sites adopt innovations developed at other institutions, they become secondary implementers. Educational innovations are often modified during secondary implementations due to both institutional differences and various constraints (Henderson and Dancy 2011). Constraints can include the ability to purchase equipment and modify organizational structures to accommodate the change (Wejnert 2002). Institutional differences mean that secondary adopters may need to make adjustments due to aspects such as class size and student population (Henderson and Dancy 2011). Regardless of institution type, instructors who adopt teaching innovations all face time constraints that hinder use (Henderson et al. 2012). With the diversity among SCALE-UP adopters, institutional differences may impact what each implementation looks like.

Training and other teaching support can ease implementation difficulties

There are significant challenges involved in making instructional changes. Some of these challenges can be minimized through training and support. For example, providing an archive of previous course materials is useful for subsequent instructors (Chasteen et al. 2011). However, simply handing over materials is rarely sufficient; instructors generally need more support (Chasteen et al. 2011).

Workshops on educational innovations can expose instructors to research-based instructional strategies and provide motivation to try these strategies (Frank et al. 2004; Henderson et al. 2012). However, in addition to providing exposure to an innovation, workshops should provide advice to help adopters overcome challenges they are likely to encounter during implementation (Henderson and Dancy 2007). One example of thorough training is at the University of Iowa. Based on faculty feedback, Florman (2014) developed comprehensive training to cover various topics in-depth, such as course transformation and technology use.

Part of this study describes how secondary sites provide training and other support and the perceived impact of that. Although the room is an important piece of implementing SCALE-UP, past studies have shown that learning gains will not increase unless the pedagogy changes to include the interactivity that the room was designed to facilitate (Cummings et al. 1999; Rogers et al. 2015). Providing training is one way to help instructors change their teaching and promote successful implementation.

Room design literature

Both K-12 and higher education research has examined issues surrounding classroom design. Although the context is different, some of the findings in the K-12 literature apply to higher education. This section provides an overview of the classroom design literature relevant to this study.

Classroom layout can impact teaching practices

Literature suggests that the physical classroom space has a critical role in changing teaching practice and subsequently, can affect, student learning (Martin 2002; Taylor 2009; Brooks 2011). For example, seating where students face one another, such as U-shape or circular configuration, more readily allows for class discussions (Rosenfield et al. 1985; Bonus and Riordan 1998), clustered desks facilitate cooperative group activities (Bonus and Riordan 1998), and classrooms where students are seated in rows result in higher levels of instructor presentation and direction (Martin 2002).

Active learning environments include strategic seating arrangements. These classrooms often include special tables to promote face-to-face interaction, as well as whiteboards, and computers. These tools can facilitate collaborative learning, help foster student-teacher relationships, and allow students to take ownership of their learning (Taylor 2009; Whiteside et al. 2009; Harvey and Kenyon 2013).

The research literature on active learning environments documents positive impacts of these spaces on attitudes and performance. Students frequently enjoy these spaces in comparison to traditional classrooms (Whiteside et al. 2009; Walker et al. 2011). Students perform better in active learning classrooms over traditional classrooms, even when controlling for factors such as ACT scores and instructor use of active learning methods (Walker et al. 2011; Cotner et al. 2013; Keiner and Gilman 2015). In other words, using active learning instructional strategies in a classroom designed for active learning is more effective than trying to use active learning in a traditional classroom designed for instructor presentation.

Some classroom designs pose challenges for activities such as test taking. Clustered desks, for example, allow for group work but would not be ideal for test taking. However, this challenge can be overcome by using temporary partitions during test time (Rogers et al. 2015). We wanted to collect information like this about challenges that secondary adopters encounter and share potential solutions.

Active learning environments are not standardized, so room characteristics and thus, their impacts, can vary. There have been efforts to create an active learning certification system similar to the LEED green building certification so implementers can understand how well their classrooms facilitate active learning (Felix and Brown 2011). The existing certification described by Felix and Brown, however, is mostly conceptual or based on action, e.g., students and instructors are able to easily interact. In this study, we hope to identify specific room elements that are helpful and unhelpful so secondary implementers who may have budget or other restrictions can prioritize their renovations.

Although the classroom layout impacts teaching practices, the instructor must be aware of the goals in their lessons and understand how the classroom design supports or hinders these goals when they set up their classrooms (Bonus and Riordan 1998; Lippman 2010). In other words, the instructor needs to know how to use the classroom. One area we were interested in exploring is how instructors learn to teach in an active learning classroom.

Technology is often not used to its fullest extent

Implementing technological innovations is often challenging. Even when technology is readily available, teachers may opt not to use it or use it in ways that do not make full use of its potential (Cuban 2001). For example, clicker technology can be used as formative feedback so the instructor can modify the lesson plan to address difficulties in real time. However, clickers are often not used in this way and instead used as a way to take attendance or give quizzes. Multiple obstacles, such as a lack of time to develop materials suitable for technology use (Cuban 2001) and the possibility of technological failures (e.g., a website that continues to crash) (Cuban 2001; Frank et al. 2004) deter teachers from using technology to its fullest extent. Since technology can be the most expensive items in the SCALE-UP room redesign, it will be important to understand how this technology is used to ensure that the investment is worthwhile.

Technology in higher education courses can be used effectively, although the use is nuanced. Students generally react positively to classroom use of laptop computers that allow for easier collaboration and channels for feedback (Barak et al. 2006). However, computer usage should be done judiciously. Instructors must recognize the limitation of technological capabilities (Lippman 2010) which can also negatively impact learning. For example, some students find laptop usage distracting and may engage in unrelated online activities (Barak et al. 2006).

Instructor decision-making about using technology is complex. Although administrators may be supportive and provide technology, instructor use of the technology often varies (Cuban 2001). Lasry et al. (2014) found that only about half of the instructors changed their teaching methods when placed in a redesigned classroom configured with technology. Instructors must see value in technology use for student learning in order for it to be adopted (Beggs 2000; Samarawickrema and Stacey 2007). Similar to adopting other educational innovations, instructors have competing responsibilities that take precedent over learning to use technology effectively (Cuban 2001). Instructors may not be willing to invest the time needed to learn the technology or to develop new materials that are compatible with the technology. Training or hiring a technology specialist can ease these burdens (Beggs 2000). In the SCALE-UP classroom implementation context, the benefits of technology alongside the challenges should be better understood in order to support secondary implementation, especially since technology can be an expensive part of renovation.

Summary

For the adoption of innovation to be successful, there should be support for those who will be using the innovation. Specific to structural educational innovations, we see that the classroom makes a difference in how instructors teach and students learn, but instructors must change their teaching in order to use the classroom's capabilities effectively. Research suggests that redesigning the classroom can help facilitate more effective interactive instruction if instructors are willing to change practice accordingly.

Research also suggests that instructors can underutilize sophisticated technology that often accompanies active learning classrooms. Similar to the general research on innovation adoption, instructors need assistance and time to develop materials suitable for technology use. These findings are relevant to SCALE-UP, as the radical overhaul of the room design suggests the need for professional development to support effective use.

Current research gap

The current body of research has some important gaps that this study addresses. By studying 21 secondary implementations of SCALE-UP, we are able to provide an in-depth look at specific aspects related to classroom design. For example, as discussed above, secondary implementers typically modify innovations due to their institutional setting and situational constraints. We will identify whether secondary implementers share similarities in their use of the rooms and typical modifications.

This study also looks at the support provided to instructors to help them use the redesigned classroom successfully. Although the relationship between the classroom environment and instructional practices is discussed in the literature, there is no mention of whether and how instructors receive professional development or other forms of support to use active learning or innovative spaces. This will help adopters know how to support the faculty that teach in these room and, hopefully, increase the likelihood of success.

Lastly, we wanted to see if classrooms have further-reaching effects on the institution and instructional practices in non-redesigned classrooms. This area is largely unexplored in prior literature.

Research questions

As mentioned previously, our main research goal is to better understand how secondary sites implement radically redesigned classrooms and support instructor use of student-centered pedagogy in these rooms. We believe this is an essential question to be asked by anyone interested in educational reform as the design of the classroom highly influences the nature of what occurs in the classroom.

Our research questions delve into descriptive aspects as well as outcomes associated with the room in order to provide recommendations to anyone interested in creating and using an active learning classroom. This study is also relevant for those interested in initiating radical, structural reforms in general.

1. How was the classroom space initiated?
   (a) Who was involved in the classroom space initiation?
   (b) Do initial teams have any subsequent impact on SCALE-UP spread?
   (c) How was the room financed?
2. What are the characteristics of the classroom space?
   (a) How did the implemented classroom characteristics compare to the recommended classroom characteristics?
   (b) What characteristics were considered helpful? Non-essential? Unhelpful?
   (c) Were additional classrooms built? If so, did subsequent classrooms differ from the initial model?
3. What training or support was offered to instructors who teach in the redesigned classroom space?
   (a) What kinds of support or training are provided?
   (b) Did implementers need to modify subsequent support and training from their initial implementation at the institution?
4. What indirect effects did the new classroom space have at the institution?

Methods

The interview participants for this study were identified from the respondents of a previous SCALE-UP-related survey that created a census of instructors who were using SCALE-UP or similar studio-style instructional strategies (Foote et al. 2014). The survey was administered between December 2012 and August 2013 and included questions about how respondents learned about SCALE-UP, room features, longevity of SCALE-UP usage, and interactions with others related to SCALE-UP. We received 659 responses out of approximately 1300 invitations sent. More information about the survey can be found elsewhere (Foote et al. 2014; Neumeyer et al. 2014).

Sample

We used survey responses to select "successful" implementations of SCALE-UP to study. For our purposes, we defined a successful SCALE-UP implementation as meeting at least one of the following requirements:

1. Multiple departments in a single institution were using SCALE-UP (i.e., high penetration within an institution).
2. Over 60 % of introductory classes in a department were taught using a SCALE-UP style pedagogy (i.e., high penetration within a department).
3. The implementation had been in place for six or more years (i.e., high longevity).
4. Interview participants were named as a source of information by many other survey participants (i.e., high degree centrality in the social network of SCALE-UP dissemination) (Neumeyer et al. 2014).

Only US-based institutions were selected in order to ensure cultural uniformity.

Additionally, a site was only considered to be a true SCALE-UP implementer if they reported the existence of a specialized room with tables to facilitate group learning. We contacted interviewees who survey respondents identified as "key contacts" about the SCALE-UP reform effort.

We contacted 63 key informants based on our criteria above, and 31 agreed to be interviewed. Five pilot interviews were used to refine the interview protocol. We eliminated five interviews because the conversation revealed the implementation did not meet our selection criteria. Our final interview sample used for analysis consisted of 21 faculty, administrators, and staff who were heavily involved with 21 unique SCALE-UP implementations. They represent 19 institutions, with two institutions having two departmental implementations that occurred independent of each other. Institutions are referred by a letter name (e.g., institution A). If two people are interviewed from the institution, they are referred to with an additional number (e.g., institution A-1).

Our sample consisted of 12 doctoral/research institutions, 6 master's colleges and universities, and 1 associate college (Carnegie Classifications 2010). Using the US Census regions, these institutions lie in the northeast ($N = 3$), south ($N = 7$), midwest ($N = 5$), and west ($N = 4$). Thirteen institutions are public, 5 private, and 1 is a community college. In this study, the interviewees discussed implementations in the following departments:

- 10 physics departments
- 3 biology departments
- 2 math departments
- 2 chemistry departments
- 2 engineering departments
- 2 multiple departments

We acknowledge that our sample is not large, and approximately 50 % of our key informants are based in physics departments. For the former limitation, we decided doing comprehensive interviews with fewer secondary implementers would provide more useful data than more interviews with less detail. The strong representation of physics departments is an artifact of studying SCALE-UP; the majority of secondary implementers are based in physics departments (Foote et al. 2014). Although this study has its limitations, the findings on how secondary implementers navigate their local settings to implement SCALE-UP do not appear to be unique to these institutions or to physics.

Interview protocol

Members of the research team (the authors) conducted semi-structured telephone interviews. We asked about room creation process (e.g., availability of funding and who was involved), room characteristics (including the original purpose of the space and usefulness of features), support/training provided, and any additional impact related to SCALE-UP. While we generally used the same interview protocol, the semi-structured nature allowed us to deviate from the protocol when the interviewee brought up an interesting point. To ensure a more uniform process, our interview protocol included multiple potential follow-up questions to explore.

Interviews were audio recorded and transcribed. This paper focuses on the classroom portion of SCALE-UP implementation, including who was involved in creating the room, sources of funding, a general description of the room, useful/not useful/non-essential room features, faculty training on using the room (e.g., professional development workshops), and additional impact of the room.

Analysis

All members of the research team worked together in an iterative process using a sub-sample of the interviews to develop a coding scheme and template for analysis. Two members of the research team then independently analyzed data using the coding scheme and guiding questions. The coding scheme was based on themes that appear in the literature, from prior research conducted in this study, and from the research team's experience. The guiding questions asked the following:

- Who was involved with obtaining a SCALE-UP room?
- How was the room funded?
- What kind of space was it (e.g., a new classroom, renovated space)?
- What is the classroom like (e.g., furnishings, room geometry, size)?
- What classroom characteristics are particularly helpful?
- What classroom characteristics are particularly unhelpful?
- What is the impact of the room on the institutional environment?
- What resources are available for faculty (e.g., professional development, curriculum support, teaching assistants)?

Emergent categories were developed from the guiding questions. Some categories were more straightforward to develop (e.g., identifying the source of funding), while others required more interpretation (e.g., whether secondary implementers truly worked in a team). These categories were refined throughout the analysis process. Coders examined each other's responses and resolved discrepancies by coming to consensus through discussion of why they interpreted the data the way they did.

Relevant categories will be introduced in the "Results" section as they become important. It is important to note that because this study used semi-structured interviews to identify emergent categories (and not a priori categories specifically asked about in the interview), the absence of an idea from a particular interviewee does not necessarily mean that this idea was not present in their SCALE-UP implementation. The interviewee may have not mentioned the item or identified it as important.

Results

This section begins with three SCALE-UP implementation stories from different types of institutions to provide some context to the results. These stories were selected because they represent similar circumstances that others in our sample have experienced. We then present the results in order of the research questions. Although some of the key findings may seem obvious, they are still important to acknowledge. SCALE-UP users have not always initially realized these key findings until much later in the process, even those in our sample identified actions and choices that are more significant in retrospect. We hope explicit acknowledgement will highlight their significance to potential secondary implementers.

Institution B is a large (over 50,000 undergraduates) research institution with a doctoral program.

Initiation: The biology department has a long history of valuing biology education, even hiring biologists who specialize in education. The interviewee was a university-level administrator who had been a tenured faculty member in institution B's biology department for many years. He felt that the biology department could improve their teaching. At the same time, the university was focusing on improving student retention. The interviewee "got together a faculty committee. We started talking about what we could do and decided that the first course of action would be to determine what were the most essential concepts that we wanted students to learn, our students to learn, during intro bio." Around the same time, the interviewee began attending national biology education research meetings. He noticed that educational resources for biology education increased, noting that the Vision and Change report (an influential biology education research report developed by the AAAS and NSF) had come out around this time. Influenced and inspired by this flurry of events, the faculty committee decided to adopt a studio-style approach.

Funding: Importantly, at this time, the university implemented program fees. The biology department applied to receive some of those fees to support the development of a SCALE-UP classroom: "We were asked to submit a proposal that had to be cleared by pretty much everyone at the university, including the students. Since I had been thinking about this stuff, we had a very mature proposal." The funding allowed them to create a classroom and hire an instructional designer.

Characteristics of classroom: For their first implementation, they renovated an unused classroom into a studio space modeled after SCALE-UP. They built an additional classroom after the first classroom was met with positive reactions. The additional classroom can accommodate 96 students and can be partitioned so that the room is split in half with each side having 48 students. The SCALE-UP room accommodates fewer students than a typical course; the large biology classes at institution B typically enroll 200–300 students but can be as large as 450. There are tables for student groups, computers, and projection screens.

Support for faculty: The implementation efforts included providing significant support to faculty teaching in the redesigned room. Besides an instructional designer hired to help "flip" classrooms, a curriculum specialist was hired to support course redesign, and a recent faculty hire runs professional development for teaching assistants.

Impact: The classroom has generated interest in active learning, both within and outside of the university: "People saw what we were doing with our intro bio and there's a lot of interest in that; there's also a lot of interest in all the community colleges in this state because they follow what we do a lot. I've done presentations to the undergraduate programs people at community colleges across the state."

Institution F is a master's level university with approximately 10,000 undergraduates.

Initiation: The interviewee from institution F had a background in physics education research and desired to teach in a more interactive fashion. The physics introductory courses had a history of high DFW rates and student complaints. This interviewee and a colleague in the physical sciences department were interested in SCALE-UP and visited NCSU to observe a class and participate in a workshop. The department chair was excited that faculty wanted to improve teaching in the department and gave permission to modify an existing classroom.

Funding: Funding for the first classroom came from dissemination funds from Beichner's NSF grant. The first classroom was created with modest changes: "They were willing to let us take a classroom and basically pull out all of the individual chairs and then put up whiteboards around the room. That's basically what we started with." After their initial classroom was created, more classrooms were needed due to increasing student population in the university. This created opportunities to have more classrooms renovated for SCALE-UP style teaching. These classrooms were funded through various channels: a colleague's overhead funds, department funds, and university funds that were allocated for furniture."

Characteristics of classroom: The classrooms have hexagonal tables, white boards, projectors, and easy access to lab equipment. They have three classrooms of differing sizes, ranging from 36 to 72 students.

Support for faculty: Although no formal training program exists, faculty members unfamiliar with SCALE-UP frequently shadow more experienced instructors by serving as a backup instructor to the more experienced instructor.

Impact: Having the classroom has encouraged colleagues in chemistry and biology to adopt active learning pedagogies in their teaching:

"Other people have started teaching in the rooms and they also saw the efficacy of having students be able to interact with each other and be able to engage the students a little bit more actively in the classroom.... they have adopted the kind of learning environment that the classroom setup supports. So there's colleagues in chemistry and in biology who routinely request the SCALE-UP classrooms when we're not actually using them."

Institution O is a doctoral-granting research university with approximately 15,000 undergraduates.

Initiation: The interviewee, a physics faculty member, was interested in SCALE-UP years before and had visited NCSU but did not believe it was possible to implement it at his university for unspecified reasons. Years later, his dean assigned the interviewee and another faculty member to investigate better teaching methods that could remedy high failure rates in an introductory course: "The dean had gotten a lot of complaints from [another department], 'cause they'd admitted [students] and they were absolutely perfect [for their major] on paper... and they weren't passing physics properly, or at an acceptable rate, so the dean charged me and a faculty member in math to research methods to approach this."

Funding: After visiting another SCALE-UP site and receiving funds from the dean for their initial room, an old classroom was converted for a pilot of the innovation. This classroom received major renovation: removing previous features of the room. The pilot classroom featured large round tables and laptops with a capacity of 42 students. One of the challenges was that the first room was too small. The pilot had good initial results so the dean provided more funding to create more classrooms.

Characteristics of classroom: The interviewee recalled that the subsequent rooms received major renovation: "Three of [our SCALE-UP rooms] started classrooms with theater style seating—it was flat, but it was that; and the other three rooms were former labs; we just took everything out. In both cases, we took everything out and rebuilt." Although subsequent classrooms were also heavily renovated, these classrooms were slightly different from the pilot classroom. They changed the tables to D-shaped tables so students could see the board and interact with one another. They added projectors to the room as well. These rooms could accommodate 42 students.

Support for faculty: Some professional development has been offered. The university provided money to bring Beichner to run a workshop. Other support offer includes shadowing, weekly SCALE-UP meetings, and undergraduate learning assistants.

Impact: The math department started using more SCALE-UP style teaching. Numerous faculty members from other departments have seen the classroom and become interested in teaching in it. As the university is growing, the department is working on creating more SCALE-UP classrooms.

Although these three implementations occurred in different ways, they have similarities, some of which are shared by the other implementations. The following sections discuss common themes by answering the research questions.

Research question #1: how was the classroom space initiated?

In order to have the SCALE-UP classroom space, adopters need to figure out logistics. At higher education institutions, this is often a collaborative decision because instructors typically share classrooms and do not have the power to renovate a classroom alone. This section delves into these aspects of SCALE-UP room implementation. In particular, we explore the important role of administrators in these implementations.

Who was involved in the classroom space initiation?

As mentioned previously, the development of SCALE-UP classroom space often involves multiple people. The types of people involved in the implementations we studied are summarized in Table 1.

Table 1 Summary of types of people involved in SCALE-UP initiation

	Initial source of information ($N = 21$)	Team creator (out of 14 institutions with teams)	Team composition (out of 14 institutions with teams)
Faculty	11	4	14
Administrator	7	7	10
University-level	4	5	8
Department chair	3	2	2
Faculty development staff	2	1	4
Non-instructional staff	–	–	3
Unknown	1	2	–

The first step in implementing a SCALE-UP room is that an individual must learn about SCALE-UP and initiate discussions about the possibility of implementing it. The implementation process often began when an individual found out about SCALE-UP and began conversations that led to the adoption of SCALE-UP as shown in the institution B and F stories. Individuals reported learning about SCALE-UP through a variety of channels, such as conferences or site visits. These "initiating" individuals held a variety of roles in the institutions we studied:

- Regular faculty ($N = 11$)
- University administrators ($N = 4$)
- Department chairs ($N = 3$)
- Faculty development staff ($N = 2$)
- Unknown ($N = 1$)

We note that the conversation starters are roughly evenly divided between regular faculty and individuals at higher levels in the institution (including department chairs, faculty development staff, and other administrators).

Although individuals started the conversations, a majority of implementations ($N = 14$) involved a team. Teams were created for a variety of reasons including generating interest from faculty and supporting staff who would undertake resolving logistical matters such as scheduling or equipment use. At institution C, a university administrator created a team for pragmatic design reasons: "[The administrator] didn't want to just [create a room] based on what one person wanted; he wanted to make sure to include it in terms of all the disciplines and different ways people might want to use it." By including representatives from multiple disciplines, the room had greater potential to serve multiple purposes and ensure instructors' needs were met. Faculty also worked together to make sure that the curriculum was suitable for the classroom.

The nature of these teams varied considerably in their creation. Teams were assembled by faculty ($N = 4$), university administrators ($N = 5$), department chairs ($N = 2$), or faculty development staff ($N = 1$). For the other teams, it is unclear how they were created. The diversity of team creators in our sample suggests that "top-down" (administrator-driven) or "bottom-up" (faculty-driven) approaches can both lead to successful team creation.

The teams varied in composition (faculty, staff, administrators) and size. All 14 teams had some faculty participation. Teams also had participation from university administrators ($N = 8$), department chairs ($N = 2$), faculty development staff ($N = 4$), and non-instructional staff, such as a technology specialist ($N = 3$). Some teams were small and strictly faculty, while others were larger and included people in different roles. For example, as shown in two of our example cases, institution F's team was a pair of faculty while institution B involved a university-level administrator (the interviewee) and multiple faculty members (those who were serving on the committee to improve biology education).

Summary In our study, both faculty members and administrators initiated discussions about developing a SCALE-UP room. These individuals did not usually work alone to develop a room; implementations typically relied on teams. These teams were most commonly created by department heads or administrators and consisted of faculty, administrators, and staff. Having the team composed of both regular faculty and administrators is likely the most effective as both groups bring their own experiences, perspectives, and abilities to inform decisions related to the reform.

Do initial teams have any subsequent impact on SCALE-UP spread?

Although the primary purpose of the team is to create the initial room, the involvement of team members may not end once the room is created. Team members may work on creating additional rooms or encourage faculty who were not on the team to use the room or active learning techniques (i.e., spread the innovation beyond immediate team).

Other faculty members or departments that were not initially involved sometimes become interested in SCALE-UP, helping the innovation diffuse or "spread" beyond the initial course or department and be used in other courses or departments. Of the five teams that mentioned spread, two faculty-created teams noted that SCALE-UP or active learning teaching techniques have been adopted by other instructors at their institution while three administrator-created teams noted spread. The presence of an administrator on the team appears to impact whether or not SCALE-UP spreads throughout a department and/or to other departments.

These initial teams also can determine who controls the space and thus, who is allowed to teach in the room. When the university schedules the space, it can become easier for instructors from any discipline to use the space. Interviewee R explains

> "[Our studio-style classrooms] are scheduled by our central classroom scheduling. Now the fact that the building is in a building that's called [biology] building, means that, means that I guess we have a little nod to priority… But other people had access to teach in it."

Other times, the department that starts the innovation has first-priority access to the space. Interviewee E-1 noted that multiple classrooms were created in his department's building and indicated that the rooms were primarily for their department's courses. Because they decided to teach all the sections of one large introductory course in the studio-style, instructors were assigned to these rooms. Subsequently, another course within their department was converted to teaching in the studio-style. This suggests that university-controlled space may be better suited for spreading SCALE-UP around the institution, while department-controlled space may be better suited for spread within the department.

Summary Having an administrator on teams can help encourage spread of SCALE-UP. University-level administrators can help spread through converting courses to use SCALE-UP or creating university-controlled spaces and allowing others outside of the department to use it.

How was the room financed?

Although the costs can vary considerably, funding is almost always needed to create a SCALE-UP room. A lack of funding for redesigning a room is a challenge (Foote et al. 2014), but as our interviewees indicate, this is a challenge that can be overcome.

Table 2 displays the different funding sources for the initial room. Most interviewees reported that funding came from the institution ($N = 14$). Within institutions, though, funding sources varied considerably with approval provided by department chairs, deans (e.g., dean of academic affairs, dean of the college), the provost, the institution's president, and facilities management. Typically ($N = 17$), this funding was used to convert existing classroom space into a SCALE-UP room and included minor renovations as well as purchasing furniture, technology, and white boards. In some cases ($N = 4$), funding for the initial SCALE-UP room occurred as part of a new building or scheduled renovation rather than a separate initiative focused only on implementing SCALE-UP.

The means of gaining approval for institutional funds varied considerably and include

Table 2 Funding sources for the initial room

Funding source	Count (N = 21)	Example source
Institutional (department and university)	14	Provost
External/government funding	4	Education improvement grant
Unknown	3	–

- Direct contact with a university-level administration ($N = 7$). Some interviewees simply had a conversation with a university-level administrator and asked that an already scheduled renovation include a studio-style classroom. One interviewee gave a presentation to the provost that featured data they had collected on learning gains from an active learning pilot classroom and were granted funds for a more suitable SCALE-UP classroom. A different interviewee sent out a general invitation on an institutional email list, inviting interested parties to her classroom to observe the active learning techniques she was using in a traditional classroom. An administrator attended one of her classes and became interested supporting these efforts.
- Contact with the department chair ($N = 3$). Department chairs sometimes helped instructors in their department obtain funds from institutional-level administration. Details were not provided.
- Using connections on a previously existing team to obtain funding ($N = 4$). Interviewees were a part of a team tasked with improving undergraduate education. They sometimes recommended SCALE-UP to achieve these goals.

As a repeating pattern, we find that there is not one way and many possible avenues can lead to success.

Although institutional funding was the most common source of funding, it was not the only source. Another funding source was external/government funding ($N = 4$). At one institution, the faculty had received an external grant prior to considering SCALE-UP and was able to use that money to redesign the classroom. Another institution partnered with the SCALE-UP developer to write a grant proposal for external funding. Similar to university funding, these funds were used to renovate existing instructional space into a SCALE-UP classroom.

In institutions where subsequent rooms were developed, funding sources were similar to the first room. In one case, an institution received financial support for subsequent SCALE-UP rooms from alumni.

Summary Our interviewees primarily funded their SCALE-UP room from the institution, drawing from different offices. There is no "right" person or office to ask for funds nor is there a "right" approach for asking; internal funding sources varied considerably from implementation to implementation. While simply asking for funding worked for some of these interviewees, others demonstrated the benefits of active learning use to argue that a more suitable classroom would be an asset for their teaching. Others were working in a team to improve undergraduate education and used the opportunity to propose SCALE-UP. If a renovation project is already scheduled with allocated funds, implementers may just need to request a SCALE-UP style renovation. We note that finding funding was not always easy for our interviewees. Identifying a receptive audience and presenting SCALE-UP as a solution to an administrator concern (e.g., high DFW rates) can help.

Research question #2: what are the characteristics of the classroom space?

When planning to develop a SCALE-UP room, it is necessary to carefully think about the characteristics of the room. This section examines the room characteristics identified by our interviewees and compares these to the room characteristics suggested by Beichner.

Initial SCALE-UP classrooms typically involved renovating existing space ($N = 17$). Classroom renovations varied in scope from adding a few pieces of equipment and furnishings to significant construction, depending on what was already available. This suggests that a classroom may only require minor modifications to be used as a SCALE-UP classroom if the classroom already has some of the suggested features.

How did the implemented classroom characteristics compare to the recommended classroom characteristics? Which classroom features are helpful? Unhelpful? Non-essential?

Implementers need to make decisions about which room features to include in a SCALE-UP room based on available resources and constraints (e.g., funding, typical class sizes). We were interested in which features were included in each of these successful implementations and how important they were to the interviewees.

Although some features are explicitly absent, some features may be present but just not mentioned by the interviewee. We did not explicitly ask the interviewees about the presence of each feature, but general questions regarding what was in their SCALE-UP rooms and what they found helpful and unhelpful. As is the case throughout this paper, it is important to keep in mind that these were open-ended interviews. Interviewees may have commented on more features if we had asked them directly.

Although not a room characteristic, three interviewees explicitly stated that having a dedicated classroom in general was helpful. For example, the interviewee from institution J explained: "it's the pedagogy that is facilitated greatly by the classrooms." The interviewee from institution R elaborated on this point: "That the space itself, and maybe I had not appreciated how much of our behavior is driven by the physical environment in which we are. And so the room itself can be a partner or a barrier in whatever it is that you want to do, and for active learning it's an enormously powerful partner." Some implicit evidence suggests that the dedicated room is helpful; one or more additional classrooms were created at 16 of the institutions, and 2 institutions indicate that they would like to have additional classrooms.

As for the details of the room, Table 3 shows the frequency of room characteristics reported by the interviewees. The categories are the recommended features as noted by Beichner on the SCALE-UP website. We included a broad "technology" category to encompass features such as computers, projection screens, and other items that are colloquially referred to as technology, because some interviewees were not specific. We note whether the specific characteristic was explicitly mentioned and also indicate how frequently the mentioned features were noted as being helpful, unhelpful, or non-essential (an item that did not hinder teaching but could be removed without affecting the use of the pedagogy).

Few features are explicitly absent. Some of these features were likely present even if they were not mentioned. For example, poor acoustics are usually noticeable because they make communication difficult, but good acoustics may go unnoticed and unmentioned by the interviewee.

Sometimes, implementers need to make deviations from the recommended features based on various factors including budget, classroom needs, and room geometry. The interviewee from institution J stated that one department deliberately chose a different table design for a combination of the aforementioned reasons:

> "There's a single screen and they set that up for a particular approach [for that department]. It's a small room and they wanted everybody focused on the same image at the same time, but they also wanted to do team-based inquiry guided learning, so they can do that at those [crescent-shaped tables], and it's not very cash heavy at all, it didn't cost much money. They decided there was this particular need served better by these tables and a front to the room."

This department demonstrates that one may be able to find a way to balance the needs of instructors with different instructional styles.

The frequency of features mentioned by interviewees is similar to previous survey data (Foote et al. 2014). The following subsections delve into the details of why interviewees perceive features as helpful or not.

Features that support collaboration are perceived as helpful Tables to promote group interactions and white boards are among the most frequently mentioned features. While many users follow the suggested large class model and use large round tables, other users choose different shapes including D-shaped tables, hexagonal tables, and cross-shaped tables.

In addition to being the most frequently named features, tables and white boards were also most frequently named as helpful. Interviewees named tables for students ($N = 7$) and whiteboards ($N = 5$) as a helpful room feature, because they help students to interact with one another. Although they are separate features, tables and white boards work in conjunction to support peer collaboration as the interviewee from institution T noted: "What people really say they love are the whiteboards and the round tables, students working in teams."

One specific benefit of the collaborative workspace is that the students can see that they are not the ones

Table 3 Current room characteristics mentioned in interviews ($N = 21$)

Feature	Explicitly present	Explicitly absent	Helpful	Unhelpful	Non-essential
Tables to promote group interactions	21	–	6	–	–
Technology[a]	21	–	3	2	2
Video screens	12	–	–	–	–
Computers for student use	10	–	–	–	–
Instructor station for use	7	–	–	–	–
Student white boards	17	–	5	–	–
Rolling, armless, un-upholstered chairs	1	–	–	–	–
Large enough room to avoid crowding, as close to square as possible	–	3	–	3	–
Adequate space between tables to facilitate instructor roaming (absolute minimum table spacing of 5′ edge to edge)	–	–	–	–	–
Good acoustics (carpeting, ceiling tile, quiet HVAC)	–	–	–	–	–

[a]We noted both the general use of technology as well as specific types of technology. Because implementers sometimes use multiple types of technology (e.g., video screens and computers for student use), the general technology category and the sum of the specific technology categories are not equal

challenged by the material, as the interviewee from institution R explained

> "That table creates a little microcosm, a supportive microcosm that helps you be part of a—you're not alone, you're not suffering alone, you're not struggling alone; you're realizing that it's a hard thing that everybody in the team is having trouble with that idea, or you know, 'I'm just as smart as everybody else' and I think there's real power in that from the student perspective."

As this interviewee suggests, the interactions can bolster student confidence and efficacy.

The table setup also benefits student-instructor interaction. Interviewee E-1 explained why tables are helpful

> "[One important feature to have is] student tables that foster peer instruction and group work and instructor access. From the instructor standpoint, when I taught SCALE-UP without the tables, it was really, really hard because I couldn't get easily to the students. It was like a gymnastic act to get into the middle of a long row to talk to a particular student or student team."

Flexible classrooms are perceived as helpful Some interviewees ($N = 4$) felt that having a flexible classroom, one in which they can rearrange all furnishings and equipment, was helpful. The interviewee from institution G liked being able to experiment with the room arrangement and recommended the following:

> "If you want faculty to innovate with set-ups in a classroom, it's got to be lightweight, something where the students themselves or the faculty can rearrange them in a couple minutes 'cause otherwise you're kind of stuck there unless you hire a crew to come in and move the tables around for you."

Beyond personal experimentation with the classroom configuration, it may be beneficial to have particular features that can be rearranged for students. The interviewee from institution N noted they designed the room to have movable smart boards: "The Smart Boards were also on movable stands, rather than attached to the walls, so they could be moved to whatever positions were suitable for the groups, while still making sure that everybody could see them."

Technology's usefulness is complicated While all interviewees noted some kind of technology was present in the rooms, it was often unclear as to whether it was helpful, non-essential, or unhelpful as either a general category and with specific types of technology (e.g., computer-based activities). Various pieces of technology were noted as helpful by three interviewees, for reasons ranging from generating faculty interest in the room and overcoming a room shape challenge to communicate with students to making some student activities easier. Some interviewees ($N = 3$) noted that they wish they had better technology in the classroom, with two who were unspecific and one who thought a remote control system to access the instructor computer would help overcome a difficult room geometry. It is interesting to note that similar to the interviewee who had communications troubles, this interviewee's use for technology was not to enhance student learning but to overcome room constraints.

However, technology is not always considered necessary in SCALE-UP classrooms. Two interviewees noted that technology was not helpful, with one due to time constraints, and two noted it was non-essential, believing that instructors can use active learning without computers.

While our results do not contradict prior research and resemble some of the challenges present in K-12 and higher education, they do suggest technology use for this style of teaching may be more related to instructor concerns or classroom layout issues rather than more directly to student engagement or learning. Technology may be more useful for student learning with better professional development.

Awkward room geometry and too small classroom size is perceived as unhelpful Few of the interviewees mentioned anything about the room size and shape. Those who did, however, noted that the room geometry was an issue ($N = 3$). Some of the rooms have layouts where students have difficulties accessing the instructor or seeing presentations, such as the L-shaped room at institution B or the long rectangular room from institution D-2. Some rooms are not large enough to accommodate as many students as the instructor would like. Although this may be an obvious issue to some, this is an issue where prospective implementers should be conscientious and perhaps advocate for a more suitable space.

Summary Having dedicated classroom space for SCALE-UP is important to encourage active learning. Although the recommended characteristics help facilitate studio-style teaching, successful SCALE-UP implementation may not need all the recommended characteristics. Deviations to the suggested model can work well as long as they are thoughtfully adapted to consider the purpose of the characteristics and the needs of the implementer.

While some deviations from the suggested room design can work, maintaining the intent of the recommended features is important. Interviewees specifically noted that features that allow for student collaboration (e.g., tables and white boards) are beneficial for both student-faculty and student-student interactions. The tables and whiteboards facilitate these interactions.

Instructors saw some value in having flexible classrooms, ones that can easily be rearranged. The flexibility appears to be for specific purpose, such as personal interest in experimenting with classroom configuration or overcoming a room shape. The authors of this paper acknowledge that these specific reasons are valuable to these users and that some features, such as chairs, benefit from mobility. However, we also note that too much flexibility means that the classroom can revert back to its original, pre-SCALE-UP state. Adopters should consider the purpose of having a flexible classroom and how flexible the classroom should be.

Technology was met with mixed results for SCALE-UP implementation. Our interviews identified that technology, in general, can help overcome difficulties in the room, but it does not seem to be the most critical aspect of a SCALE-UP room. For example, if the room has a poor layout, technology may be almost imperative to facilitate interaction. However, in many cases, it appears possible to develop a successful room with minimal technology.

Classroom size and geometry can be a hindrance if the room is too small or makes accessing students difficult. Because most SCALE-UP implementations happen in renovated classrooms, users may not have control over the geometry or size. When possible, as noted by Beichner, the room should be as close to square-shaped as possible so that the instructor and other staff can access all students easily.

Were additional classrooms built? If so, did subsequent classroom differ from the initial model?

Sites that begin with one SCALE-UP classroom often build additional classrooms so more instructors can teach using active learning techniques. We were interested in whether secondary adopters made any modifications to subsequent classrooms (e.g., choosing a different layout or different furnishings) and if so, why.

The majority of sites ($N = 16$) built additional rooms. They generally did not make major changes to their initial room design, suggesting that the design of the initial rooms were considered to be sufficient. When differences in subsequent rooms occurred, they often arose because of local logistics of new rooms to be renovated, such as size or shape rather than because features of previous rooms were deemed inadequate.

One implementer did intentionally change the initial room design in subsequent classrooms. The interviewee from institution Q did not have an ideal initial classroom due to institutional constraints. Students sat at long lab benches around the room. Upon institution Q's administration obtaining money for SCALE-UP rooms, they were able to renovate classrooms. The interviewee, comparing the new space to the previous room, remarked

> "It was night and day. The old one, some of the students were facing in the wrong direction. They really couldn't get together as groups and we didn't have much in the way of technology in the room. The new ones are really nice."

The newer classrooms had major improvements that made the classroom look like a typical SCALE-UP room. Subsequent classrooms contained tables for students to easily work in groups and technology (computers, lab equipment) that allowed for the student groups to work concurrently, without waiting for another group to complete their work. Institution Q's changes to the classroom speak to the importance of having furniture that allows for group work and how technology can be used effectively.

Summary Subsequent rooms are typically similar to initial rooms. This suggests that institutions are happy with their initial room designs and perhaps can be attributed to careful planning and use of resources such as those by Beichner on the SCALE-UP website, which all interviewees had access to, or through interacting with a SCALE-UP user. Knowledge is not enough, however, if the implementers cannot obtain key pieces such as suitable furniture.

Research question #3: what training or support was offered to instructors who teach in the redesigned classroom space?

Professional development has been emphasized in other work in order to ease the challenges instructors face in teaching in an unfamiliar style (Cummings et al. 1999; Rogers et al. 2015). As SCALE-UP is a departure from traditional teaching, instructors may be unsure how to change their practice and feel disoriented in the classroom. We were interested in the ways that instructors at these successful implementations learn how teach effectively in the room and what kinds of support (e.g., teaching assistants) are available and helpful. In this section, we examined the kinds of professional development and support that are offered to the instructors who use these rooms as well as why implementers offer training.

What kinds of support or training are provided?

Fourteen implementations mentioned offering training for users of the SCALE-UP room. The interviewee from institution O pointed out that active learning techniques may not have been experienced by instructors in any context: "you have to learn a different set of teaching skills [to teach using SCALE-UP] than probably you were exposed to as a student." The interviewee from institution R observed that lack of training prevented SCALE-UP use at a different institution: "I was at one place where the room was not used most of the time. They had invested a whole bunch of money, but the faculty weren't trained to use it yet. That to me just seems really not a good idea." Similarly, the interviewee from institution P preemptively created a professional learning community to support faculty teaching.

Training can help screen potential users of the room. The faculty member from institution T observed the need for instructor training for this reason: "We wanted to know why they needed that space. It's a huge capital investment so we wanted to know that whoever was teaching in there was converting their courses appropriately." Institution T requires that instructors apply to use the room and are trained.

The types of professional development offered at the 14 institutions that discussed professional development in the interviews include the following:

- Formal training programs ($N = 6$)
- Instructor shadowing ($N = 5$) and
- Informal training programs (often organized by the implementer) ($N = 3$)

At most institutions, training is optional ($N = 11$), while for others training is required in order to use the room ($N = 3$).

Formal training consisted of structured activities, such as the professional learning community at institution P or workshops. The length of formal training in our case studies varied from a 1-day session to multiple sessions over an academic semester. For example, institution U offers a weeklong training prior to the beginning of the academic year. The interviewee from institution U described

> "I would actually sit [the faculty] through my own [weekly studio course]. Teaching them what the class should look like, I kind of modeled the best practices and taking them through that. They actually would spend time working in groups completing these new labs, learning how to use the software, learning how to use the sensors, going through all of that process. I would have them write reflections at the end of the day, I would have them work together in groups, and all, any of the techniques I was using, I wrapped that into the course to help them teach them about the new technologies available in the room, the new lab equipment, what this should look like."

Shadowing, a specific type of informal training, entails observing a current instructor and occasionally, assisting with classroom activities once the novice instructor feels more comfortable. An example of shadowing is what institution H does

> "The best plan is that they come into my class and they spend the semester with me and see how it goes. I would hand off my stuff to them, and they would do it. So that's kind of the training program, if you will, it's a loose program. So there's no rigorous training, there's no boot camp to go through. We don't... leave someone to sink or swim; that would be bad."

Informal training can include unstructured faculty mentoring. For example, an experienced instructor might guide a novice instructor. Instructors may chat about teaching in the SCALE-UP room and offer advice. These conversations may lead to an informal learning community for instructor, where instructors troubleshoot and problem solve. This was the case with interviewee D-1's efforts to offer support for instructors. Faculty started by sharing course material, but then they became part of a "collaborative of people sharing new ways that they've tried to get across a concept or new ways of approaching a laboratory or how to integrate the laboratory with the concepts so they share all kinds of materials."

These three types of professional development suggest that there are multiple ways that instructors can become familiar with SCALE-UP. Although they may take different formats, the information may not be radically different. For example, the shadowing at institution H and the formal training at institution U both expose novice users to what the classroom and teaching in the classroom look like.

Although the implementers who offered professional development focused on completely inexperienced SCALE-UP instructors, continued professional development may also help. The interviewee from institution U noted that some instructors enroll in training more than once

> Some people might have even gone through the experience twice because "Oh, I'm not teaching it in the fall but who knows, I might be doing it in the spring," and so they would ahead and go through the workshop. And then they would go through the workshop again, [with the mindset of] "Okay, I've got a feel now but let's dig a little bit deeper."

Simply revisiting the material may be enough for faculty to gain more out of the material.

Professional development of undergraduate and graduate teaching assistants Because SCALE-UP entails a high-level student-instructor interaction, we were interested in what types of additional teaching staff is available to help with numerous groups and how this teaching staff is prepared to teach in the classroom. As our interviewees have indicated, training is necessary for instructors teaching in these classrooms. Is it also necessary for teaching assistants?

Approximately half of these institutions use undergraduate or graduate teaching assistants to support instruction in the SCALE-UP rooms ($N = 10$). All of the undergraduate teaching assistants ($N = 5$) are called learning assistants, and the majority ($N = 4$, with 1 unclear) adopted the University of Colorado's Learning Assistant model, which includes a pedagogy course for their training.

Extra teaching staff helps ensure more students receive the help they need, as described by the interviewee from institution C

> "One of the things we did when we did the large classrooms was we also included learning assistants, undergraduates, to help out with the group work and just be a bigger presence in the classroom to move around and handle those large numbers of students, help assist the faculty member with answering questions and things like that."

The learning assistants, who often have previously taken the course in which they work, serve a unique role in the classroom. They are able to act as role models for the students currently enrolled in the course and help them adjust to SCALE-UP, as the interviewee from institution R observed

> "I think that having the reality of somebody who's been through this class before and has learned to, has figured out how to learn well in that modality and has gone through the frustration, 'cause students are very frustrated that they aren't just lectured to and entertained; we found that early on to be very helpful in helping students come to grips with having to do something in class rather than just sit there. "

Although learning assistants are enrolled in a pedagogy course, they may receive additional training to support classroom activities. According to interviewee E-2, the institution has begun to create increasingly structured training materials to encourage faculty instructors and undergraduate assistants to use inquiry-based methods

> "We developed guiding questions that we would prepare our people with, both our faculty and our undergraduates, so that when students got stuck, rather than drifting toward just telling them what to do, they had more and more tools for helping the students push into a discovery of their own."

Although relatively rare ($N = 2$) in the cases examined in this study, training may be important to train graduate teaching assistants as well. The interviewee from institution Q explained why the institution felt teaching assistants needed additional training

> "It took us a while to realize that the graduate students needed training. We talked to them. We had some really two brief orientation sessions at the beginning of the year. But I want to say that we frankly were a little bit remiss, I guess, in not giving them more introduction into what it was we were trying to do."

At institution T, graduate students meet with the faculty instructors. She notes that these meetings depend on the faculty; some faculty may not provide any training for their graduate teaching assistants.

Summary Our interviewees found that professional development was necessary for faculty teaching in these rooms. Training can help instructors who are unfamiliar with SCALE-UP learn to teach in the room effectively and feel more confident in their ability to do so. Our interviewees demonstrate that professional development does not have to take one form, but there are common threads of showing novice SCALE-UP instructors how to teach in the classroom.

Like faculty, undergraduate and graduate student teaching assistants also benefit from professional development. If a department or institution adopts a learning assistant program, some of the training in active learning techniques may already be provided. Developing guides with examples of what questions to ask students may also be useful. In the case of institution Q, providing information on SCALE-UP through a short orientation is a small but perhaps important step.

Did implementers need to modify subsequent support and training from their initial implementation at the institution? Similar to why we were interested in whether modifications were needed for subsequent rooms, we were interested in whether implementers changed the professional development that they offered. Changes can provide insight to any challenges that the implementers found with their initial training offering or give clues as to what information and training should be included.

Of the 14 implementations providing professional development, only seven did from the beginning. The other seven added professional development, with two interviewees noted that this was done based on a recognized need. For example, one interviewee began weekly meetings when he realized other instructors were not using the room effectively. Another interviewee discussed adding training, because the instructors who would be using the room requested training. The motivations for adding training are unclear for the other five implementers, but some of these implementers were initially the only person teaching in the classroom. Perhaps they realized how daunting teaching in such a room could be and sought to lower the learning curve for subsequent users.

Research question #4: what indirect effects did the new classroom space have at the institution?

SCALE-UP focuses on activities and teaching within courses. In our interviews, we noted additional indirect benefits to institutions that developed a SCALE-UP room. Frequent themes included institutional pride (the institutions use the classroom as a positive symbol to show guests) and expanded active learning techniques beyond courses taught in the SCALE-UP room.

Institutions use the room to promote their image

Four institutions report that the SCALE-UP room is a source of institutional pride. Administration likes to show off the room to prospective students and other guests, for example, on a campus tour to prospective students or alumni.

The room can also ignite interest for alumni to donate. One institution was able to attract alumni support to fund further SCALE-UP construction. Interviewee E-2 described how this happened

> "While classes were in session, we'd invite [alumni or esteemed visitors] into our classes, but if classes weren't in session, we would hold a class for other people so they could see what we were doing. It resulted in additional support coming from the alumni base. Partially the idea was [to engage] the donors who aren't really interested in building a new building, and donors that aren't really interested in a statue or whatever. Some of those donors will be really interested in supporting a learning space, especially if they see the way that it works. That was another thing that was a conscious effort on our part to attract more money, more people, more converts to the movement, as it were."

Building and using the room encouraged active learning techniques more broadly

Eleven interviewees observed an increased interest in reformed teaching from other faculty or themselves, including an increase in teaching workshop attendance. Some of this may be creating an awareness of active learning techniques by offering professional development. The interviewee from institution L noticed that knowledge about science teaching varies from instructor to instructor: "I did a couple sessions myself on how do you teach active learning, how do you teach active, some of those people were already doing that, some people had some things to learn." While the provided professional development is primarily to help instructors learn how to use the room, there is greater benefit of faculty broadening their teaching repertoire.

This increased interest can change their instructional practices in classes that are not taught in the SCALE-UP classroom. Teaching in the SCALE-UP room is not always possible because of space (e.g., laboratory safety restrictions) and scheduling restrictions. Three interviewees said they started teaching their traditional courses differently, and three interview participants said they have more of a personal interest in generally using active learning techniques. The interviewee from institution F described the impact of teaching in the room on her teaching practice beyond teaching in the special rooms

> "I would say that like say, for example, in my upper division classes, I use a lot of the same kinds of techniques. I very rarely talk for very long, you know, so I really try as much as I can to make the students active in class in a variety of different ways... I taught a lecture-based physical science course for non-majors... using all the same methods and techniques in that class as well. For me personally, it doesn't make any sense to me to just try to talk to people and think that they're going to get it, you know?"

This suggests that teaching in the room can be transformative for the instructor.

Summary The SCALE-UP room can be leveraged to engage multiple populations and support institutional concerns outside of teaching. These include recruiting students and seeking funding from alumni. A SCALE-UP room also has additional benefits for teaching practice. Our findings suggest that the classroom can support the spread of active learning teaching techniques to other faculty and other courses taught in more traditional rooms. The presence of the classroom can aid the development of an institutional culture that is invested in teaching reforms.

Discussion

Our ultimate goal was to study successful implementations in order to offer guidance to those seeking to implement a

SCALE-UP-like reform at their own institution. Although each of the 21 SCALE-UP implementations we studied had unique initiation and implementation stories, we saw patterns that provide useful information for either future implementations or those wanting to improve current implementations. These data contribute to the current body of research providing insight on why and how secondary implementers modify the SCALE-UP innovation, what support can help instructors effectively use the room, and what additional impacts these classrooms can have on institutions and instructional practice. Below, we highlight and discuss recommendations that came from our analysis of these cases. While in many ways these recommendations may appear obvious, we are aware of many reform efforts that do not follow them.

Recommendation 1: initiate the reform as a team

As described above, all of the successful implementations we studied were the result of working with others. Many of these included a diverse group of individuals. This finding is in alignment with the finding that successful implementation should take place in a supportive environment (Klein and Sorra 1996; Zhu and Engels 2013) and that collaboration tends to be more successful than individuals attempting to implement an innovation (Zhu and Engels 2013).

A team approach (in contrast to the individual superhero model which we anecdotally find common in reform efforts) appears to have numerous benefits. Namely, we identified three primary benefits

1. Garnering interest across the department and university for building, supporting, and using a SCALE-UP room. Team members may have strong relationships with key administrators or access to resources. Interviewee E-1's initial classroom was funded because of help from his department chair asking the provost: "Our department chair was good at negotiating, you know, 'you give me this I'll give you that' kind of thing."
2. Creating a room that is serviceable for multiple users. Our interviewee from institution C pointed out that including perspectives from different disciplines can help create a room that suits multiple needs. Other users, regardless of discipline, may have preferences as well. This may help encourage more users for the room.
3. Receiving input from support staff to ensure smooth operations. Besides faculty, there are others involved with the day-to-day operations of a course. SCALE-UP usage often means staff may have to change their current systems. The interviewee from institution D identified seeking the technical staff's involvement, because they would have to "...do the nuts and bolts of putting these laboratories together."

Recommendation 2: include an administrator (departmental or institutional) on the team. Involvement of an administrator from the beginning can increase the likelihood that the implementation spreads to include more departmental courses and/or spreads to include more departments

Wejnert (2002) identified that the inability to modify organizational structures is a constraint to educational innovations. Our work may have found a way to mitigate this constraint. While administrators cannot completely overhaul the structure, they are positions to make changes as we saw in our data. Having an administrator on the team has clear benefits as administrators have the most control over university structures such as funding, scheduling, and professional development support. As we noted, most rooms in this study were built using internal funds that were provided by the administration. In short, getting administrative buy-in is important and getting buy-in is easier if administrations are part of the reform initiation team. By including an administrator from the beginning, the administrator likely will have better understanding of the innovation and its potential to improve student learning. At institution O, the dean asked our interviewee to seek out a solution for high failure rates in an introductory class. The dean was able and willing to invest more money into creating more classrooms after the initial classroom demonstrated promising results. The lack of buy-in from an administrator can also be issue for even simple changes, as interviewee from institution G saw: "I mean literally for, like, from 2002 until around 2000, let's say, 2008, I kept saying let's move them around and the chair just didn't do it."

In addition to increasing access to resources, administrators can help to spread the innovation through and across departments. For example, they can facilitate the collection of feedback to ensure rooms are built suitably for multiple disciplines as described above. Administrators can also facilitate spread by assigning others to the space or deciding to convert multiple traditional classrooms into university-controlled spaces available to faculty in other departments. Having multiple classrooms and multiple instructors using the classrooms may also help sustain innovation use. Multiple classrooms mean more instructors can access the innovation, and multiple instructors using the innovation means that the continued use does not rely on one individual.

Recommendation 3: persist in your search for funding to build a room and think creatively

Potential SCALE-UP adopters are often concerned about how to pay for a room. The perceived belief that funding is impossible leads efforts to cease. While we agree that funding is necessary and sometimes difficult to obtain, the stories of the implementers in this study demonstrate that it is not impossible and that it can be obtained through creativity and perseverance.

We note that there was no clear pattern of how funding was obtained, rather implementers found a variety of solutions. The funding sources ranged from alumni funds to grants to different institutional units, and the ways the sources were approached ranged from simple conversations to presentation to receiving help from one's department chair. This finding is reminiscent of Henderson and Dancy's (2011) finding that secondary implementers may need to make adjustments to educational innovations for their institution's characteristics. Those interested in obtaining a room should consider their institution and adjust accordingly when crafting their requests for funding. Knowing whom and how to ask is dependent upon the local situation.

Recommendation 4: be creative and resourceful in looking for classroom space

SCALE-UP rooms can be created from many different types of classroom space. Our interviewees' initial classrooms had many different formats, ranging from space in a new building to rearranging a pre-existing classroom and adding a few key pieces. This suggests that there is not one "right" type of space and that implementers should not feel that creating a SCALE-UP room involves heavy construction. The literature broadly finds that innovations are customized to local conditions (Henderson and Dancy 2011); the choice in classroom space is a reflection of local conditions. If there are opportunities to choose the space, issues such as whether students can see the instructor should be considered.

It is important to stay up-to-date with the institution's plans. Perhaps construction projects for new or renovated space can accommodate a SCALE-UP room. Otherwise, be aware of the possibilities of currently existing space. There may be classrooms available that require few modifications to work for a SCALE-UP room.

Recommendation 5: when designing a room, give priority consideration to features that facilitate collaboration and enable flexibility

Implementers, faced with constraints and their own unique outlook, may wonder how essential it is to follow all suggested features. No two implementations among our successful sites were identical, with the implication being that some modification is fine. However, two features rose to the top of those mentioned by implementers as being most helpful: those that facilitate collaboration and those that enable flexibility.

Despite differences in the details, all of the SCALE-UP rooms were designed to facilitate peer-peer and peer-instructor interaction and many mentioned this explicitly as a helpful feature. Studio-style reforms were created to foster collaboration (Beichner 2014), so it was not surprising that special tables and whiteboards were seen as helpful. However, we have seen attempts (with poor results) to implement SCALE-UP philosophy without these structures in place (i.e., trying to make it work in a traditional lecture hall with the chairs bolted down). Our interviewees highlight that collaborative classroom features are a priority for success. As described by the interviewee from institution R in the "How did the implemented classroom characteristics compare to the recommended classroom characteristics? Which classroom features are helpful? Unhelpful? Non-essential?" section, the collaborative features are not just about ensuring students understand the concepts but also helping students recognize they are not the only ones who do not understand the material.

Along these same lines, having flexible arrangements in the room was reported helpful. Every instructor has their own unique ways of teaching and having an adaptable classroom space encourages a wider range of individuals to use the space. It also helps them maximize the impact of their unique teaching style.

Finally, we note the mixed response to the helpfulness of technology. While most interviewees did not go into detail about specifics, technology was not named as a must-have for the classroom activities. The literature provides some possibilities as to why technology is not critical, ranging from instructors not using technology well or not modifying their teaching to incorporate it (Cuban 2001; Lasry et al. 2014) to unreliable technology (Cuban 2001; Frank et al. 2004). Some of the helpful aspects of technology were circumstantial, e.g., to help mitigate less ideal classroom environment such as room shape. One interviewee indicated it was helpful for getting faculty interested in teaching in the classroom but non-essential for classroom activities. This indicates that technology can be helpful, but that if space and/or finances are an issue, it is likely that SCALE-UP can be implemented successfully without it. Technology is just a tool after all, and in and of itself does not dictate the benefit of its use.

Recommendation 6: incorporate professional development into any implementation of SCALE-UP

The literature demonstrates a clear need for professional development when adopting innovations (Cummings et al. 1999; Chasteen et al. 2011; Florman 2014; Rogers et al. 2015). Our interviewees supported the need for professional development as evidenced by both the statements they made directly claiming professional development was important as well as the fact that half of the sites started without it but then added it as they recognized its importance.

Even for experienced and highly competent instructors, teaching in a SCALE-UP type classroom is a novel experience that requires new skills and support. Expecting instructors to enter a new classroom without any support learning to teach in the new environment is less likely to lead to a successful outcome. It can be particularly problematic if an instructor has a bad experience in the reform environment and then turns away from this type of teaching and/or makes negative comments about the experience to other colleagues. Instructors are more likely to have positive experiences, to keep teaching in this style, and to help spread the reform when they receive professional development.

Recommendation 7: make the SCALE-UP classroom visible to improve teaching across the university and to increase sustainability of the room

As mentioned above, our analysis indicates that a highly visible room advertises active learning techniques and increases instructor interest in active learning techniques. This leads some instructors to use reformed pedagogies in non-SCALE-UP rooms. Thus, the benefits of SCALE-UP extend beyond the immediate active learning classroom. Even if it does not specifically lead to increased SCALE-UP usage, it can lead to improved teaching in other classes.

An additional benefit of a visible classroom is that it looks impressive. We found that several institutions use rooms to attract and impress prospective students and alumni, for example, as part of the campus tour. This likely benefits the sustainability of SCALE-UP on the campus, as it becomes a part of the institution's identity. Interestingly, the room for one of our abandoner case was in a building that was not typically used by the implementer's department. Encouraging administration to show off the classroom to gain support for the room and SCALE-UP, implementers can suggest that the room is a featured destination for guests on tours or for meetings to be held in the room.

Conclusions

Despite our efforts, we found only one definite abandoner when there are 259 known SCALE-UP secondary implementers from the past 20 years. In contrast, approximately one third of all faculty who try a research-based instructional strategy will eventually abandon it (Henderson et al. 2012). Why does SCALE-UP achieve a higher rate of sustainability? While we cannot definitely answer this question, we can offer educated hypotheses and suggest future research.

Before embarking on this study, we knew SCALE-UP has positive results (i.e., documented learning gains, retention rates) and that faculty typically enjoy teaching in this environment, but is that enough to create sustainable change? While this is true, it is also true of other reforms that are more frequently abandoned. So we believe this is a necessary but not sufficient for high sustainability.

We hypothesize that radical, structural changes associated with SCALE-UP increase sustainability. Specifically, the team effort needed to implement the structural changes required to redesign a classroom space. As presented and discussed above, fully implementing a SCALE-UP reform typically involves a team effort, often with administrators on board. By the time SCALE-UP is implemented, there usually have been many conversations among many individuals with different perspectives, motivations, and interests. We believe these discussions (and likely debates, compromises, etc.), which may seem difficult at the time, eventually pay off with more buy-in across parties in the long run. This investment across different levels of an institution likely protects the reform even if the situation changes.

We also hypothesize that SCALE-UP is protected against abandonment because once an investment is made, it would require significant effort to undue the reform. Just time and money are required to put SCALE-UP into place (discussions and buy-in among different parties, funding, etc.); effort would be required to revert back to traditional instruction. Our lack of SCALE-UP abandoners supports this hypothesis. Although getting a SCALE-UP room is not a trivial undertaking for many secondary implementers, their efforts are rewarded in having a sustained, significant change that will be around for many years.

The implication of this is of great importance for anyone interested in sustained use of research-based instructional strategies (RBIS). The building of and use of a SCALE-UP classroom appears to be an effective reform strategy for sustainability, in addition to positive impacts on student learning. Not only does creating a classroom supports the spread of the innovation but it also encourages non-users of the classroom to integrate more RBIS in their teaching as well. We offer that if a change agent is interested in bringing about sustained change that spreads over time, creating a SCALE-UP type classroom is likely to be a worthwhile focus.

In trying to summarize how to successfully build and use a SCALE-UP classroom, we found that there is no one story, rather successful implementation happened in a variety of ways. While the stories share common themes, the adopters at each institution take different paths to implementation. The rooms deviate from the NCSU model, adapting to the instructor, the institution, and available resources. This is not a negative aspect, but rather a strength that indicates productive customization. It is important that the implementations maintain the intent of the classroom space: to keep an environment where students can easily collaborate.

Ultimately, having classroom space that is conducive to SCALE-UP style teaching is a huge asset to institutions that are moving toward SCALE-UP or other types of active learning teaching. The space's impact can reach beyond the SCALE-UP classroom, opening instructors to possibilities and transforming how they approach their teaching. Despite the differences among classroom space initiation, classrooms themselves, and professional development, secondary adopters retain the core ideas behind SCALE-UP and still reap benefits from the implementation. We also see SCALE-UP rooms used by institutions to symbolize their commitment to innovative teaching.

Competing interests
The authors declare that they have no competing interests.

Authors' contributions
AVK conducted some of the interviews and led the analysis of data for the article. KTF conducted some of the interviews, worked on the analysis, and provided edits. CH and MD conducted some of the interviews and provided feedback throughout the process. RB provided feedback throughout the process. All authors approved the final draft.

Acknowledgements
This project is supported by NSF: 1223405, 1223564, 1223405.

Author details
[1]Department of Physics, Western Michigan University, 1903 West Michigan Ave, Michigan 49008, USA. [2]Department of Physics, University of Auckland, Auckland 1010, New Zealand. [3]Department of Physics, 2000 Colorado Ave, Boulder, CO 80309-0390, USA. [4]Department of Physics, North Carolina State University, 421 Riddick Hall, Campus Box 8202, Raleigh, NC 27695-8202, USA.

References
Barak, M, Lipson, A, & Lerman, S (2006). Wireless laptops as means for promoting active learning in large lecture halls. *Journal of Research on Technology in Education, 38*(3), 245–263.

Beggs, TA (2000). Influences and Barriers to the Adoption of Instructional Technology. In *Proceedings of the Mid-South Instructional Technology Conference*. Murfreesboro: Middle Tennessee State University. (ERIC Document Reproduction Service No. ED 446 764).

Beichner, R (2008). The SCALE-UP project: a student-centered active learning environment for undergraduate programs. *Invited paper for the National Academy of Sciences*. Retrieved May 2, 2016 from http://publish.illinois.edu/disruptivespaces/files/2014/07/SCALE-UP-Paper1.pdf.

Beichner, RJ (2014). History and evolution of active learning spaces: history and evolution of active learning spaces. *New Directions for Teaching and Learning, 2014*(137), 9–16.

Beichner, R (2015). Room design. Retrieved May 3, 2016, from https://scaleupserver.physics.ncsu.edu/wiki/pages/42x7D5E3/Room.

Beichner, RJ, Saul, JM, Abbott, DS, Morse, J, Deardorff, D, Allain, RJ, … & Risley, JS (2007). The student-centered activities for large enrollment undergraduate programs (SCALE-UP) project. *Research-Based Reform of University Physics, 1*(1), 2–39.

Bonus, M, & Riordan, L (1998). *Increasing student on-task behavior through the use of specific seating arrangements. (Report no. PS026868)*. Chicago: Saint Xavier University.

Brooks, DC (2011). Space matters: the impact of formal learning environments on student learning. *British Journal of Educational Technology, 42*(5), 719–726.

Carnegie classifications. (2010). Retrieved May 26, 2015, from http://carnegieclassifications.iu.edu/

Chasteen, SV, Perkins, KK, Beale, PD, Pollock, SJ, & Wieman, CE (2011). A thoughtful approach to instruction: course transformation for the rest of us. *Journal of College Science Teaching, 40*(4), 70–76.

Cooke, NJ, & Hilton, ML (Eds.). (2015). *Enhancing the effectiveness of team science*. Washington: National Academies Press.

Cotner, S, Loper, J, Walker, JD, & Brooks, DC (2013). It's not you, it's the room—are the high-tech, active learning classrooms worth it? *Journal of College Science Teaching, 42*(6), 82–88.

Cuban, L (2001). *Oversold and underused: Reforming schools through technology, 1980-2000*. Cambridge: Harvard University.

Cummings, K, Marx, J, Thornton, R, & Kuhl, D (1999). Evaluating innovation in studio physics. *American Journal of Physics, 67*(S1), S38–S44.

Czujko, R, Redmond, K, Sauncy, T, & Olsen, T (2014). *Equipping physics majors for the STEM workforce*. College Park: AIP Statistical Research Center.

Dori, YJ, Hult, E, Breslow, L, & Belcher, JW (2007). How much have they retained? Making unseen concepts seen in a freshman electromagnetism course at MIT. *Journal of Science Education and Technology, 16*(4), 299–323.

Felix, E, & Brown, M (2011). The case for a learning space performance rating system. *Journal of Learning Spaces, 1*(1), 1–9.

Florman, JC (2014). TILE at Iowa: adoption and adaption. *New Directions for Teaching and Learning, 137*, 53–59.

Foote, KT, Neumeyer, X, Henderson, C, Dancy, MH, & Beichner, RJ (2014). Diffusion of research-based instructional strategies: the case of SCALE-UP. *International Journal of STEM Education, 1*(1), 1–18.

Frank, KA, Zhao, Y, & Borman, K (2004). Social capital and the diffusion of innovations within organizations: the case of computer technology in schools. *Sociology of Education, 77*(2), 148–171.

Harvey, E, & Kenyon, M (2013). Classroom seating considerations for 21st century students and faculty. *Journal of Learning Spaces, 2*(1). Retrieved May 2, 2016 from http://libjournal.uncg.edu/jls/article/view/578/454.

Henderson, C, & Dancy, MH (2007). Barriers to the use of research-based instructional strategies: the influence of both individual and situational characteristics. *Physical Review Special Topics - Physics Education Research, 3*(2), 1–14.

Henderson, C, & Dancy, M (2011). *Increasing the impact and diffusion of STEM education innovations*. Commissioned paper for National Academy of Engineering Forum—the impact and diffusion of transformative engineering education innovations, New Orleans, LA, Feb. 7–8, 2011. Washington, DC: National Academy of Engineering.

Henderson, C, Dancy, M, & Niewiadomska-Bugaj, M (2012). Use of research-based instructional strategies in introductory physics: where do faculty leave the innovation-decision process? *Physical Review Special Topics - Physics Education Research, 8*(2), 1–15.

Keiner, LE, & Gilman, CS (2015). Implementation of interactive engagement teaching methods in a physical oceanography course. *Journal of College Science Teaching, 45*(2), 70–78.

Klein, KJ, & Sorra, JS (1996). The challenge of innovation implementation. *Academy of Management, 21*(4), 1055–1080.

Lasry, N, Charles, E, & Whittaker, C (2014). When teacher-centered instructors are assigned to student-centered classrooms. *Physical Review Special Topics - Physics Education Research, 10*, 1–9.

Lippman, PC (2010). Can the physical environment have an impact on the learning environment? *CELE Exchange, Centre for Effective Learning Environments*, 1–6. Doi: 10.1787/20727925

Martin, SH (2002). The classroom environment and its effects on the practice of teachers. *Journal of Environmental Psychology, 22*, 139–156.

Narum, JL (2013). Student-centered active learning environment with upside-down pedagogies (SCALE-UP). In *Planning for Assessing 21st Century Spaces for 21st Century Learners* (pp. 86–87).

Neumeyer, X, Foote, K., Beichner, R, Dancy, M, & Henderson, C (2014). Examining the diffusion of research-based instructional strategies using social network analysis: a case-study of SCALE-UP. In *ASEE Annual Conference and Exposition, Conference Proceedings*. Washington, DC: American Society for Engineering Education

President's Council of Advisors on Science and Technology. (2010). Prepare and inspire: K-12 education in science, technology, engineering, and math (STEM) for America's future. Report to the president. Washington, DC: Executive Office of the President

Rogers, MM, Keller, LD, Crouse, A, & Price, MF (2015). Implementing comprehensive reform of introductory physics at a primarily undergraduate

institution: a longitudinal case study. *Journal of College Science Teaching, 44*(3), 82–90.
Rosenfield, P, Lambert, NM, & Black, A (1985). Desk arrangement effects on pupil classroom behavior. *Journal of Educational Psychology, 77*(1), 101–108.
Samarawickrema, G, & Stacey, E (2007). Adopting Web-Based Learning and Teaching: A case study in higher education. *Distance Education, 28*(3), 313–333.
Taylor, SS (2009). Effects of studio space on teaching and learning: preliminary findings from two case studies. *Innovative Higher Education, 33*(4), 217–228.
Walker, BJD, Brooks, DC, & Baepler, P (2011). Pedagogy and space: empirical research on new learning environments. *Educause Quaterly, 34*(4), 1–24.
Wejnert, B (2002). Integrating models of diffusion of innovations: a conceptual framework. *Annual Review of Sociology, 28*, 297–326.
Whiteside, AL, Jorn, L, Duin, AH, & Fitzgerald, S (2009). Using the PAIR-up model to evaluate active learning spaces. *Educause Quarterly, 32*(1), 1–16.
Zhu, C, & Engels, N (2013). Organizational culture and instructional innovations in higher education: perceptions and reactions of teachers and students. *Educational Management Administration & Leadership, 42*(1), 136–158.

Permissions

All chapters in this book were first published in IJSE, by Springer; hereby published with permission under the Creative Commons Attribution License or equivalent. Every chapter published in this book has been scrutinized by our experts. Their significance has been extensively debated. The topics covered herein carry significant findings which will fuel the growth of the discipline. They may even be implemented as practical applications or may be referred to as a beginning point for another development.

The contributors of this book come from diverse backgrounds, making this book a truly international effort. This book will bring forth new frontiers with its revolutionizing research information and detailed analysis of the nascent developments around the world.

We would like to thank all the contributing authors for lending their expertise to make the book truly unique. They have played a crucial role in the development of this book. Without their invaluable contributions this book wouldn't have been possible. They have made vital efforts to compile up to date information on the varied aspects of this subject to make this book a valuable addition to the collection of many professionals and students.

This book was conceptualized with the vision of imparting up-to-date information and advanced data in this field. To ensure the same, a matchless editorial board was set up. Every individual on the board went through rigorous rounds of assessment to prove their worth. After which they invested a large part of their time researching and compiling the most relevant data for our readers.

The editorial board has been involved in producing this book since its inception. They have spent rigorous hours researching and exploring the diverse topics which have resulted in the successful publishing of this book. They have passed on their knowledge of decades through this book. To expedite this challenging task, the publisher supported the team at every step. A small team of assistant editors was also appointed to further simplify the editing procedure and attain best results for the readers.

Apart from the editorial board, the designing team has also invested a significant amount of their time in understanding the subject and creating the most relevant covers. They scrutinized every image to scout for the most suitable representation of the subject and create an appropriate cover for the book.

The publishing team has been an ardent support to the editorial, designing and production team. Their endless efforts to recruit the best for this project, has resulted in the accomplishment of this book. They are a veteran in the field of academics and their pool of knowledge is as vast as their experience in printing. Their expertise and guidance has proved useful at every step. Their uncompromising quality standards have made this book an exceptional effort. Their encouragement from time to time has been an inspiration for everyone.

The publisher and the editorial board hope that this book will prove to be a valuable piece of knowledge for researchers, students, practitioners and scholars across the globe.

List of Contributors

Douglas B Clark, Pratim Sengupta, Mario M Martinez-Garza and Stephen S Killingsworth
College of Education, Vanderbilt University, Box 230, 230 Appleton Place, Nashville, Tennessee 37203-5721, USA

Corey E Brady
School of Education and Social Policy, Northwestern University, Annenberg Hall, 2120 Campus Drive, Evanston, Illinois 60208, USA

Lyn D English
Faculty of Education, Queensland University of Technology, Victoria Park Road, Kelvin Grove, Brisbane, Queensland, 4059, Australia

Jane M Watson
Faculty of Education, University of Tasmania, Private Bag 66, Hobart, Tasmania 7001, Australia

Şenay Purzer
School of Engineering Education, Purdue University, Wang Hall 4545, 516 Northwestern Avenue, West Lafayette, IN 47906, USA

Molly Hathaway Goldstein and Robin S Adams
School of Engineering Education, Purdue University, Armstrong Hall, 701 West Stadium Avenue, West Lafayette, IN 47906, USA

Charles Xie and Saeid Nourian
The Intelligent Learning Environments Laboratory, The Concord Consortium, 25 Love Lane, Concord, MA 01742, USA

Aikaterini Bagiati
MIT-SUTD Collaboration Office, Massachusetts Institute of Technology, Cambridge, MA, 02139, USA

So Yoon Yoon
Texas A&M Engineering Experiment Station, Texas A&M University, College Station, TX 77843, USA

Demetra Evangelou
Department of Education Sciences in Early Childhood, Democritus University, Alexandroupolis 69100, Greece

Alejandra Magana
Computer and Information Technology Department, Purdue University, West Lafayette, IN 47907, USA

Garene Kaloustian
Department of Education, Lebanese American University, Beirut, Lebanon

Jiabin Zhu
Graduate School of Education, Shanghai Jiao Tong University, Shanghai City, P. R. China

Lyn D. English
Faculty of Education, Queensland University of Technology, S Block, Victoria Park Road, Kelvin Grove, Brisbane, Queensland 4059, Australia

Kevin Mulqueeny and Victor Kostyuk
Reasoning Mind, 2000 Bering Drive, Suite 300, TX,77057, Houston

Ryan S. Baker and Jaclyn Ocumpaugh
Teachers College, Columbia University, 525 West 120th Street, NY,10027, New York

Andrzej Sokolowski
Department of Mathematics and Science, Lone Star College, Tomball, TX 77375, USA

Yeping Li
College of Education and Human Development, Department of Teaching Learning and Culture, Texas A&M University, College Station, TX 77843-4225, USA

Victor Willson
College of Education and Human Development, Department of Educational Psychology, Texas A&M University, College Station, TX 77843-4225, USA

Wendy R Aaron
College of Education 204E Furman Hall Oregon State University, Corvallis, OR 97330, USA

Patricio G Herbst
School of Education 610 East University Ave. University of Michigan, Ann Arbor, MI 48109-1259, USA

Alan H. Schoenfeld
School of Education, University of California, EMST, Tolman Hall # 1670, Berkeley, CA 94720-1670, USA

Mike Thomas and Bill Barton
Department of Mathematics, The University of Auckland, Private Bag 92019, Auckland 1142, New Zealand

Jesse L. M. Wilkins
School of Education/Teaching and Learning, War Memorial Hall, RM 300C, Virginia Tech, 370 Drillfield Drive, Blacksburg, VA 24061, USA

Hamsa Venkat
Wits School of Education, University of the Witwatersrand, Johannesburg, South Africa
Wits School of Education, University of the Witwatersrand, Johannesburg, South Africa and Jönköping University, Jönköping, Sweden

Meixia Ding
Temple University, 436 Ritter Hall, 1301 Cecil B. Moore Avenue, Philadelphia, PA 19122-6091, USA

Alexis V. Knaub and Charles Henderson
Department of Physics, Western Michigan University, 1903 West Michigan Ave, Michigan 49008, USA

Kathleen T. Foote
Department of Physics, University of Auckland, Auckland 1010, New Zealand

Melissa Dancy
Department of Physics, 2000 Colorado Ave, Boulder, CO 80309-0390, USA

Robert J. Beichner
Department of Physics, North Carolina State University, 421 Riddick Hall, Campus Box 8202, Raleigh, NC 27695-8202, USA

Index

A
Active Learning Spaces, 182, 202-203

Animation, 89, 108, 112-113, 115-116, 118

Awareness, 7, 22-25, 37-39, 41, 50, 122, 129, 132, 134-136, 152-153, 156-157, 159, 164, 198

B
Blended Learning, 77-79, 82-83, 88-90

C
Classroom Design, 182, 185-186

Classroom Instruction, 77, 82, 85, 106, 168, 170, 178

Classroom Scenario, 108, 112

Classrooms, 1, 19-20, 24, 26, 42, 52, 55, 68, 77, 83, 85-86, 88, 90-91, 104, 109-111, 113, 117-119, 137, 139, 148, 154-155, 162, 167, 182-187, 189-195, 197, 199-200, 202

Computer-aided Design, 42-43, 46, 53

Computers, 19, 85, 91-92, 94-97, 100, 103-107, 115, 123, 185-186, 189, 193-195

Conceptual Integration, 1-3, 5, 12, 18

Conjecturing, 108-110, 112-115, 117-119

Content Knowledge, 3, 24, 54, 71, 103, 119, 123, 133, 136, 140-141, 147, 152, 154-156, 163-165, 167, 169, 171, 173, 175, 177, 179-181

Curriculum Documents, 23, 74

D
Decision-making, 43, 48-50, 52, 94, 111, 121-126, 128-130, 134, 137, 186

Design Processes, 42, 49-50, 52-53

Designer Learns, 43

Designing Games, 1, 10, 18

Digital Games, 1-3, 5-7, 9-11, 13, 15-21

Disciplinary Integration, 1, 3, 5, 7, 9, 11, 13-19, 21

E
E-learning, 77, 79, 81, 83, 85, 87, 89-90, 105

Early Engineering, 54, 63, 68

Educational Software, 10, 20, 78, 89-90

Educational Systems, 54-57

Elementary School, 22-23, 25, 27, 29, 31, 33, 35, 37, 39-41, 75, 88, 93, 106, 136, 138-139, 141, 143, 145, 147, 149, 162, 180

Energy3d, 42, 46-48, 52

Engaged Concentration, 77-78, 82-88

Engineering, 42-47, 49-69, 71-76, 78, 89, 105, 187, 202

Engineering Design, 42-45, 47, 49-53, 72-73, 75

Engineering Education, 42, 52-57, 59-60, 62, 64, 67-69, 71-72

Evaluation, 41, 60, 64-66, 89-90, 101, 138, 149-150, 162

Explorations, 91-95, 97, 99, 101-105

F
Fourth-grade Students, 22, 75

Fundamental Mathematical Ideas, 163-165, 168-170, 179-180

G
Game Play, 3, 5, 7, 9-12, 14-18

Geometry, 24, 40-41, 49, 92, 95, 99-103, 105-106, 108-113, 117-120, 140, 193-195

Graphical Representations, 12, 22, 25

H
Human Knowledge, 1-2

I
Informed Design, 42, 44-45, 48-50, 52

Instructional Design, 19-20, 77, 79

Interdisciplinary, 69-71, 73, 75

International Comparison, 54, 57

Intervention, 24, 60, 74, 116, 137, 148

Intuitive Thinking, 7-8

Iteration, 24

L
Languages, 54, 56-58, 60-64, 66-67

Learning, 1-5, 7-13, 15-21, 23-24, 26, 28, 38, 40-45, 47-48, 50, 52-57, 59-63, 65, 67-79, 81-83, 85, 87-96, 98-107, 109, 117, 119-121, 126, 130, 134-139, 141, 149-150, 152-156, 162-172, 174-175, 177-187, 189-199, 201-203

Learning Design, 44

Learning Experience, 69

Learning Goals, 9, 18, 183-184

Learning Outcomes, 24, 60, 67, 69, 74-75, 78, 88, 90, 106

Learning Technologies, 1

Linear Measurement, 22-24, 28-29, 37

M
Manipulating, 1, 4, 16-18, 153

Mathematical Beliefs, 138-141

Mathematical Disposition, 138-139, 141, 147

Mathematical Practices, 130, 151-157, 159-162

Mathematics Curriculum, 24, 39, 75, 83, 93, 107, 138, 140, 146, 149-150

Mathematics Education, 20, 40-41, 68-69, 75-76, 94, 105-108, 119, 126, 128, 135-139, 148-151, 153, 162, 164, 177, 180-181

Measurement, 20, 22-33, 35-41, 89-91, 139-150

Meta-analysis, 19, 21, 72, 75, 91, 93-97, 99, 101, 103-107

Methods Course, 163-164, 167-170, 172, 177, 179

Middle-school Mathematics, 77, 79, 81, 83, 85, 87, 89

Modifying Education Innovation, 182

Multidisciplinary, 53, 69-70, 149-150

N

Navigation, 5, 7-8, 15

O

Open Educational Resources Teacher Preparation, 54

Open Web Resources, 54-55

P

Partial Recognition, 24

Policy Developers, 69-70

Prek-12 Engineering, 54-57, 59-63, 65, 67

Prek-12 Stem, 54, 56, 61

Preservice Elementary Teachers, 163, 165, 167, 169, 171, 173, 175, 177, 179-181

Primary Mathematics, 151, 154-155, 180-181

Problem Solving, 3, 7, 18-20, 40-41, 43, 45, 52-53, 75-76, 90-107, 153, 162, 167, 177, 179, 183

Q

Quantitative Literacy, 138-143, 145-150

R

Re-designing, 7

Retention, 22, 37, 39, 106, 183, 188, 201

S

Scale-up, 182-202

School Curricula, 39, 71

Science Education, 1, 3, 5, 9, 19-21, 42, 52-53, 59, 62, 64-66, 75, 93, 107, 119, 149, 202

Science Learning, 1, 3, 5, 7, 9, 11, 13, 15, 17-21, 42, 44, 50, 52-53, 90

Scientific Expertise, 1-2, 17

Scientific Inquiry, 16, 21, 42-44, 52, 72, 93-94, 98, 105

Solar Energy, 42, 46, 49

Specialized Content Knowledge, 163-165, 167, 169, 171, 173, 175, 177, 179, 181

Standards-based Mathematics Curricula, 138-139, 141, 143, 145, 147, 149-150

Statistical Investigations, 22-23

Statistical Thinking, 22-23, 25-27, 29, 31, 33, 35, 37, 39, 41

Stem Education, 52, 55-56, 61, 68-77, 202

Stem Integration, 53, 65, 68-72, 74-76

Stem Research, 69, 71

Student Achievement, 91, 94-96, 102-106, 150

Students, 2-12, 14-30, 32-50, 52-55, 59-63, 65-68, 70-75, 77-79, 81-96, 98-119, 121-125, 127-132, 134-136, 138-150, 155, 159, 162, 164-167, 169-170, 172, 177-186, 189-190, 193-195, 197-198, 200-203

Students' Game Play, 7, 10

Students' Progress, 16, 22

Studio-style Instruction, 182-183

Surge's Motion, 7, 12

T

Teacher Preparation, 54, 68

Teachers' Perceptions, 68, 108-113, 115, 117-119

Technological, 18, 42, 53-54, 57, 59, 64-65, 75, 82, 94, 106, 115, 186

Time On-task, 77, 85, 88

Trade-offs, 42-47, 49-50, 52

Transdisciplinary Integration, 69

Troubleshooting, 43, 45, 49, 90

V

Variation, 22-41, 58, 73-74, 96, 162

Videotapes, 73, 121